AUDITORY DISORDERS

AUDITORY DISORDERS
A MANUAL FOR CLINICAL EVALUATION

Susan Jerger / James Jerger

Baylor College of Medicine
Texas Medical Center, Houston

Foreword by
Bobby R. Alford, M.D.
Professor and Chairman
Department of Otorhinolaryngology and Communicative Sciences
Baylor College of Medicine
Texas Medical Center, Houston

Little, Brown and Company · Boston

Library of Congress Catalog Card No. 81-80010

ISBN 0-316-46140-7

Printed in the United States of America

HAL

Cover design by Betsy Hacker

To Scott Jerger

CONTENTS

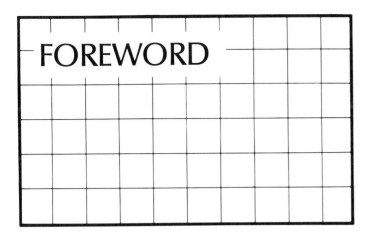

FOREWORD

In this book, Susan and James Jerger have captured the very essence of what is known today about the hearing assessment of auditory disorders. The contents of this volume reflect their dedicated pursuit of the meaningful evaluation of hearing function in health and disease. The organization of the book into specific chapters that deal with disease problems or disorders is a unique way to present the fine points in audiology that contribute to disease recognition and evaluation. The annotated text presentation should enhance substantially the accessibility of the subject matter.

That an otolaryngologist was asked to write the foreword for this book highlights the partnership that has evolved between otolaryngology and audiology. This professional relationship has led to an interdependence in the clinical setting that has provided many advances in the understanding of ear disease and specifically auditory disorders.

This excellent book will be referred to often by everyone interested in hearing and will be a reference source for future research.

Bobby R. Alford

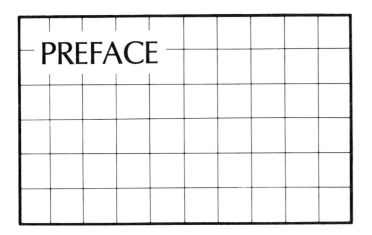

PREFACE

This book catalogs the patterns of audiometric test results that audiologists and otologists may expect to encounter in evaluating the various clinical entities collectively comprising auditory disorders. We confine our attention, in this volume, primarily to the clinical entities of adults. However, we plan a subsequent volume devoted to the auditory disorders of children.

HISTORICAL PERSPECTIVE

The variety of audiometric patterns encountered in clinical evaluation derives, in large measure, from the differing roles played by the various structures of the auditory system in the transformation, transduction, coding, transmission, and decoding of the auditory signal. Ernst Weber was perhaps the first investigator to encounter this differential symptomatology when he noted, in 1834, that bone-conducted signals were referred to the poorer ear in conductive hearing loss. Only 21 years later, in 1855, Heinrich Rinne described a method for quantifying air-bone gap by comparing the duration of perception by air conduction to the duration of perception by bone conduction.

For almost a century, these two tuning fork tests, Weber and Rinne, remained the cornerstones of diagnostic audiometry. They provided the fundamental test results for differentiating conductive from sensorineural hearing loss. From today's perspective it is apparent that each test was ideally suited to this task in the sense that it addressed the unique function of the middle ear mechanism: its transformer action in matching the impedance of the fluid medium within the cochlea to the air medium outside the cochlea. When this transformer action is altered, the result must necessarily be a marked reduction in sensitivity to air-conducted as compared to bone-conducted signals (Rinne test) and as an enhancement of sensitivity to bone-conducted signals (Weber test).

The first half of the twentieth century saw the invention of the vacuum tube, the development of the electric audiometer and an explosive increase in studies of auditory sensitivity. There was little further progress, however, in diagnostic audiometry. It was not until 1948 that the next milestone in differential symptomatology occurred. In that memorable year, Dix, Hallpike, and Hood, in England, published, in the Proceedings of the Royal Society, their now famous observation that loudness re-

cruitment, as measured by the alternate binaural loudness balance (ABLB) test, was characteristically positive in patients with Meniere's disease, but characteristically negative in patients with eighth nerve tumor.

To be sure, the phenomenon of loudness recruitment was already well known. From the middle of the nineteenth century, otologists recognized that hypersensitivity to loud sounds often accompanied hearing loss. Moreover, the phenomenon had been studied at some length by E. P. Fowler, Sr., in the period 1928 to 1937. But Dix, Hallpike, and Hood were the first to assign correct topical significance to the symptom by showing its unique correspondence with cochlear site.

The next decade saw the development of a multitude of procedures designed to measure loudness recruitment indirectly. Intensity and frequency discrimination, masking of tones by noise, adaptation, and fatigue were all investigated exhaustively in an attempt to exploit the differential diagnostic potential suggested by the work of Dix, Hallpike, and Hood. Investigators reasoned that an indirect test of loudness recruitment, not dependent on interaural asymmetry like the ABLB test, would be a valuable tool in differentiating cochlear and eighth nerve site. As a corollary to this axiom, the ABLB test result was regarded as the validation yardstick against which to evaluate the efficacy of each new procedure.

One of the few positive rewards from this flurry of investigation was the growing realization that loudness recruitment, per se, was not the parent phenomenon distinguishing cochlear from eighth nerve site, but only one of many possible manifestations of cochlear disorder based on a more general or "parent" phenomenon relating to disorders in the transduction and biological amplification processes.

One important consequence of this development was the realization that the ultimate validating criterion of a proposed diagnostic procedure was not how well it agreed with ABLB in detecting loudness recruitment but how well it actually predicted site of lesion. Before this important conceptual breakthrough occurred, there had been a good deal of nonproductive theoretical conjecture on the relations or lack of relations among various psychoacoustic measures and loudness recruitment. When it was finally recognized, however, that the goal was not to predict loudness recruitment but to predict site of disorder, a more appropriate conceptual framework, based on the relation between symptomatology and function, could be developed.

The decade of the 1960s saw three parallel lines of activity in diagnostic audiometry: (1) the evaluation of abnormal adaptation as a phenomenon unique to retrocochlear, and especially eighth nerve, site; (2) the development of new speech audiometric measures to differentiate peripheral from central auditory disorders; and (3) the development of instrumentation for impedance audiometry.

Abnormal adaptation, like loudness recruitment, was a phenomenon well known to nineteenth century otologists. Its full exploitation as a differentiating symptom, however, awaited the development of sufficiently sophisticated electronic instrumentation. Bekesy's self-recording audiometer, introduced in 1947, opened the door to this new and exciting avenue of investigation by providing a unique tool for the precise study of temporal changes in auditory sensitivity to sustained stimulation. The initial report in 1952, by Reger and Kos, of progressive threshold adaptation in a patient with retrocochlear disorder initiated a series of studies in the late 1950s and early 1960s, documenting the unique correspondence between abnormal adaptation and retrocochlear, especially eighth nerve, site.

Although a number of nineteenth and early twentieth century otologists, especially in Germany, experimented with the diagnostic potential of speech audiometry, the important breakthrough came in 1955 when Bocca and his colleagues, in Italy, showed how speech signals could be used to identify temporal lobe disorder. This pioneering work stimulated an important body of research throughout the world in the 1960s, aimed at the development of materials and techniques for exploiting the diagnostic potential of speech audiometry. As a result of this work, speech audiometry has become one of our most important techniques for identifying and evaluating central auditory disorders and for differentiating peripheral from central site.

Impedance audiometry was pioneered in the Scandinavian countries. Following the now-classic 1946 monograph of Metz, a number of investigators in Denmark and Sweden developed and refined tympanometry and acoustic reflex measurement. It was not until the late 1960s that clinical impedance audiometry reached the United States. During the 1970s, however, its use became widespread to the point that it is now considered an integral part of the basic audiometric evaluation. It is probably fair to say that no new testing technique has had such a profound effect on audiologic practice since the development of the electric audiometer itself.

Finally, the 1970s saw the development of another powerful new technique: auditory brain stem response (ABR) audiometry. Sohmer and Feinmesser, in Israel, and Hecox and Galambos, in the United States, were among the first to point out the potential value of the auditory brain stem response in audiologic evaluation, especially in testing babies and young children. During the past several years, the importance of this new technique has been revealed in virtually every type of auditory disorder from the middle ear to the brain stem.

The addition of impedance and ABR audiometry to the audiologic evaluation has greatly refined and extended the scope of diagnostic evaluation. We can now differentiate, relatively successfully, among five potential sites of disorder: the middle ear, the cochlea, the eighth nerve, the brain stem auditory pathways, and the auditory cortex in the temporal lobe. The approach to each is characterized by a unique testing strategy.

THE TEST BATTERY APPROACH

As the tools of audiologic evaluation became more sophisticated, there was a parallel development in the concept of a test battery approach to assessment. As clinicians experimented with various combinations of tests, they found that whereas a single test, sensitive to disorder at one site, might have a certain given effectiveness, a combination of two or more tests, each sensitive to a different site of disorder, often led to a more accurate site prediction.

Today's approach to the test battery concept is based on three considerations. First, the choice of appropriate tests often depends on the degree of sensitivity loss. The acoustic reflex, for example, is quite sensitive to eighth nerve disorder when sensitivity loss is mild or moderate, but often becomes ambiguous when sensitivity loss is too great. The Bekesy tracing, on the other hand, is less sensitive to eighth nerve site than the acoustic reflex when the loss is mild or moderate, but continues to be applicable and useful as sensitivity loss becomes more severe. Thus, whereas one test may excel for some loss ranges, a different test may be more appropriate for other ranges.

A second factor leading to the test battery concept is the fact that some tests are more structure-specific than others. A suitable test battery can exploit such differences to achieve quite specific site localization. The auditory brain stem response, for example, is generated by a series of relatively specific structures in the eighth nerve and caudal brain stem. The acoustic reflex depends partly on a subset of the same structures that mediate the ABR and partly on other structures in the brain stem. While individual abnormalities on these two tests are each relatively site-specific, a consideration of the combination of abnormalities on the two-test battery can lead to even more precise site localization.

Finally, different combinations of tests are often dictated by the chief complaint or by the audiologist's working hypothesis. When a functional problem is suspected, for example, the optimal test battery may be quite different from the combination of tests appropriate for differentiating cochlear from eighth nerve site.

In general, however, the selection of an appropriate test battery follows a rational course based on sequential findings. The basic data of the diagnostic audiometric evaluation are the pure tone air conduction threshold levels, the results of impedance (immittance) audiometry, and the results of basic speech audiometry. If all three results are within normal limits, the patient may be classified as *audiometrically normal.*

If air conduction levels are abnormal, and any aspect of impedance audiometry is abnormal, one is obliged to pursue the possibility of a middle ear site. The appropriate test battery would include one or more of the following procedures: (1) bone conduction audiometry, (2) SAL audiometry, (3) audiometric Weber test, or (4) audiometric Bing test (occlusion index). The purpose of this unique test battery is to confirm the presence of conductive loss and to quantify the magnitude of the conductive component. This is usually feasible only to the extent that the non-test ear can be successfully masked to exclude its participation.

If air conduction levels are abnormal and impedance results are normal, then the loss is, in all probability, sensorineural. The appropriate test battery for further diagnostic site differentiation now depends upon the degree of air conduction sensitivity loss. For relatively mild loss, the optimal test battery includes (1) auditory brain stem response (ABR) audiometry, (2) speech audiometry, and (3) acoustic reflex measures. In the case of relatively severe loss of air conduction sensitivity, the optimal test battery includes (1) Bekesy-type threshold tracing, (2) Bekesy-type comfortable loudness (BCL) tracing, and (3) threshold and/or supra-threshold tone decay test (TDT or STAT).

These procedures, while not as sensitive to early retrocochlear disorder as ABR, acoustic reflex, and speech audiometry, are less influenced by degree of loss. They may be successfully employed, therefore, over a wider range of hearing loss conditions.

The combination of relatively normal pure tone sensitivity and abnormal speech audiometric results signifies the high probability of a central auditory disorder, either in the brain stem auditory pathways or at a higher cortical level.

For suspected central lesions, a useful test battery includes (1) ABR, (2) acoustic reflex, and (3) speech audiometry (monaural in presence of competition and binaural-dichotic).

ABR and acoustic reflex measures are quite sensitive to involvement of specific structures in the caudal brain stem, and monaural speech testing in the presence of competition is sensitive to any retrocochlear disorder, but especially the brain stem pathways. The binaural-dichotic procedures, on the other hand, are relatively more sensitive to disorders at the temporal lobe level.

By the judicious use of this test battery approach, it has been possible to achieve, in recent years, relatively precise site localization of a wide variety of auditory disorders.

SENSITIVITY AND SPECIFICITY

Still another parallel development, especially during the 1970s, was increased sophistication in the evaluation of test effectiveness. Early test developers were concerned primarily with *hit rate*; i.e., the extent to which the test correctly identified disorder at a particular site. At first there was little appreciation of the equally important *false-alarm* rate; i.e., the extent to which the test incorrectly identified disorder at a particular site.

Contemporary workers, however, have a keener appreciation of the concepts of "sensitivity" and "specificity" as equally important dimensions of test performance. A particular procedure is no longer regarded as necessarily effective simply because it has high sensitivity. We have learned to ask what is its specificity as well, and we have come to appreciate the bitter, often frustrating, truth: that sensitivity and specificity are forever intertwined, that they are inseparable cohabitants of the diagnostic arena, and that we purchase improvement in one only at the expense of the other. Appreciation of these fundamentals and of the costs and values associated with various joint outcomes has greatly increased sophistication in the evaluation of test efficacy.

In this book, we have relied on these various principles to define profiles of the various clinical entities of auditory disorder. A separate chapter is devoted to each entity. In each chapter we present the clinical picture from two points of view: (1) the expected pattern of test results commonly associated with the disorder, and (2) the variability likely to be encountered over a series of patients exhibiting the entity. In addition, we have attempted, wherever feasible, to include data on the distribution and prevalence of the disorder, as well as unique factors characterizing its clinical appearance.

In order to use the book most effectively, we suggest that the reader first consult the chapter dedicated to a particular entity, in order to gain an overview of the disorder and the procedures appropriate to its evaluation, and then consult the glossary for more specific descriptions of unfamiliar terms and tests.

No book of this scope can possibly aspire to a comprehensive treatment of all the tests and procedures that have been advocated or are in current use among audiologists. Nor would such comprehensive treatment serve a useful purpose. The overlap and duplication among innumerable tests, and confusion in interpretation, would mitigate the value of such an approach.

In the present volume we have attempted only to present what we hope is a reasonably balanced approach to site localization that we have found useful in our own clinical work.

S.J./J.J.

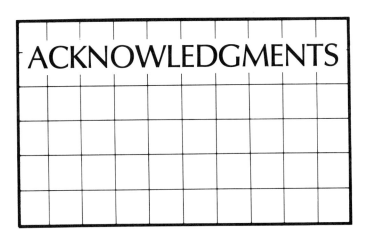

ACKNOWLEDGMENTS

This book would not have been possible without the help of our friends, particularly,

Bobby R. Alford, M.D.

. . . for professional support and friendship.

Mrs. E. O. Wood and Mrs. Imogene Childress

. . . for personal support and kindness.

Susan Lewis

. . . for editorial assistance and encouragement.

Kim Kulik, Susan Lewis, Monica Pacelli,
and Sue Ellen Ruggles

. . . for research assistance and for refusing to settle for less than the best.

Our sincere thanks.

KEY TO SYMBOLS

PURE TONE AUDIOMETRY

	Unmasked	Masked
Air Conduction	○	●
Bone Conduction	△	▲
SAL	◇	

	Crossed	Uncrossed
Acoustic Reflex	⊠	□

SPEECH AUDIOMETRY

	Unmasked	Masked
PB	○	●
SSI (in quiet)	△	▲
SSI (with competing message)	□	■

AUDITORY DISORDERS

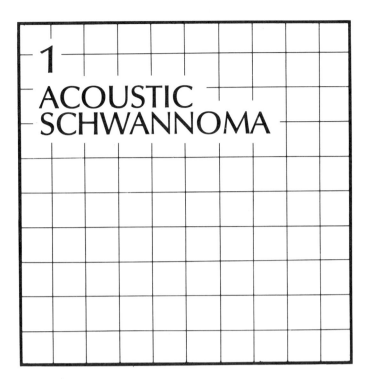

1
ACOUSTIC SCHWANNOMA

1. Acoustic Schwannomas . . . occur in about 8.7 persons per 1000 . . . may be referred to as *acoustic neurinomas, neurilemmomas,* or *neuromas* . . . may be classified as intracanalicular (within the internal auditory canal) or extracanalicular (extending or arising outside the internal auditory canal) . . . comprise 8% to 10% of intracranial neoplasms . . . account for 70% to 80% of cerebellopontine angle neoplasms.

2. The occurrence of bilateral acoustic Schwannomas is usually associated with von Recklinghausen's disease (multiple neurofibromatosis).

3. Although symptoms generally occur in a well-defined pattern as described, variations in the clinical course may occur in many individuals.

DESCRIPTION

Acoustic Schwannomas are tumors that arise from the neurilemmal sheath, the sheath of Schwann, of the eighth cranial nerve. Characteristically, the tumor arises within the internal auditory canal from the vestibular portion of the eighth nerve. As the tumor increases in size, it may extend medially from the internal auditory meatus into the cerebellopontine angle. Symptoms are due to compression, atrophy and invasion of the auditory and vestibular nerve trunks, interference with the blood supply to the cochlea, biochemical disturbances of the cochlear fluids, pressure on adjacent cranial nerves, and/or compression or displacement of adjacent brain stem structures.[1]

PATIENT CHARACTERISTICS

Onset of symptoms is usually between 30 and 50 years of age. Approximately 55% to 65% of patients are female. The tumor is unilateral in about 95% of patients.[2]

CLINICAL COURSE

Progressive, unilateral sensorineural hearing loss. The onset of hearing loss is characteristically insidious, but may be abrupt in about 4% of persons. The loss is preceded or accompanied by tinnitus in more than 80% of individuals. Dizziness or unsteadiness may be observed in about 65% of persons. A sensation of pressure or fullness within the ear may be reported by many patients.

The clinical symptomatology reported by patients with acoustic Schwannomas generally occurs in a predictable sequence of symptoms. With rare exceptions, the first sign of an acoustic Schwannoma is hearing loss and/or tinnitus. Hearing complaints are characteristically accompanied by other symptoms in the following order: ". . . labyrinthine symptoms; suboccipital discomfort; incoordination and staggering gait; involvement of other cranial nerves; headaches, vomiting, and papilledema; and dysarthria, dysphagia, and respiratory difficulties" (Bebin, 1979, p. 72). A well-defined sequence of developing abnormalities is attributed to the predictable anatomic growth and progression of the disease process.[3]

The treatment of acoustic Schwannomas generally involves surgery. In some patients, however, the tumor may recur after surgical intervention.

SITE OF DISORDER

Eighth nerve. Secondary sites may be the cochlea or the brain stem.

GENERAL AUDIOLOGIC PATTERN

The distinguishing signs of acoustic Schwannoma are primarily based on the phenomenon of abnormal adaptation. Patients generally show an inability to sustain response to a continuous pure tone signal. Usually, abnormal symptoms are more apparent at suprathreshold levels than at threshold or near-threshold levels. This latter observation implies that the most sensitive indices of eighth nerve disorder are tests involving relatively high suprathreshold intensities (i.e., PI functions, acoustic reflexes, etc.).

Impedance results typically show normal, type A, tympanograms, normal static compliance measures, and elevated or absent acoustic reflex thresholds. The reflex pattern based on crossed vs uncrossed reflex thresholds is characterized by a diagonal configuration. Reflexes are abnormal with sound to the affected ear and normal with sound to the unaffected ear. One exception involves patients with acoustic reflexes at relatively

4. At frequencies of 2000 Hz and above, the diagnostic value of the reflex decay phenomenon is compromised by a high incidence of false positive results in otherwise normal ears.

normal HLs on both ears. In those patients, if the reflex eliciting signal is sustained over time in the affected ear, reflex amplitude generally shows pronounced decay. The presence of reflex decay is a strong indication of eighth nerve site at frequencies below 2000 Hz.[4]

Pure tone sensitivity results generally, but not invariably, show unilateral or asymmetric bilateral sensorineural loss with a sloping audiometric contour (greater loss in the high frequency region than in the low frequency region). Speech intelligibility scores may be normal or disproportionately reduced relative to the degree of pure tone sensitivity loss. In contrast to the pronounced variability of maximum intelligibility scores, however, the shape of the PI function for speech materials is usually abnormal (the rollover phenomenon).

If reflexes are abnormal and/or the PI function shows rollover or disproportionately reduced maximum intelligibility performance, further tests for the diagnostic evaluation of eighth nerve site are indicated.[5] Appropriate tests may include Bekesy and BCL audiometry, STAT, TDT, and ABR audiometry.

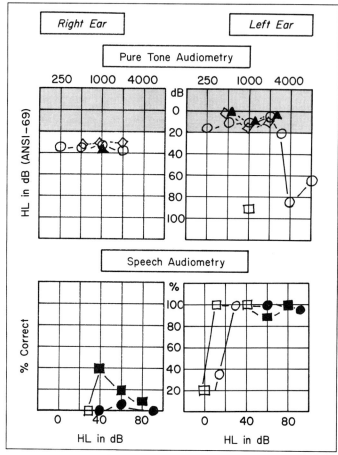

Case 1-1A

Illustrative Patients

CASE 1. A 38-YEAR-OLD MALE WITH A 3-CM ACOUSTIC SCHWANNOMA OCCUPYING THE RIGHT POSTERIOR FOSSA SPACE. SURGICAL FINDINGS NOTED THAT A SMALL PORTION OF THE TUMOR EXTENDED INTO THE RIGHT INTERNAL AUDITORY CANAL. A PORTION OF THE TUMOR WAS ADHERENT TO THE BRAIN STEM.

History

The patient complains of a hearing loss and "stopped-up" feeling in the right ear for the past 6 weeks. The hearing loss followed an acute episode of right ear pain. Presently, the patient notices numbness and weakness on the right side of his face. He does not report tinnitus or dizziness. He has a history of noise exposure in the military service. The patient does not have any hearing complaints about the left ear.

Otorhinolaryngologic evaluation and a general physical examination are within normal limits except for decreased hearing on the right ear and decreased sensation on the right side of the face. Facial nerve studies

are consistent with lower motor neuron involvement. Neurologic examination reveals involvement of cranial nerves five through ten on the right. EEG findings and routine laboratory studies are normal.

Results of computerized axial tomographic (CT) scanning, right carotid and left vertebral angiography, and lumbar pneumoencephalography indicate the presence of an elipsoidal extraaxial neoplasm at the right cerebellopontine angle cistern centered opposite the meatus of the right internal auditory canal. The fourth ventricle chamber is rotated and elevated.

Results

The audiogram (Case 1-1A) on the right ear shows a mild sensorineural loss through 2000 Hz and a profound sensorineural loss above 2000 Hz. On the left ear, the audiogram shows normal sensitivity through 3000 Hz and a severe sensorineural loss above 3000 Hz. The PTA scores (Case 1-1B) are 37 dB HL on the right ear and 10 dB HL

5. A critical distinction must be made between *type* of auditory disorder (acoustic Schwannoma) and *site* of auditory disorder (eighth nerve). Auditory tests may identify the site of disorder, but not the type of disorder. For examples of other types of disorder that may also be associated with eighth nerve site, see Chapter 5, Diabetes Mellitus; Chapter 7, Facial Nerve Disorders; Chapter 12, Intracranial Tumors Affecting the Central Auditory System; Chapter 15, Multiple Sclerosis; and Chapter 22, Sudden (Idiopathic) Sensorineural Hearing Loss.

In a series of approximately 800 patients with complete neuro-otologic evaluations and surgically confirmed acoustic tumors, audiologic test results provided the only evidence of the eighth nerve disorder in 2% of individuals (Sheehy, 1976).

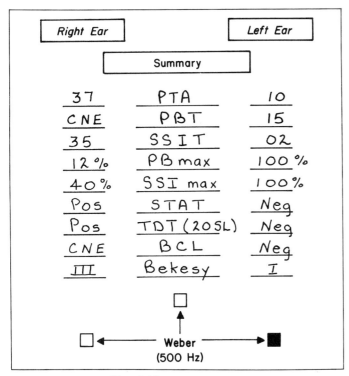

37	PTA	10
CNE	PBT	15
35	SSIT	02
12 %	PBmax	100 %
40 %	SSImax	100 %
Pos	STAT	Neg
Pos	TDT (20SL)	Neg
CNE	BCL	Neg
III	Bekesy	I

Case 1-1B

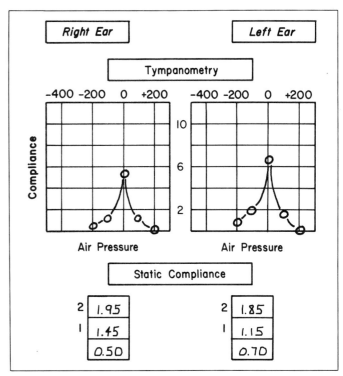

Case 1-1C

6. Notice that bone conduction sensitivity on the right ear is not plotted at 500 and 2000 Hz. At these frequencies, a plateau could not be defined and all bone conducted signals were referred to the non-test ear, even with maximum masking. In this circumstance, SAL audiometry provides valuable information about the degree of conductive component on the right ear.

on the left ear. SAL audiometry and bone conduction testing (Case 1-1A) do not show a conductive component on either ear.[6] The Weber test (Case 1-1B) at 500 Hz lateralizes to the left ear.

On the right ear, the PI-PB and PI-SSI functions (Case 1-1A) show reduced maximum intelligibility scores. The PB max score is 12%; the SSI max score is 40%. Additionally, the PI-SSI function shows the rollover effect. Performance declines from 40% at 40 dB HL to only 10% at 80 dB HL. The SSIT score (Case 1-1B) on the right ear is 35 dB HL. Poor maximum intelligibility scores preclude measurement of PI-PB rollover and a PBT score on the right ear.

On the left ear, the PI-PB and PI-SSI functions (Case 1-1A) are normal. The PB max and SSI max scores are 100%. The PBT, 15 dB HL, and SSIT, 2 dB HL (Case 1-1B) are consistent with pure tone sensitivity results.

Impedance audiometry (Case 1-1C) shows normal, type A, tympanograms and normal static compliance measures bilaterally. Crossed and uncrossed acoustic reflexes (Case 1-1A) are absent with sound to the right ear. With sound to the left ear, crossed reflexes are absent at all frequencies. The uncrossed reflex at 1000 Hz in the

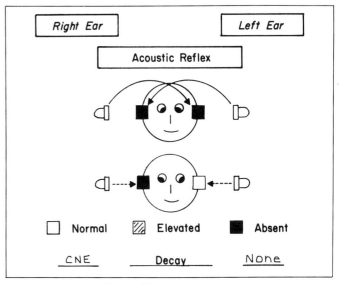

Case 1-1D

7. The L-shaped reflex pattern, in and of itself, is diagnostically nonspecific. The L-shaped pattern may reflect a right middle ear disorder, an intraaxial brain stem disorder eccentric to the right, or a right combined seventh and eighth nerve

left ear is within normal limits, however. The reflex pattern at 1000 Hz (Case 1-1D) is characterized by an inverted L-shaped pattern. Only the uncrossed reflex on the left ear is normal; all other reflexes are absent. The reflex pattern indicates a combined probe effect (vertical pattern) and sound effect (diagonal pattern) on the right ear.[7] On the right ear, the absence of reflexes precludes measurement of reflex decay. On the

4

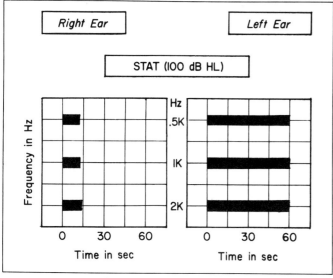

Case 1-1E

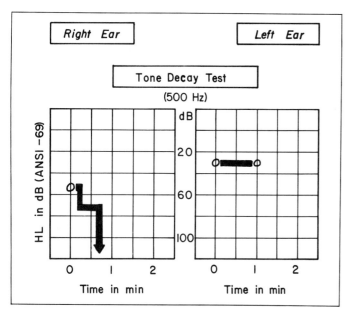

Case 1-1F. *20 dB SL modification.*

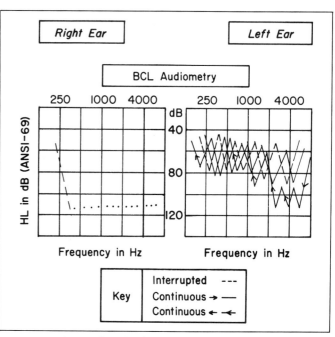

Case 1-1G

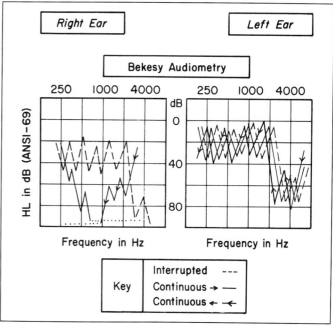

Case 1-1H

disorder. In this patient, a middle ear site is ruled out by SAL, bone conduction, and Weber tests. A brain stem site is considered unlikely since abnormal symptoms are not observed on the left, contralateral, ear. The remaining possibility is a combined seventh and eighth nerve disorder. This result is consistent with auditory test re-

left ear, uncrossed reflex decay is not observed at 1000 Hz.

The STAT (Case 1-1E) shows abnormal adaptation on the right ear. The patient stopped responding to STAT signals in less than 15 seconds at all test frequencies. On the left ear, the STAT test is negative.

The modified TDT (20 dB SL) shows abnormal adaptation on the right ear. The patient's responses at 500 Hz (Case 1-1F) and 1000 Hz decayed beyond equipment limits in less than 1 minute. On the left ear modified TDT results are normal at all frequencies.

sults and the patient's history of right facial weakness and numbness.

The BCL audiogram (Case 1-1G) on the right ear cannot be classified. The patient reported that sounds at equipment limits were never comfortably loud. BCL results on the left ear are negative.

The Bekesy audiogram (Case 1-1H) on the right ear is a type III tracing. A discrepancy between continuous forward and continuous backward tracings is observed. The Bekesy audiogram on the left ear is a type I

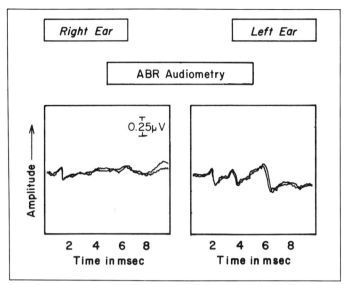

Case 1-1I

tracing with no forward-backward discrepancy.

Case 1-1I shows the ABR waveform on both ears to click signals of 100 dB HL. The response on the right ear shows a well-defined peak I wave with no identifiable later waves (II through V). The latency of peak I is within the normal range. This result, combined with the absence of subsequent waves, is consistent with right retrocochlear disorder. The waveform on the left ear shows well-formed peak I, III and V waves. The latency of all peaks, however, is delayed about 0.6 msec relative to the normal range. The delay is consistent with the presence of a severe high frequency sensitivity loss (Case 1-1A). The I-V interwave latency is normal (4.0 msec).

Impression

RIGHT EAR: Mild sensorineural loss through 2000 Hz; profound sensorineural loss above 2000 Hz. Diagnostic test results are consistent with combined eighth and seventh nerve disorder. An eighth nerve abnormality is indicated by the observation of abnormal adaptation on STAT, TDT, and Bekesy audiometry; abnormal ABR results; reduced maximum speech intelligibility scores, abnormal rollover of the PI-SSI function; and absent acoustic reflexes with sound to the right ear. A seventh nerve site is suggested by absent acoustic reflexes with probe to the right ear.

LEFT EAR: Sensitivity within normal limits through 3000 Hz; severe sensorineural loss above 3000 Hz. Results are consistent with the patient's history of noise exposure.

CASE 2. A 23-YEAR-OLD FEMALE WITH A 3-CM ACOUSTIC SCHWANNOMA ON THE RIGHT.

Surgical Findings

An extracanalicular neoplasm was found. The tumor was adjacent to the normal-appearing internal auditory meatus.

History

The patient reports a gradually increasing hearing loss in her right ear for approximately 4 months. She also complains of constant high pitched tinnitus in the right ear. She has particular difficulty understanding people on the telephone with her right ear. The patient denies dizziness, headaches, light-headedness, and facial weakness. She has no hearing complaints about her left ear.

General physical examination, otolaryngologic evaluation, and neurologic studies are within normal limits except for eighth nerve involvement on the right and a parotid mass on the left side of the neck. Other cranial nerve, brain stem, and cerebellar functions appear to be normal. Skull x-rays and polytomes of the internal auditory canals do not demonstrate any abnormality. There is no evidence of meatal enlargement or of skeletal erosion or destruction. A right vertebral angiogram shows a large neoplasm lying between the medial portion of the right petrous bone and the adjacent right lateral pons and inferior right cerebellar hemisphere.

Results

On the right ear the audiogram (Case 1-2A) shows normal sensitivity except for a mild sensorineural loss at 2000 Hz. On the left ear, sensitivity is within normal limits at all frequencies. The PTA scores (Case 1-2B) are 13 dB HL on the right ear and −4 dB HL on the left ear. On both ears, bone conduction sensitivity is superimposed on air conduction results.

Speech audiometry (Case 1-2A) on the right ear shows reduced maximum intelligibility scores and substantial rollover for both PI-PB and PI-SSI functions. The PB max is 72%; the SSI max is 70%. The PBT score, 21

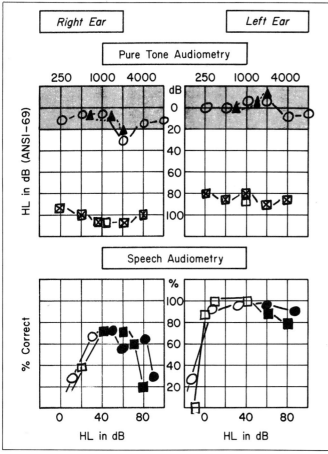

Case 1-2A

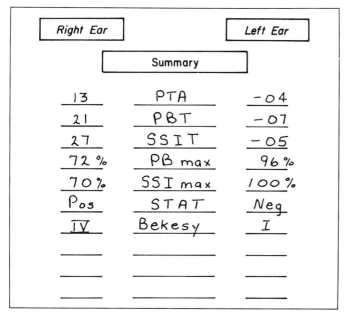

Case 1-2B

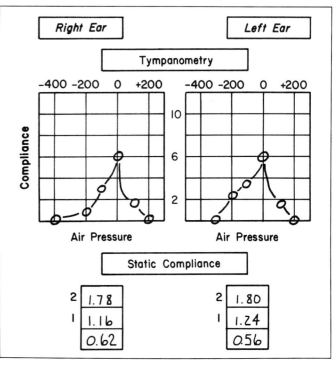

Case 1-2C

8. Notice that the relation between pure tone sensitivity and the SSIT in this patient is in the opposite direction from the pure tone vs speech threshold relation usually found in functional disorders. Remember in retrocochlear patients, speech thresholds, especially in the presence of a competing message, may be poorer than pure tone thresholds. Conversely, in functional patients, speech thresholds are usually better than voluntary pure tone responses. Contrast results in this patient with results in patient 3, Chapter 8, Functional Hearing Disorders.

9. On the right ear, notice that reflex thresholds at 250, 500, and 4000 Hz are within the "limits" of the normal range. However, in this patient,

dB HL (Case 1-2B), is in agreement (± 10 dB) with pure tone sensitivity on the right ear. The SSIT (27 dB HL), however, is elevated with respect to average pure tone sensitivity.[8]

The PI-PB function (Case 1-2A) on the left ear is normal. PB max is 96% correct. The PI-SSI function on the left ear shows normal maximum intelligibility score (100%) and slight rollover. Speech thresholds (Case 1-2B) on the left ear agree with pure tone sensitivity results. The PBT is −7 dB HL; the SSIT is −5 dB HL.

Impedance audiometry (Case 1-2C) shows normal, type A, tympanograms and normal static compliance measures bilaterally. Crossed and uncrossed acoustic reflexes (Case 1-2A) are elevated at 1000 and 2000 Hz with sound to the right ear and present at normal HLs at all frequencies with sound to the left ear. The reflex pattern (Case 1-2D) is characterized by a diagonal configuration.[9]

The reflex decay test on the right ear shows positive reflex decay at 500 Hz (Case 1-2E) and 1000 Hz. Reflex decay was not observed on the left ear at 500 Hz or 1000 Hz. SPAR measures (Case 1-2D) predict mild to moderate sensitivity loss on the right ear and normal sensitivity on the left ear.

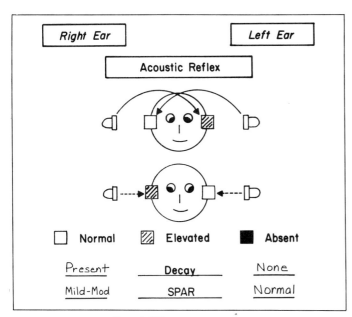

Case 1-2D

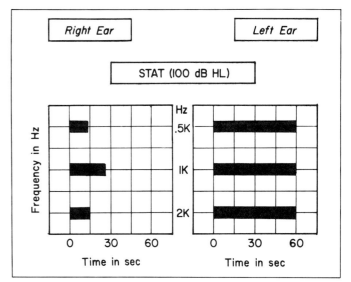

Case 1-2F

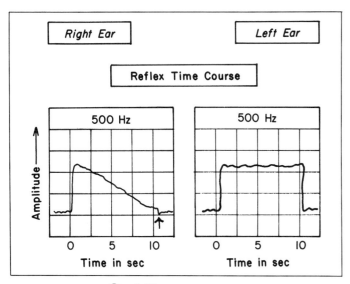

Case 1-2E

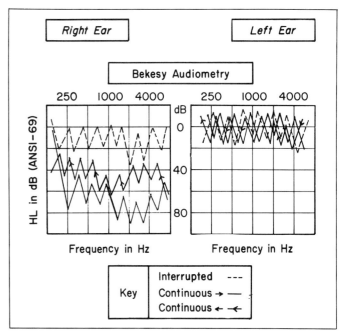

Case 1-2G

a more sensitive interpretation of threshold measures may be gained by comparing results on the right ear to thresholds on the left, normal, ear. In comparison to reflex thresholds on the normal control ear, all reflex thresholds on the right ear are elevated.

10. The interrupted vs continuous relation on Bekesy audiometry shows abnormal adaptation.

The STAT test (Case 1-2F) shows abnormal adaptation on the right ear at all test frequencies. No abnormal adaptation is observed on the left ear at any frequency. Bekesy audiometry (Case 1-2G) on the right ear shows a type IV threshold tracing with a significant forward-backward discrepancy.[10] Bekesy results on the left ear show a type I tracing with interweaving forward and backward continuous tracings.

Case 1-2H shows the ABR waveform on both ears to clicks at 80 dB HL. On the left ear all component waves appear at normal latencies. The I-V interwave interval is within the normal range (4.1 msec). On the

This finding is a strong presumption of eighth nerve site. In this circumstance, the continuous backward tracing is not really necessary. Generally, the purpose of the continuous forward vs backward relation is to sensitize the Bekesy technique when the forward continuous tracing is not abnormal.

right ear all waves are observed, but the IV-V complex is delayed relative to wave I. The I-V interwave latency is abnormal (4.7 msec). An abnormal interwave interval is consistent with right retrocochlear disorder.

Impression

RIGHT EAR: Sensitivity within normal limits with the exception of mild sensorineural loss at 2000 Hz. Diagnostic test results are consistent with eighth nerve site. Eighth nerve disorder is indicated by abnormal adaptation on STAT and Bekesy audiometry, ab-

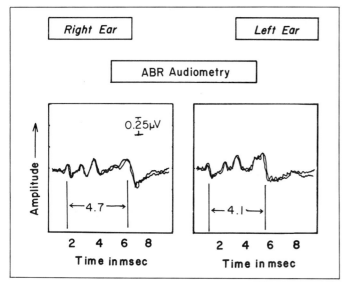

Case 1-2H

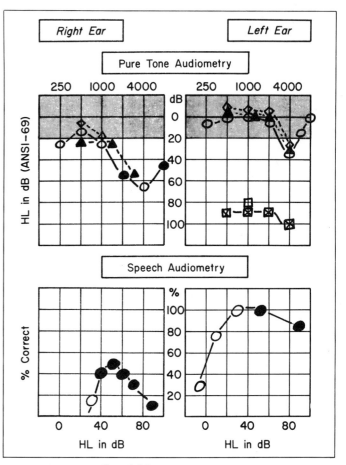

Case 1-3A

normal results on ABR audiometry, elevated acoustic reflexes, abnormal reflex decay with sound to the right ear, reduced maximum speech intelligibility scores, and unusual rollover of the PI functions on speech audiometry.

LEFT EAR: Normal.

CASE 3. A 22-YEAR-OLD MALE WITH A 4-CM ACOUSTIC SCHWANNOMA ON THE RIGHT.

Surgical Findings

The tumor was noted to extend into the tentorial notch and impinge on the brain stem.

History

The patient has noticed gradually increasing hearing loss in the right ear for approximately 4 years. He reports a constant high pitched tinnitus in the right ear for the last 3 years. His primary hearing complaint is difficulty understanding in noisy situations. He has not experienced any dizzy spells. He has a history of noise exposure from machinery and from hunting. The patient has no hearing complaints about his left ear.

General physical examination and oto-rhinolaryngologic evaluation are unremarkable except for hearing loss on the right ear. Hypocycloidal laminagraphy and posterior fossa myelography show evidence of an extracanalicular tumor at the meatus of the right internal auditory canal and adjacent cerebellopontine angle cistern.

11. In the differentiation of eighth nerve and intraaxial brain stem disorders, asymmetric pure tone sensitivity results on the two ears is a vote for eighth nerve site. Notice that all three patients in this chapter have asymmetric hearing sensitivity. For an example of the symmetric pure tone results characterizing most patients with intraaxial brain stem disorders, see patients 3 and 4, Chapter 12, Intracranial Tumors Affecting the Central Auditory System.

Results

The audiogram (Case 1-3A) on the right ear shows a mild sensorineural loss through 1000 Hz and a moderate sensorineural loss above 1000 Hz. Pure tone sensitivity on the left ear is within normal limits with the exception of a mild sensorineural loss at 4000 Hz.[11] The PTA scores (Case 1-3B) are 32 dB HL on the right ear and 1 dB HL on the left ear. SAL audiometry (Case 1-3A) does not show a conductive component on either ear. Bone conduction measures are superimposed on air conduction thresholds on both ears.

The PI-PB functions (Case 1-3A) are normal on the left ear but show substantial rollover on the right ear. The PB max scores are 100% on the left ear and 48% on the right ear. The PBT scores, 35 dB HL on the right ear and 0 dB HL on the left ear (Case 1-3B), agree with average pure tone sensitivity.

Impedance audiometry (Case 1-3C) shows normal, type A, tympanograms and normal static compliance measures on both

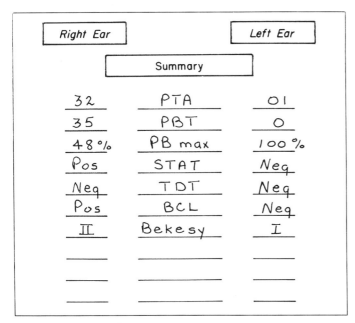

Case 1-3B

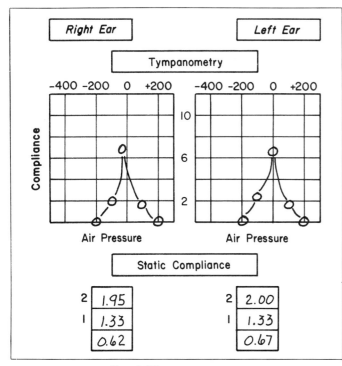

Case 1-3C

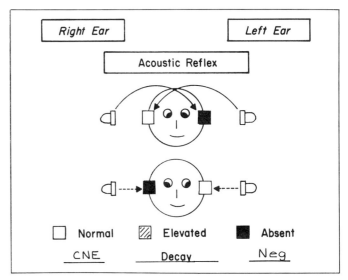

Case 1-3D

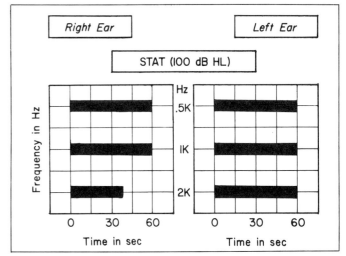

Case 1-3E

ears. Crossed and uncrossed acoustic reflexes (Case 1-3A) are absent at all frequencies with sound to the right ear and present at normal HLs with sound to the left ear. The reflex pattern (Case 1-3D) is characterized by a diagonal (sound effect) configuration. Absent reflexes on the right ear preclude measurement of reflex decay. On the left ear, the reflex decay test at 500 and 1000 Hz is negative.

12. Notice that suprathreshold vs threshold test results in this patient show striking differences. Threshold results (TDT and Bekesy audiometry) consistently yield false negative findings. In contrast, suprathreshold results (STAT and BCL) consistently identify the presence of eighth nerve disorder.

The STAT test (Case 1-3E) is positive on the right ear at 2000 Hz only. STAT results are negative at all frequencies on the left ear. The TDT results are normal on both ears at 500, 1000, and 2000 Hz (Case 1-3F). BCL audiometry (Case 1-3G) yields a positive pattern on the right ear and negative results on the left ear. Conventional threshold Bekesy audiometry (Case 1-3H) shows a type II tracing on the right ear with no forward-backward discrepancy. Bekesy audiometry on the left ear shows a type I tracing.[12]

Case 1-3I shows the ABR waveform on both ears to click signals at 100 dB HL. On the left ear all waves are present at normal latencies. On the right ear, however, no repeatable wave can be observed. Abnormal results on the right ear can be interpreted

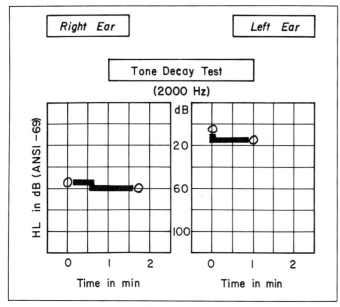

Case 1-3F

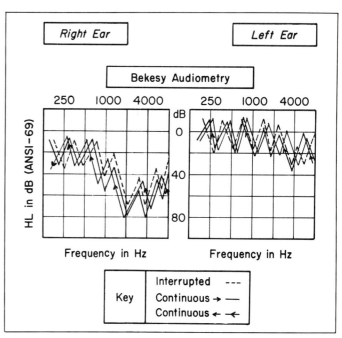

Case 1-3H

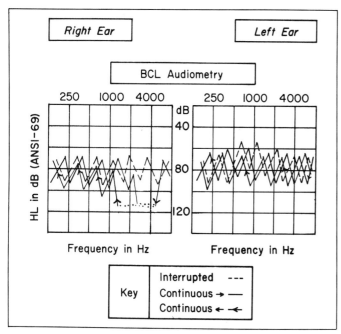

Case 1-3G

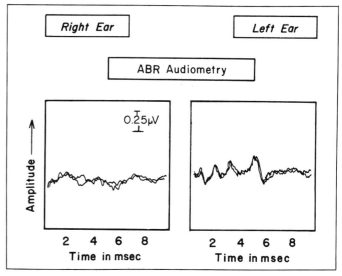

Case 1-3I

only in relation to the audiometric contour (Case 1-3A). In the case of a purely cochlear disorder, the presence of a moderate high frequency sensitivity loss would affect the latency of all components and would probably eliminate the early waves (I, II, and III). However, a wave V response would be expected. Consequently, the absence of all waves from the right ear is considered a retrocochlear sign.

Impression

RIGHT EAR: Mild sensorineural loss through 1000 Hz; moderate sensorineural loss above 1000 Hz. Diagnostic test results are consistent with eighth nerve site. Eighth nerve disorder is indicated by abnormal adaptation on STAT and BCL testing; absent acoustic reflexes with sound in the right ear, abnormal ABR audiometry, reduced maximum speech intelligibility performance; and abnormal rollover on the PI-PB function.

LEFT EAR: Normal sensitivity with the exception of a mild sensorineural loss at 4000 Hz.

Results are consistent with the patient's history of noise exposure.

COMMENT

Findings in these three patients emphasize the importance of suprathreshold auditory tests in the evaluation of eighth nerve site. More specifically, in two patients (Cases 1-1B and 1-2B), both threshold and suprathreshold measures showed abnormal adaptation. However, in one patient (Case 1-3B), threshold vs suprathreshold testing revealed striking differences. Specifically, for this latter patient, threshold measures were consistently negative; suprathreshold measures were consistently positive for eighth nerve site. This finding suggests that auditory test batteries for the detection of eighth nerve disorder should always include suprathreshold test measures.

SELECTED READINGS

Bebin, J. Pathophysiology of Acoustic Tumors. In W. House and C. Luetje (eds.), *Acoustic Tumors*. Vol. 1: *Diagnosis*. Baltimore: University Park Press, 1979. Pp. 45–83.

Dublin, W. *Fundamentals of Sensori-neural Auditory Pathology*. Springfield, Ill.: Thomas, 1976. Pp. 157–173.

Igarashi, M. Pathology of the Inner Ear Endorgans. In J. Minkler (ed.), *Pathology of the Nervous System* (vol. 3). New York: McGraw-Hill, 1972. Pp. 2856–2879.

Jerger, J., and Jerger, S. Diagnostic Audiology. In D. Tower (ed.), *The Nervous System*. Vol. 3: *Human Communication and Its Disorders*. New York: Raven Press, 1975. Pp. 199–205.

Jerger, J., and Mauldin, L. Prediction of sensori-neural hearing level from the brain stem evoked response. *Arch. Otolaryngol.* 104:456, 1978.

Nager, G. Acoustic neurinomas. Pathology and differential diagnosis. *Arch. Otolaryngol.* 89:252, 1969.

Neely, J., Alford, B., Templeton, T., and Neblett, C. Clinical correlates of neoplastic involvement of the eighth cranial nerve in man. *Surg. Forum* 28:508, 1977.

Perez de Moura, L. Inner ear pathology in acoustic neurinoma. *Arch. Otolaryngol.* 85:125, 1967.

Sheehy, J. Treatable sensorineural hearing impairment. *J. Otolaryngol. Soc. Austral.* 4:3, 1976.

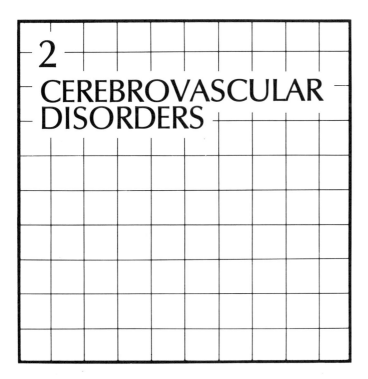

2
CEREBROVASCULAR DISORDERS

DESCRIPTION

Cerebrovascular disease (CVD) refers to pathologic conditions involving the blood vessels of the brain. Blood vessel abnormalities may include weakening or rupture of vessel walls, failure of systemic circulation, vasospasms, and occlusion by thrombus or embolus. Consequences of blood vessel disease may include intracranial hemorrhage and ischemia.

Cerebrovascular disorders may be transient or permanent. Some medical disorders associated with CVD are atherosclerosis, hypertensive arteriosclerosis, aneurysms, trauma, and developmental anomalies, such as arteriovenous (AV) malformations.[1]

PATIENT CHARACTERISTICS

Approximately 80% of patients are 65 years of age or older. In general, the sex prevalence for CVD varies with age, from approximately 65% males in young and middle-aged adults to about 50% males in elderly persons. Two types of CVD present exceptions to this general sex ratio, however. One exception is that, for all age groups, transient ischemic attacks occur twice as frequently in males as in females. The other unusual finding is that aneurysms of the internal carotid region and aneurysmal subarachnoid hemorrhages occur more frequently in females. For the latter

condition, the female-male ratio is about 1.4 : 1.

CLINICAL COURSE

Neurologic symptoms in CVD vary considerably, depending on the location and size of the lesion. Subjective auditory complaints are rarely observed. Symptoms characteristically include hemiplegia, numbness, dizziness/vertigo, diplopia, impaired vision, sensory deficits, tinnitus, dysarthria, headache, mental impairment, ataxia, vomiting, and aphasia.[2]

Onset of symptoms may be insidious or instantaneous.[3] Duration of symptoms may vary from permanent impairment to transient conditions with no sustained neurologic sequelae. Treatment may involve drug therapy, rehabilitation therapies, and/or surgical management.

SITE OF DISORDER

Central auditory system. Two primary exceptions to this site of disorder occur, however, depending on the anatomical site of the lesion and the state of recovery. One exception involves patients with normal auditory function and no apparent involvement of the brain stem or temporal lobe auditory areas. The other exception concerns patients with vertebral basilar disease involving the internal auditory artery. In these patients, sudden sensorineural hearing loss may occur. Symptoms accompanying the hearing loss may include tinnitus, vertigo, nausea, and vomiting.[4]

GENERAL AUDIOLOGIC PATTERN

Pure tone sensitivity results usually show normal hearing or a sensorineural loss consistent with the patient's age. Impedance measures are generally within normal limits. One exception to this observation concerns patients with CVD involving the brain stem auditory pathways. In these patients, acoustic reflex measures may be abnormal. Reflex abnormalities are typically characterized by horizontal or inverted L-shaped patterns.

Speech intelligibility scores for PB words are usually normal or consistent with pure tone sensitivity results. An exception to this observation may involve patients with aphasia who cannot perform the required

1. The prevalence of CVD varies as a function of age. Annual incidence rates range from about 1 per 100,000 for individuals less than 35 years of age to about 840 per 100,000 for individuals 65 to 74 years of age. An average incidence rate is about 200 per 100,000 annually. Transient cerebrovascular episodes may be referred to as transient ischemic attacks, transient vascular insufficiency, carotid artery insufficiency, and vertebral basilar artery insufficiency.

2. Of individuals with CVD, 10% to 40% have aphasia.

3. A sudden, dramatic onset of neurologic deficits may be termed *stroke* or *cerebrovascular accident (CVA)*.

4. Of the arterial systems supplying intracranial structures, the temporal, frontal and parietal lobes are primarily supplied by the carotid artery system. In contrast, the inner ear, the brain stem, and a small portion of the temporal lobe are primarily nourished by the vertebral basilar artery system.

Of patients with vertebral basilar insufficiency, approximately 1.5% notice a change in hearing (see Chapter 22, Sudden [Idiopathic] Sensorineural Hearing Loss).

13

verbal repetition task. In contrast to typically normal findings on unaltered speech tasks, performance on degraded speech tasks is usually abnormal. Generally, patients with CVD involving the brain stem auditory pathways show consistently depressed performance for difficult monotic speech tasks, such as the SSI procedure in the presence of an ipsilateral competing message. Patients with CVD at the level of the temporal lobe, on the other hand, usually show greater performance deficits for difficult dichotic speech messages, such as the SSI procedure in the presence of a contralateral competing message. In patients with aphasia, pronounced performance deficits for both degraded monotic and dichotic listening tasks may be observed.

The ear yielding the abnormal auditory findings may vary. For example, patients with aphasia or with auditory disorders at the level of the brain stem characteristically show depressed performance on both ears. In contrast, patients with temporal lobe auditory disorders without aphasia primarily show performance deficits on the ear contralateral to the affected side of the brain.

Other abnormalities may include deficits on temporal order tasks, loudness discrimination tasks, and threshold duration functions.[5]

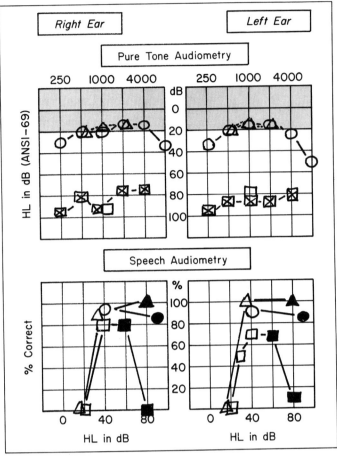

Case 2-1A

5. For further discussion of the clinical manifestations of central auditory disorder, see Chapter 12, Intracranial Tumors Affecting the Central Auditory System.

Illustrative Patients

CASE 1. A 48-YEAR-OLD FEMALE WITH A 3-CM SACCULAR ANEURYSM ATTACHED TO THE SUPRACLINOID PORTION OF THE RIGHT INTERNAL CAROTID ARTERY.

A thrombosed segment of the aneurysm elevates the right middle cerebral artery. The aneurysm has produced hydrocephalus involving both lateral ventricles.

History

The patient was hospitalized for evaluation of headache and visual disturbances. The patient complains of three severe headaches during the last year. The headaches consist of intense pulsatile pain localized in the right supraorbital region. The headaches are preceded by blurring of vision in the right eye. There is no family history of migraine.

Approximately 1 year ago, the patient began to experience blank spaces (negative scotoma) in her vision to the right. Recently,

6. Verbalization of pure tone sensitivity results presents a choice between borderline normal vs sensorineural classifications. The sensorineural category was preferred in this instance because the audiometric contour is not normal. Notice that sensitivity is better in the mid frequency area than in the low or high frequency regions. A rising-sloping configuration is a consistent observation in patients with central auditory lesions.

she has been noticing negative scotoma in her left eye also. For the past 4 months, the patient reports episodes of disorientation and increasing short-term memory difficulties. She has no specific sensory or motor complaints. In particular, she has no noticeable hearing difficulties.

Results

The audiogram (Case 2-1A) shows a mild sensorineural loss on both ears.[6] The PTA scores (Case 2-1B) are 18 dB HL on the right ear and 17 dB HL on the left ear. Unmasked bone conduction thresholds (Case 2-1A) are superimposed on air conduction thresholds.

The PI-SSI function (Case 2-1A) shows reduced maximum intelligibility scores and severe rollover on both ears. SSI max scores are 80% on the right ear and 70% on the left ear. A PI function for SSI materials in quiet is normal on both ears. Maximum scores for the SSI-quiet procedure are 100% bilaterally. PB word testing at high intensity levels

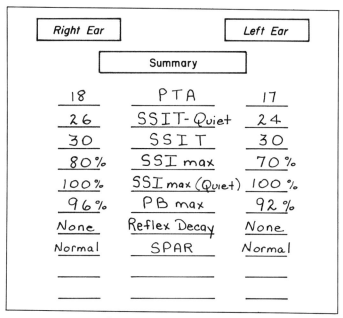

Right Ear		Left Ear

	Summary	
18	PTA	17
26	SSIT-Quiet	24
30	SSIT	30
80%	SSI max	70%
100%	SSI max (Quiet)	100%
96%	PB max	92%
None	Reflex Decay	None
Normal	SPAR	Normal

Case 2-1B

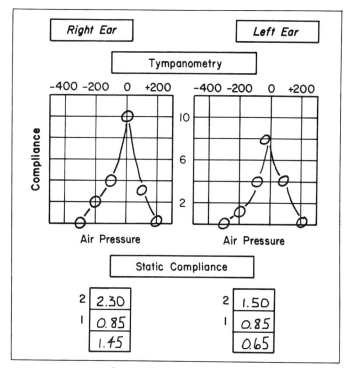

Case 2-1C

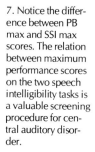

7. Notice the difference between PB max and SSI max scores. The relation between maximum performance scores on the two speech intelligibility tasks is a valuable screening procedure for central auditory disorder.

8. In retrocochlear disorders, unusually poor speech thresholds may be found on degraded speech tasks (see patient 2, Chapter 1, Acoustic Schwannoma). Remember, in contrast to the SSI-quiet function, the PI-SSI function is obtained with a competing message in the background.

shows normal intelligibility scores and no significant rollover. PB max scores are 96% on the right ear and 92% on the left ear.[7]

Speech thresholds (Case 2-1B) for the SSI-quiet procedure agree (± 10 dB) with average pure tone sensitivity results. SSIT-quiet scores are 26 dB HL on the right ear and 24 dB HL on the left ear. Speech thresholds for the PI-SSI function are slightly elevated on both ears. SSIT thresholds are 30 dB HL on each ear.[8]

Impedance audiometry (Case 2-1C) shows normal, type A, tympanograms and normal static compliance measures on both ears. Crossed and uncrossed acoustic reflex thresholds (Case 2-1A) are present at normal HLs on both ears. Reflex decay (Case 2-1B) is not observed at 500 or 1000 Hz on either ear. SPAR measures predict relatively normal sensitivity bilaterally.

Impression

Very mild sensorineural loss on both ears. Impedance audiometry is consistent with normal middle ear function bilaterally. The difference between PB max and SSI max scores and rollover of PI-SSI functions suggest central auditory disorder. Further diagnostic auditory testing for the differentiation of brain stem and temporal lobe sites could not be carried out due to the patient's physical malaise.

9. Notice the normal, bilaterally symmetric, pure tone sensitivity results in this patient. In the differentiation of brain stem and eighth nerve disorders, this pattern of pure tone sensitivity results is consistent with a brain stem site.

CASE 2. A 64-YEAR-OLD FEMALE WITH VERTEBRAL BASILAR ARTERY INSUFFICIENCY SYNDROME.

History

The patient was referred to the Audiology Service with complaints of tinnitus and a "pounding" sound in both ears. She has noticed the ear noises for the past 3 months. During this time period, she also experienced attacks of episodic vertigo. The frequency of attacks was approximately once a week. Recently, the patient also noticed decreased visual acuity.

Results

The audiogram (Case 2-2A) shows normal pure tone sensitivity bilaterally.[9] The PTA scores (Case 2-2B) are 8 dB HL for the right ear and 10 dB HL for the left ear. Speech audiometry (Case 2-2A) shows normal PI-PB functions on both ears. PB max scores are 92% for the right ear and 96% for the left ear. PBT scores (Case 2-2B) on both ears agree with pure tone sensitivity results. The PBT scores are 7 dB HL on the right ear and 14 dB HL on the left ear.

Impedance audiometry (Case 2-2C) shows normal tympanograms and normal static compliance measures bilaterally. On

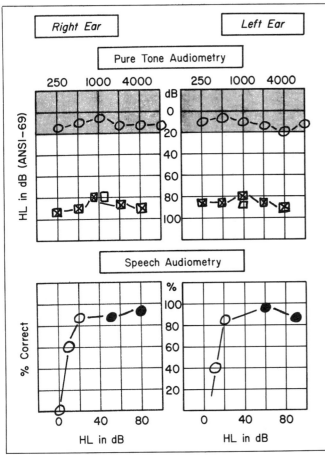

Case 2-2A

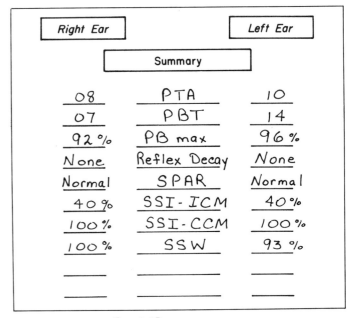

Case 2-2B

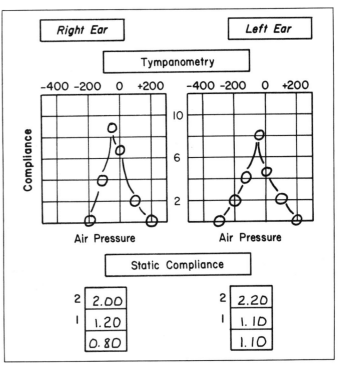

Case 2-2C

10. On the left ear, notice the performance dip at 0 dB MCR (Case 2-2D). Some individuals report that 0 dB MCR is an unusually difficult listening task because the target and the competition are presented at the same intensity level. Consequently, listeners do not have loudness cues to aid in differentiating the target from the competing background.

both ears, crossed and uncrossed acoustic reflexes (Case 2-2A) are present at normal HLs with no reflex decay. SPAR results (Case 2-2B) predict normal sensitivity in each ear.

SSI-ICM scores (Case 2-2D) show depressed performance on both ears. Average SSI-ICM performance (Case 2-2B) is 40% on both ears.[10] In contrast to SSI-ICM performance, SSI-CCM performance (Case 2-2D) is unimpaired on either ear. SSI-CCM scores (Case 2-2B) are 100% at all test conditions.

SSW results (Case 2-2B) are within normal limits for all test conditions on both ears. Performance scores for the competing condition are 100% for the right ear and 93% for the left ear.

Impression

Pure tone sensitivity is within normal limits bilaterally. Impedance audiometry is consistent with normal middle ear function on both ears. Diagnostic test results indicate a central auditory disorder involving the brain stem auditory pathways. A brain stem site is

supported by the observation of SSI-ICM performance deficits in the presence of normal SSI-CCM performance.

CASE 3. A 24-YEAR-OLD FEMALE WITH CEREBROVASCULAR DISEASE OF THE RIGHT FRONTAL-TEMPORAL-PARIETAL AREA. Angiography showed ischemic area involving the right frontal-temporal-parietal region. Cerebral edema and hydrocephalus within at

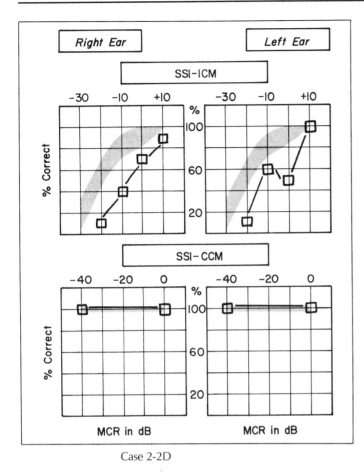

Case 2-2D

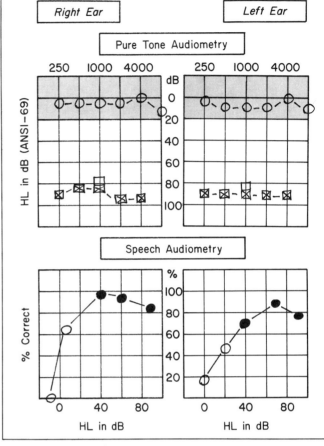

Case 2-3A

least the right lateral ventricle were also observed. EEG results showed a focus of abnormal activity in the right occipito-temporal region.

History

The patient was admitted to the hospital after intermittent fainting spells for the previous 6 hours. During the patient's school years, she received three severe blows to the head that resulted in unconsciousness. Two years ago, she experienced seizure episodes during her eighth month of pregnancy. The seizures were apparently controlled by drug therapy.

For the past 3 months, she complains of recurrent headaches and difficulty in speaking. She also notices a problem understanding people in some situations. She has particular difficulty using the telephone on the left ear.[11]

Results

The audiogram (Case 2-3A) shows normal pure tone sensitivity on both ears. PTA

11. The "telephone sign" is a helpful indicator of central auditory disorder. The telephone presents a degraded (filtered) speech message to listeners. Consequently, some patients with central auditory problems may notice a hearing problem for the first time when using a telephone on the affected ear.

12. Notice the unusually slow rise to maximum performance on the left ear. At 40 dB HL, for example, performance on the left ear is about 25% poorer than results on the right ear. In view of the normal pure tone sensitivity, asymmetric speech intelligibility results suggest central auditory disorder.

On the left ear, a speech threshold from the PI-PB function may not be determined by the 50% intelligibility level due to the abnormally slow rise to maximum performance. In this circumstance, the PBT is determined by the 25% correct point.

scores (Case 2-3B) are 5 dB HL on the right ear and 10 dB HL on the left ear.

The PI-PB functions (Case 2-3A) show maximum intelligibility scores of 96% on the right ear and 88% on the left ear. The degree of rollover is within normal limits on both ears. PBT scores (Case 2-3B), 0 dB HL on the right ear and 5 dB HL on the left ear, agree with pure tone sensitivity results on both ears.[12]

Impedance audiometry (Case 2-3C) shows normal, type A, tympanograms and normal static compliance measures bilaterally. Crossed and uncrossed acoustic reflexes (Case 2-3A) are present at normal HLs on both ears. Reflex decay testing (Case 2-3B) at 500 and 1000 Hz was normal bilaterally.

SSI-ICM performance (Case 2-3D) is slightly below the normal range on the right ear and depressed at all MCRs on the left ear. Average performance scores (Case 2-3B) are 53% on the right ear and 40% on the left ear. SSI-CCM performance (Case

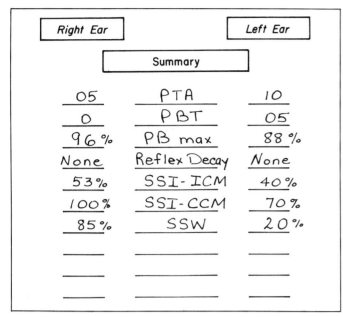

Case 2-3B

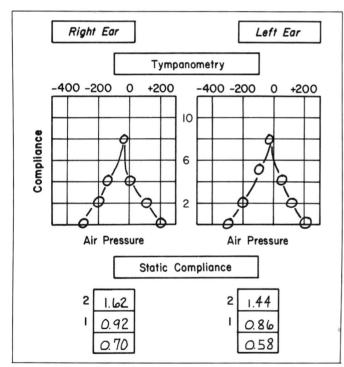

Case 2-3C

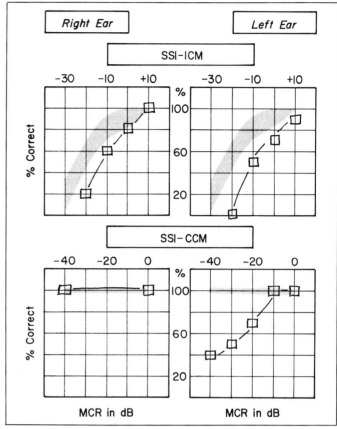

Case 2-3D

2-3D) is normal on the right ear, but shows substantial performance deficits on the left ear. Average performance scores (Case 2-3B) are 100% on the right ear and 70% on the left ear.

SSW results (Case 2-3B) for the competing condition showed a large difference between ears. Average performance for the competing monosyllables was 85% on the right ear but only 20% on the left ear.

13. In this patient, performance deficits were observed on the left ear, the ear contralateral to the right temporal lobe disorder. However, consistent left ear deficits may also be found in patients with left temporal lobe site (see patient 2, Chapter 12, Intracranial Tumors Affecting the Central Auditory System).

Impression

Pure tone sensitivity is within normal limits bilaterally. Impedance audiometry is consistent with normal middle ear function on each ear. Diagnostic test results are consistent with temporal lobe site. A temporal lobe site is supported by the observation of a large performance deficit on the competing condition of the SSW test and by a relatively more severe deficit for the SSI-CCM procedure than for the SSI-ICM task. All abnormal auditory findings are observed on the left ear.[13]

CASE 4. A 42-YEAR-OLD MALE WITH APHASIA FOLLOWING A SUBARACHNOID HEMORRHAGE.

History

At hospitalization, the patient reported a history of aphasia and right hemiplegia. Two months ago, he experienced severe generalized headache, stiffness of the neck, and a brief loss of consciousness. Ten days later, he suddenly became comatose and was unconscious for several days. Upon regaining consciousness, he had aphasia and right hemiplegia. He was in Singapore dur-

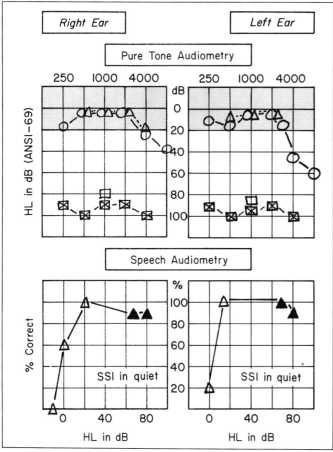

Case 2-4A

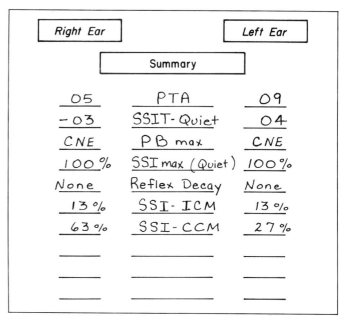

Case 2-4B

ing this period and medical records are unavailable.

At the present admission 2 months post-trauma, the patient had regained the use of his right arm and leg. However, a right-sided weakness was noted. Brain scan indicated decreased blood flow in the left middle cerebral artery. EEG findings showed a focus of intermittent slow activity in the left temporal region.

Speech pathology evaluation at this time noted expressive aphasia, verbal apraxia, and deficits in auditory and visual receptive skills. The patient is right-handed.

Presently, the patient is having difficulty understanding other people, particularly in crowds or in noisy places. Prior to the aphasia, he did not notice any hearing problems on either ear.

Results

The audiogram (Case 2-4A) shows normal sensitivity on both ears through 3000 Hz, then a moderate, bilateral, sensorineural loss. Unmasked bone conduction thresholds

14. Notice that results in this patient are consistent with a generalized language disorder associated with damage to the hemisphere dominant for speech.

are superimposed on air conduction. The PTA scores (Case 2-4B) are 5 dB HL on the right ear and 9 dB HL on the left ear.

PI-PB testing (Case 2-4B) could not be carried out due to the patient's limited expressive language ability. A PI function for SSI materials in quiet (Case 2-4A) is normal on both ears. Maximum scores for the SSI-quiet procedure (Case 2-4B) are 100% bilaterally.

Speech thresholds (Case 2-4B) for the SSI-quiet procedure agree (± 10 dB) with average pure tone sensitivity results. SSIT-quiet scores are −3 dB HL on the right ear and 4 dB HL on the left ear.

Impedance audiometry (Case 2-4C) shows type A tympanograms, normal static compliance measures, and normal crossed and uncrossed acoustic reflexes (Case 2-4A) on both ears. Reflex decay testing (Case 2-4B) is normal on both ears.

The SSI-ICM and SSI-CCM procedures (Case 2-4D) show pronounced performance deficits on both ears. Average SSI-ICM scores (Case 2-4B) are 13% on both ears. Average SSI-CCM scores are 63% on the right ear and 27% on the left ear.[14]

Impression

Normal pure tone sensitivity in both ears through 3000 Hz, then a moderate, bilateral, sensorineural loss. Impedance audiometry is consistent with normal middle ear function bilaterally. Results of diagnostic

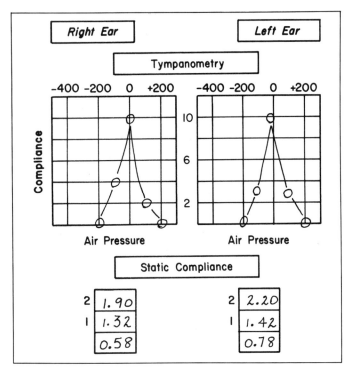

Case 2-4C

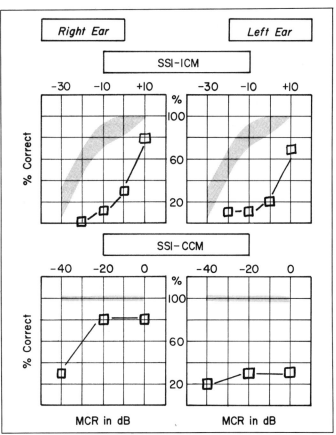

Case 2-4D

speech audiometry are consistent with the presence of aphasia.

COMMENT

With the exception of the patient with aphasia, findings in these cases illustrate the normalcy of routine audiologic measures in patients with CVD. For example, in the first three patients, pure tone sensitivity results (Cases 2-1A, 2-2A, and 2-3A) were essentially normal; maximum intelligibility scores for PB words (Cases 2-1A, 2-2A, and 2-3A) were relatively unimpaired; and impedance measures (Cases 2-1A, 2-1C, 2-2A, 2-2C, 2-3A, and 2-3C) were within normal limits.

In addition to normal routine auditory test results, the patients' histories are essentially negative for subjective hearing disorder. For example, none of the first three patients complained of noticeable hearing difficulties. Even with structured questioning, only patient 3 admitted difficulty in understanding people, particularly on the telephone.

These observations stress the importance of a screening procedure for central auditory disorder in patients with normal findings on routine pure tone and PB word tests. Results in patient 1 (Case 2-1A) highlight the importance of a central screening measure. This patient was too ill for complete diag-

nostic evaluation. However, a quick evaluation of performance with the PI-SSI procedure yielded striking evidence of retrocochlear abnormality.

SELECTED READINGS

Burns, R. A. Basilar-vertebral artery insufficiency as a cause of vertigo. *Otolaryngol. Clin. North Am.* 6:287, 1973.

Fisher, C. M., Mohr, J. P., and Adams, R. D. Cerebrovascular Diseases. In M. Wintrobe, G. Thorn, R. Adam, E. Braunwald, K. Isselbacher, and R. Petersdorf (eds.), *Principles of Internal Medicine* (7th ed.). New York: McGraw-Hill, 1974. Pp. 1743–1779.

Ginsberg, M., and Reivich, M. Cerebrovascular Pathophysiology. In D. Tower (ed.), *The Clinical Neurosciences.* New York: Raven Press, 1975. Pp. 157–166.

Kurtzke, J. *Epidemiology of Cerebrovascular Disease.* New York: Springer-Verlag, 1969.

Toole, J., and Patel, A. Applied Anatomy of Brain Arteries. In J. Toole and A. Patel (eds.), *Cerebrovascular Disorders.* New York: McGraw-Hill, 1967. Pp. 1–25.

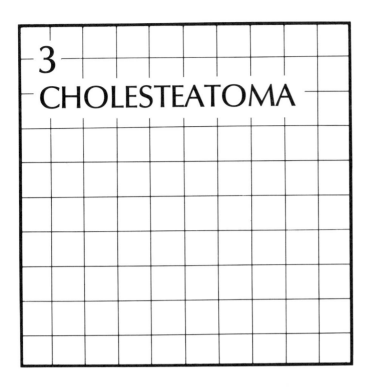

3
CHOLESTEATOMA

DESCRIPTION

1. The term *cholesteatoma* derived from the belief that cholesterol was a primary component of this cyst. Today, many people consider the term a misnomer.

The prevalence of cholesteatoma in a white, middle-class population is about 6 per 100,000 individuals. The prevalence varies as a function of age, with a peak rate in the 10 to 30-year-old group (Harker, 1977).

In a series of 50 children with suppurative chronic mastoiditis, cholesteatoma occurred in 73% of persons (Rambo, 1972).

Congenital cholesteatomas account for 0.2% to 1.5% of all intracranial tumors and about 6% of cerebellopontine angle tumors (Nager, 1975).

Cholesteatoma may be referred to as *epidermoid cholesteatoma* or *keratoma* and may be called *pearl tumor* because of a lustrous pearl-like color.

Cholesteatoma is a cystic mass that may occur within the middle ear and other pneumatized areas of the temporal bone. As a general rule, cholesteatomas develop as a complication of recurrent or chronic middle ear infection. Retraction or perforation of the tympanic membrane usually accompanies the formation of cholesteatoma. On rare occasions, however, cholesteatomas may occur with no apparent predisposing middle ear abnormality. A possible danger of cholesteatoma involves erosion of important otologic or cranial structures, i.e., destruction of the ossicular chain, fistulization or invasion of the bony labyrinth, erosion of the fallopian canal, etc.[1]

PATIENT CHARACTERISTICS

Cholesteatomas may be congenital (about 2%) or acquired (about 98%) (Cody, 1977). The onset of symptomatology may occur at any age. A qualification to this observation, however, involves patients with congenital cholesteatomas. In these patients, the peak age of the onset of symptoms is about 15 years (Paparella and Rybak, 1978). The characteristic age at which a congenital cholesteatoma is diagnosed may vary depending on whether the tumor is located within the middle ear space or arises in the petrous pyramid (Derlacki, 1973). More

specifically, patients with congenital cholesteatomas originating in the middle ear and mastoid areas characteristically are diagnosed between 3 and 14 years of age. In contrast, patients with congenital cholesteatomas originating in the petrous pyramid generally are diagnosed between 35 and 55 years of age. Cholesteatomas may be unilateral or bilateral. Cholesteatoma is predominantly a disease of males; 80% of congenital cholesteatomas and 63% of acquired cholesteatomas occur in males (Cody, 1977).

CLINICAL COURSE

Progressive conductive hearing loss. The onset of the loss is characteristically insidious. The patient may complain of earache, tinnitus, and a foul-smelling discharge from the ear. Exceptions to this pattern occur, however, depending on the size and location of the cholesteatoma. For example, patients with cholesteatomas in the attic area may have normal hearing and no apparent disorder of the middle ear vibratory system. Another exception involves patients with cholesteatomas that have invaded the bony labyrinth, the internal auditory canal, or the cerebellopontine angle. In these patients, symptoms may include sensorineural hearing loss and facial palsy.

In general, cholesteatomas develop slowly over a period of years. However, in the presence of active infection, cholesteatomas may develop more rapidly. Treatment may include surgical removal of the cholesteatoma. In some patients, however, cholesteatomas may recur after surgical intervention.

SITE OF DISORDER

Middle ear and external ear systems. On rare occasions, the cochlea and/or eighth nerve may be involved.

GENERAL AUDIOLOGIC PATTERN

Pure tone sensitivity results generally show a conductive hearing loss. The degree of loss varies, however, depending on the site and size of the cholesteatoma. On occasion, either a sensorineural loss or normal pure tone sensitivity may occur. Speech intelligibility scores are usually within normal limits.

Impedance results vary depending on the

nature and extent of ossicular chain involvement. For example, if the cholesteatoma produces slight pressure upon the ossicular chain, the impedance data may reflect a fixation pattern. The tympanogram may be a shallow, type A, shape; static compliance measures may be slightly reduced; and acoustic reflex thresholds may be elevated. If, however, the tumor envelops the ossicular chain, impedance results may reflect a mass effect. The tympanogram may be a type B shape, static compliance may be below normal limits, and reflexes may be absent. Finally, if the cholesteatoma erodes through the ossicular chain, a discontinuity pattern may result. Findings may be characterized by an unusually deep tympanogram, static compliance above the normal range, and elevated or absent acoustic reflexes.[2]

One exception to the above findings involves patients with cholesteatomas that have eroded the ossicular chain. Sometimes, in these patients, the tumor itself may form a functional connection between the ossicles. In this circumstance, a rounded tympanogram and surprisingly little air-bone gap may be observed.

Illustrative Patients

CASE 1. A 31-YEAR-OLD MALE WITH A CHOLESTEATOMA ON THE RIGHT EAR.

Surgical Findings

The cholesteatoma originated in the attic and extended down into the middle ear to the level of the incudostapedial joint. The tympanic membrane was almost totally absent.

History

The patient complains of intermittent middle ear infections and fluctuating hearing loss in his right ear for 19 years. He reports a chronic tympanic membrane perforation for at least 15 years. The patient does not report tinnitus or dizziness. At the present time, he thinks his hearing in both ears is good.

Results

The audiogram (Case 3-1A) shows a mild conductive loss on the right ear and normal sensitivity on the left ear. PTA scores (Case 3-1B) are 17 dB HL on the right ear and −2 dB HL on the left ear. Bone conduction and

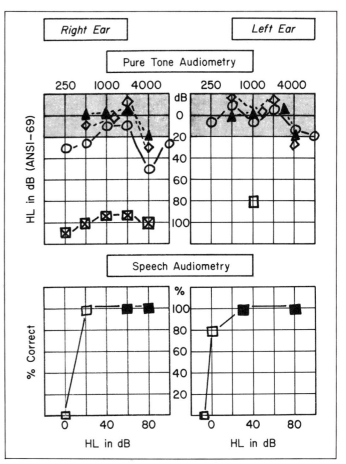

Case 3-1A

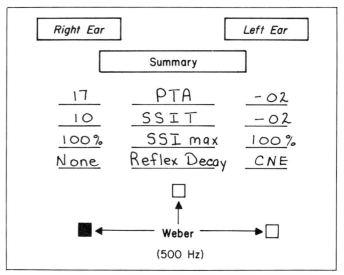

Case 3-1B

SAL audiometry (Case 3-1A) on the right ear show a conductive component of about 10 to 20 dB. On the left ear, bone conduction and SAL results are superimposed on air conduction.

The Weber test (Case 3-1B) at 500 Hz

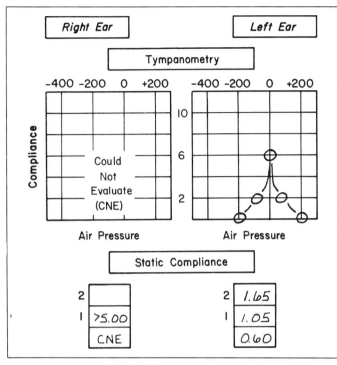

Case 3-1C

3. On the static compliance box for the right ear, notice how large the first measurement is. Remember, to determine static compliance, two volume measurements are made. The first measurement represents the volume of the closed cavity in the external ear canal. In patients with intact tympanic membranes (TMs), external canal volumes range from about 0.5 to 1.5 cc. (For example, notice the normal value on the left ear.) On the right ear, a perforation of the TM is indicated by the abnormally large external canal volume measurement and the large difference between canal volumes on the ears.

In patients with perforations of the TM, Eustachian tube function should be routinely assessed.

lateralizes to the right ear. The Bing test (not shown) at 500 Hz shows no occlusion effect on the right ear. On the left ear, an occlusion effect of 20 dB is observed.

PI-SSI functions (Case 3-1A) are normal on both ears. Maximum SSI scores are 100% bilaterally. SSIT scores (Case 3-1B), 10 dB HL on the right ear and −2 dB HL on the left ear, agree with average pure tone sensitivity.

Tympanometry and static compliance measures (Case 3-1C) on the right ear could not be obtained due to the perforated tympanic membrane.[3] Neither positive nor negative pressure could be maintained in the right ear. This finding suggests a patulous Eustachian tube. On the left ear, the tympanogram is a normal, type A, shape. Static compliance is within normal limits. With one exception, crossed acoustic reflexes on the right ear and uncrossed acoustic reflexes on the left ear are present at HLs within the normal range. The exception notes the elevated crossed reflex threshold on the right ear at 250 Hz.[4] No reflex decay (Case 3-1B) was observed at 500 or 1000 Hz on the right ear. Acoustic reflex measures with sound to the left ear and probe tip in the right ear could not be obtained.

4. In interpreting acoustic reflexes, data are described in relation to a normal range. However, in this patient, a more sensitive interpretation of reflex thresholds may be gained by comparing reflexes on the right ear to reflexes on the left, normal, ear. In comparison to reflexes on the normal control ear, reflexes at 1000 Hz on the right ear are elevated approximately 15 dB, instead of within normal limits. Elevated reflexes on the right ear are consistent with mild conductive loss.

5. Notice the complementary nature of SAL and bone conduction (BC) tests. On the right ear, BC results at 500 Hz could not be obtained. Even with maximum masking, all signals were heard in the non-test ear. In this circumstance, SAL results provided valuable information about the presence of a mild conductive disorder. However, on the left ear, an SAL threshold could not be defined at 1000 Hz. With the SAL noise, the patient's air conduction threshold was beyond equipment limits, indicating a conductive component of more than 55 dB. In this situation, BC testing defined the degree of conductive loss more precisely.

6. Bing results on the right ear would have been helpful in cross-checking the presence of a low frequency conductive component. However, results at 500 Hz were unobtainable because

Impression

RIGHT EAR: Mild conductive loss. Impedance audiometry is consistent with a perforation of the tympanic membrane.

LEFT EAR: Normal pure tone sensitivity. Impedance audiometry indicates normal middle ear function.

CASE 2. A 41-YEAR-OLD MALE WITH BILATERAL CHOLESTEATOMAS.

Surgical Findings

On the right ear, a cholesteatoma consumed Prussak's space and extended into the epitympanum. The cholesteatoma was lateral to the body of the incus.

On the left ear, extensive cholesteatoma occupied the superior mesotympanum, epitympanum, antrum, and periantrum space. In addition, the cholesteatoma had eroded part of the external auditory canal. The head of the malleus appeared fixed. The incus and part of the stapes were absent.

History

The patient reports frequent episodes of otorrhea, ear pain, and fluctuating hearing loss during childhood. He remembers more trouble on the left ear than on the right ear. He has experienced no pain or otorrhea for the past three years. However, for the last several months, his hearing on the left ear has been getting progressively worse.

Results

The audiogram (Case 3-2A) shows pure tone sensitivity within normal limits on the right ear with the exception of a mild loss at 8000 Hz. However, bone conduction and SAL audiometry on the right ear show a conductive component, at all frequencies, of 5 to 15 dB. On the left ear, the audiogram shows a moderate conductive loss.[5] PTA scores (Case 3-2B) are 13 dB HL on the right ear and 42 dB HL on the left ear.

The Weber test (Case 3-2B) at 500 Hz lateralizes to the left ear, the ear with the greatest conductive component. The Bing test (not shown) at 500 Hz shows no occlusion effect on the left ear. On the right ear, Bing results at 500 Hz could not be obtained.[6]

The shape of the PI-SSI functions (Case 3-2A) is normal on both ears. The SSI max scores (Case 3-2B) are 100% on the right ear

24

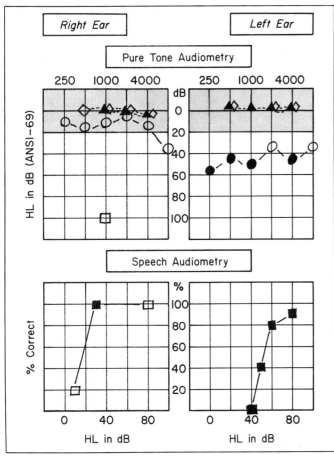

Case 3-2A

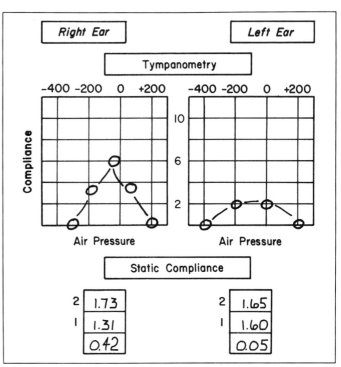

Case 3-2C

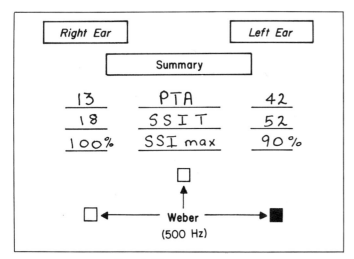

Case 3-2B

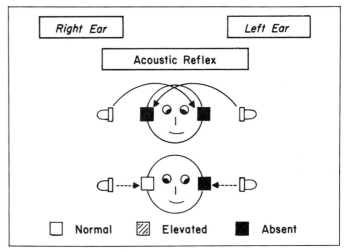

Case 3-2D

the left ear could not be adequately masked.

7. Notice that speech results on the right ear at 80 dB HL are not recorded with a

and 90% on the left ear. SSIT scores (Case 3-2B) agree with pure tone sensitivity results. SSIT scores are 18 dB HL on the right ear and 52 dB HL on the left ear.[7]

Tympanometry and static compliance measures (Case 3-2C) are within normal limits on the right ear. On the left ear, how-

masked symbol. A speech signal to the right ear of 80 dB HL may be heard in the left ear at about 40 dB HL due to crossover. In this patient, masking out the crossed speech signal on the left ear is a problem. The masking noise presented to the left ear by air conduction is attenuated by the large conductive component.

ever, the tympanogram is a rounded, type B, shape and static compliance is abnormally low. Crossed and uncrossed acoustic reflexes (Case 3-2A) are absent with sound to the left ear. With sound to the right ear, crossed reflexes are absent at all frequencies, but the uncrossed reflex at 1000 Hz is within normal limits. The reflex pattern (Case 3-2D) is characterized by an inverted L-shaped configuration. Results suggest a combined probe effect (vertical pattern) and sound effect (diagonal pattern) on the left ear.

Theoretically, the remaining masking noise may be insufficient to mask out a crossed speech signal of 40 dB HL.

Impression

RIGHT EAR: Pure tone sensitivity within normal limits with the exception of a mild loss at 8000 Hz. Bone conduction and SAL audiometry, however, suggest a mild, primarily low frequency, conductive component. Tympanometry, static compliance, and the uncrossed acoustic reflex at 1000 Hz are within normal limits.

LEFT EAR: Moderate conductive loss. Impedance results are consistent with a middle ear disorder characterized by reduced mobility of the ossicular chain.

SELECTED READINGS

Ballenger, J. J. *Diseases of the Nose, Throat and Ear.* Philadelphia: Lea & Febiger, 1977. Pp. 828–832; 858–884.

Cody, D. The Definition of Cholesteatoma. In B. McCabe, J. Sade, and M. Abramson (eds.), *Cholesteatoma: First International Conference.* Birmingham, Ala.: Aesculapius, 1977. Pp. 6–9.

Derlacki, E. L. Congenital cholesteatoma of the middle ear and mastoid. *Arch. Otolaryngol.* 97:177, 1973.

Friedmann, I. *Pathology of the Ear.* London: Blackwell, 1974. Pp. 83–103.

Harker, L. Cholesteatoma: An Incidence Study. In B. McCabe, J. Sade, and M. Abramson (eds.), *Cholesteatoma: First International Conference.* Birmingham, Ala.: Aesculapius, 1977. Pp. 308–309.

Nager, G. Epidermoids involving the temporal bone: Clinical, radiological and pathological aspects. *Laryngoscope* 85 (Suppl. 2):1, 1975.

Neely, J. G. *Treatment of Uncomplicated Aural Cholesteatoma (Keratoma).* American Academy of Ophthalmology and Otolaryngology, 1977.

Paparella, M., and Rybak, L. Congenital cholesteatoma. *Otolaryngol. Clin. North Am.* 11: 113, 1978.

Rambo, J. Surgical Treatment of Chronic Otitis. In A. Glorig and K. Gerwin (eds.), *Otitis Media: Proceedings of the National Conference. Callier Hearing and Speech Center.* Springfield, Ill.: Thomas, 1972. P. 207.

Schecter, G. A review of cholesteatoma pathology. *Laryngoscope* 79:1907, 1969.

Schuknecht, H. *Pathology of the Ear.* Cambridge: Harvard University Press, 1974. Pp. 196–197; 225–228.

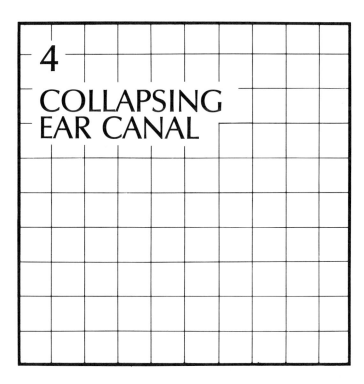

4
COLLAPSING EAR CANAL

DESCRIPTION

1. Estimates of the prevalence of collapsing ear canal range from 0.1% to 4%. The former percentage is based on individuals between 17 and 25 years of age who failed an audiometric screening test at 20 dB HL. The latter percentage describes a typical audiology case load.

Permanent meatal collapse may be referred to as prolapsed ear canal.

Collapsing ear canal refers to a narrowing or closure of the external auditory meatus. In general, collapsing ear canal is produced when unusual pressure compresses the pinna against the side of the head. During audiometric testing, for example, meatal collapse may be observed when earphones are placed on the auricles. In contrast to temporary meatal closure, however, permanent stenosis of the external auditory canal may occur. Permanent stenosis characteristically results from traumatic or inflammatory causes.[1]

PATIENT CHARACTERISTICS

Collapsing ear canals may occur in patients of any age. However, about one-third of patients are 65 years of age or older. In general, patients with collapsing ear canals may have unusually small, narrow canal openings; protruding pinnas; exceptionally large, lop ears; or abnormally flaccid, pliable canals. Collapsing ear canals may be unilateral or bilateral. A sex ratio is not reported.

CLINICAL COURSE

An apparent, erroneous conductive hearing loss. The "loss" may be superimposed on normal hearing or any type of hearing disor-

der. If the ear canal collapse is a result of earphone pressure against the pinna, rather than a permanent condition, the apparent degree of loss and the patient's subjective degree of handicap may be discrepant. If auditory canal stenosis is a permanent disorder, treatment may involve surgical intervention.

SITE OF DISORDER

External auditory canal.

GENERAL AUDIOLOGIC PATTERN

The erroneous air conduction loss produced by collapsing ear canal varies substantially. On the average, collapsing ear canal produces an air conduction threshold shift of about 10 to 15 dB. In individual patients, however, the effect of collapsing ear canal on air conduction thresholds may vary from about 5 to 50 dB. Variation seems related to the amount of occlusion produced by the collapsing meatus.

In addition to variation in degree of air conduction loss, the audiometric configuration associated with collapsing ear canal also varies. As a general rule, auditory canal stenosis causes greater high frequency loss, particularly in the 2000 Hz region, than low frequency loss. However, any audiometric contour may occur.

2. Supraaural or doughnut cushions may produce meatal collapse more readily than circumaural earphone cushions.

3. Remember, before the uni-box or horizontal configurations are interpreted as a retrocochlear sign, false elevation of crossed reflex thresholds due to occlusion of the ear canal must be carefully evaluated.

Another characteristic of air conduction results in patients with collapsing ear canal may be unusual threshold variability. Variability may be especially apparent if the earphone headband tension has been readjusted or if the earphones have been removed and replaced.[2]

Impedance results in collapsing ear canal characteristically show elevated crossed acoustic reflexes with sound to the affected ear. In contrast, uncrossed acoustic reflexes are typically normal. This unusual difference between crossed and uncrossed reflexes yields a false uni-box or horizontal reflex pattern.[3]

Speech audiometry may also reflect unusually poor speech threshold measures due to collapsing ear canal. Maximum intelligibility scores, however, are generally not affected. Intelligibility scores are usually consistent with the true organic cochlear sensitivity.

In contrast to speech thresholds, acoustic

reflexes, and air conduction measures, bone conduction thresholds are typically unaffected by ear canal collapse.

CLINICAL RESOLUTION OF COLLAPSING EAR CANAL

4. In routine clinical practice, two criticisms of the insert approach may be encountered. One is that inserts should not be placed into an ear canal without direct medical supervision. The other is that some inserts may modify ear canal resonance characteristics, thus altering threshold sensitivity results.

At least three different approaches are available for obtaining ear canal patency during audiometric testing. In one approach, a small tube or speculum may be inserted into the ear canal.[4] An alternative solution involves placing a tightly rolled pad of gauze behind the pinna before earphone placement. A third, less effective, approach is to obtain air conduction results with the earphone held in very light contact with the pinna. For frequencies above 1000 Hz, a hand-held earphone may be sufficient. For frequencies below 1000 Hz, however, inadequate coupling between the ear and the earphone will affect sensitivity measures.

Illustrative Patients

CASE 1. A 6-YEAR-OLD FEMALE WITH BILATERAL COLLAPSING EAR CANALS.

History

5. Language problems are being increasingly reported in children with chronic middle ear disorders during the years critical for learning speech and language.

The patient has a history of chronic serous otitis media, recurring episodes of external otitis, and recurrent bronchitis. Two years ago, the patient had a tonsillectomy and adenoidectomy. Polyethylene (PE) tubes were placed into both tympanic membranes at surgery. One year ago, a speech pathology evaluation noted language delay. Results were characterized by reduced auditory comprehension, a verbal expressive language disorder, and inconsistent vocal resonance problems.[5]

Presently, the patient is admitted to the hospital for meatoplasty. At admission, physical examination noted low set ears and stenosis of both external canals.

Results

6. Notice the difference between ears on air conduction tests with and without tubing. At 2000 Hz, for example, the right ear improved 40 dB, but the left ear changed only 10 dB.

The audiogram (Case 4-1A) shows air conduction test results with and without tubing inserted into the external auditory canal. Without tubing (dashed lines), threshold levels are approximately 53 dB HL on the right ear and 35 dB HL on the left ear. With tubing inserted into the ear canal to maintain patency, however, air conduction sensitivity improved.[6] With tubing, PTA scores

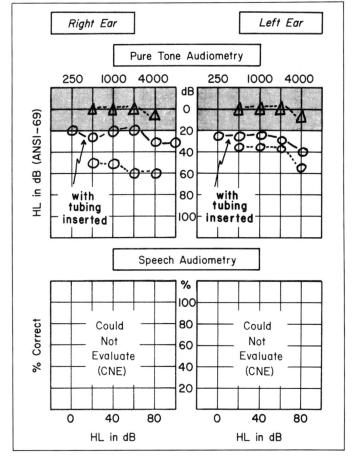

Case 4-1A

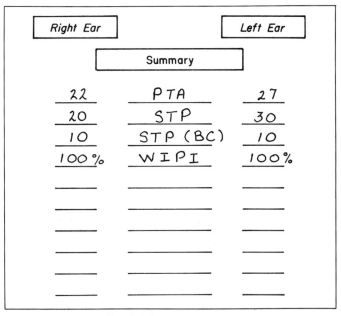

Case 4-1B

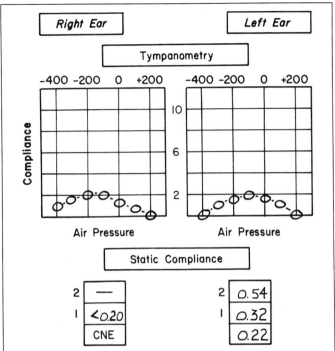

Right Ear		Left Ear

Tympanometry

Case 4-1C

ear. For example, the canal volume on the right ear is below measurable limits (<0.20). In comparison, the canal volume on the left ear is noticeably larger. Remember, air conduction tests with and without tubing (Case 4-1A) also suggested more severe collapse on the right ear than on the left ear.

7. Notice bone conduction results for pure tone vs speech signals. Pure tone bone conduction thresholds (Case 4-1A) are not specific to either ear. In this patient, pure tone thresholds in the presence of masking noise simply could not be reliably obtained. In contrast, bone conduction thresholds for speech signals in masking noise (Case 4-1B) were easily obtained on both ears. Speech bone conduction thresholds were important in documenting a conductive component on each ear.

8. External auditory canal volume measurements (the first number in the static compliance box) indicate more collapse on the right ear than on the left

(Case 4-1B) are 22 dB HL on the right ear and 27 dB HL on the left ear. Unmasked bone conduction thresholds (Case 4-1A) are within normal limits at all frequencies.

On both ears, speech audiometry (Case 4-1B) yields 100% correct performance at 70 dB HL for the word intelligibility by picture identification (WIPI) test. PI functions for PB-K words (Case 4-1A) could not be obtained due to the patient's verbal expressive language delay (see History). Spondee thresholds obtained with selected pictures (STP) (Case 4-1B) agree with pure tone air conduction and bone conduction results. With tubing, air conduction spondee thresholds are 20 dB HL on the right ear and 30 dB HL on the left ear. Bone conduction spondee thresholds (Case 4-1B) are 10 dB HL on each ear.[7]

Impedance audiometry (Case 4-1C) shows type B tympanograms on both ears. Static compliance could not be obtained on the right ear. On the left ear, static compliance was below normal limits.[8] Crossed (with tubing) and uncrossed acoustic reflexes were absent at equipment limits at all frequencies on both ears.

Impression

Auditory test results were obtained with tubing inserted into both external auditory

canals to maintain patency. Results indicated a mild conductive loss on both ears. Impedance audiometry was consistent with bilateral middle ear disorder characterized by extremely reduced mobility of the ossicular chain.

Case 2. A 57-Year-Old Female with Stenosis of Left External Auditory Canal.

History

Fifty-one years ago, the patient had a mastoidectomy performed on the left ear. After the operation, collapse of the left external auditory canal was noted. During the past several years, the left meatal stenosis has been getting worse. Presently, the patient complains of difficulty with wax and water collecting in the left ear canal. She reports a gradually increasing hearing problem on the left ear. She has no complaints about her right ear.

Surgical Findings

Stenosis of the left external auditory canal was corrected with a meatoplasty. At surgery, middle ear exploration revealed a small otosclerotic focus involving the footplate of the stapes. Inspection of other middle ear structures was within normal limits.

Results

On the right ear, the audiogram (Case 4-2A) shows normal pure tone sensitivity with the exception of a mild loss at 8000 Hz. On the left ear, the audiogram shows a mild conductive loss. However, results were obtained without resolution of the collapsing ear canal.

PTA scores (Case 4-2B) are 11 dB HL on the right ear and 25 dB HL on the left ear. Bone conduction and SAL results (Case 4-2A) on the right ear are superimposed on air conduction. On the left ear, bone conduction and SAL measures show a conductive component of approximately 25 dB.

Weber results at 500 Hz (Case 4-2B) are consistently heard on the left ear. The Bing test at 500 Hz (not shown) on the right ear shows an occlusion effect of 10 dB. On the left ear, however, there is no difference between occluded and unoccluded results.

PI-SSI functions (Case 4-2A) show maximum intelligibility scores of 90% on both ears. PB word testing (Case 4-2B) at high intensity levels shows normal (100%)

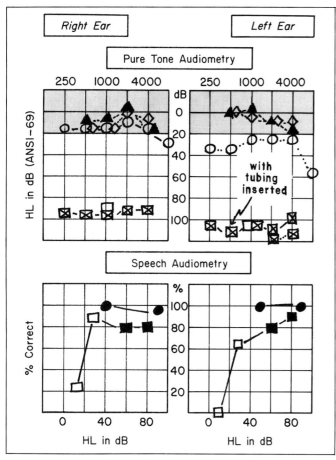

Case 4-2A

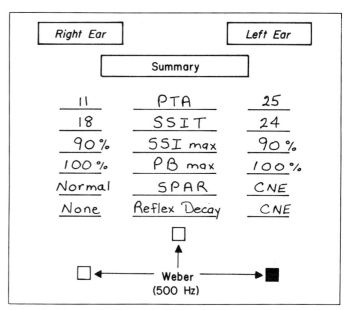

Case 4-2B

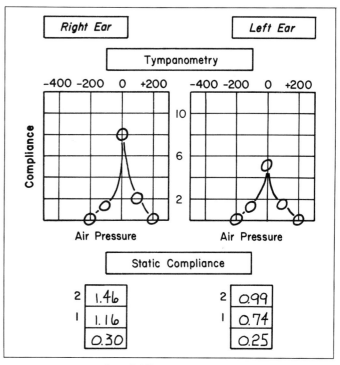

Case 4-2C

9. Notice the difference between maximum performance on PB and SSI procedures. A mild PB vs SSI discrepancy is consistent with the patient's age.

10. Notice how shallow the left tympanogram is in comparison to the right tympanogram. At surgery, mild otosclerosis was found on the left ear.

11. In this patient, notice that reflex abnormalities on the left ear are related to a sound effect. For example, with probe to the left ear (sound to the right ear) crossed reflexes are present at normal HLs. With sound to the left ear,

maximum performance scores bilaterally. No significant rollover is observed on either ear.[9]

Speech thresholds for the PI-SSI functions agree with pure tone sensitivity results on both ears. SSIT scores without tubing (Case 4-2B) are 18 dB HL on the right ear and 24 dB HL on the left ear.

Impedance audiometry (Case 4-2C) shows normal, type A, tympanograms and low static compliance measures on both ears.[10] Crossed and uncrossed acoustic reflexes (Case 4-2A) on the right ear are present at normal HLs. Without tubing, crossed acoustic reflexes with sound to the left ear (dashed line) are absent at 250, 500, and 1000 Hz and elevated at 2000 and 4000 Hz. With tubing (solid line), however, crossed reflex thresholds on the left ear improve 10 to 15 dB at all frequencies. Uncrossed reflexes at 1000 Hz on the left ear are present at 105 dB HL.[11]

SPAR measures (Case 4-2B) on the right ear predict normal sensitivity. Reflex decay

however, crossed and uncrossed reflexes are elevated relative to results on the right ear. A sound effect on the left ear suggests that the probe tip (uncrossed mode) and the tubing (crossed mode) did not sufficiently overcome the attenuation produced by the ear

testing on the right ear is within normal limits. SPAR and reflex decay measures on the left ear were not evaluated because of reflex threshold variability with sound to the test ear.

Impression

RIGHT EAR: Pure tone sensitivity within normal limits with the exception of a mild loss at 8000 Hz. Impedance audiometry indicates normal middle ear function.

canal collapse. Remember, in conductive loss, abnormal sound conditions and normal probe conditions may occur for two types of disorders: collapsing ear canal and ossicular chain discontinuity with a functional connection (see patient 2, Chapter 6, Discontinuity of the Ossicular Chain).

LEFT EAR: Mild conductive hearing loss. However, most or all of the conductive component may be due to stenosis of the external auditory canal. Impedance audiometry shows a relatively shallow, type A, tympanogram and elevated crossed and uncrossed acoustic reflexes with sound to the left ear. Significant middle ear dysfunction is unlikely due to the normal reflex thresholds with probe to the left ear and sound to the right ear. Further, if air conduction thresholds are corrected by the threshold shift observed for reflexes with and without tubing, then air conduction thresholds are essentially superimposed on bone conduction measures at frequencies above 500 Hz.

COMMENT

Results in the present patients illustrate the desirability of obtaining auditory measures with and without the effect of the collapsing ear canal counteracted. In clinical practice, for example, auditory test results may be viewed from two different approaches. One orientation revolves primarily around rehabilitative information. Toward this goal, the degree of impairment produced by ear canal collapse may be critical. For example, if the collapse is permanent and severe, the degree of auditory handicap experienced by the patient in everyday life may be substantially influenced. If, on the other hand, the collapse is associated with pinna compression, situational problems, such as talking on the telephone, may be troublesome for the patient.

Another orientation, however, is directed primarily toward diagnostic information. Of primary importance in this circumstance is documenting the degree and site of auditory disorder. Results in patient 1 (Case 4-1A) with and without tubing illustrate the reality of combined sites of disorder. In this patient, both an external ear and middle ear disorder were documented.

In short, auditory test results with and without the ear canal collapse resolved may yield important diagnostic information about the possibility of combined sites of auditory disorder. Failure to identify and resolve effects of collapsing ear canal can lead to inappropriate management.

SELECTED READINGS

Bess, J. C. Ear canal collapse. *Arch. Otolaryngol.* 93:408, 1971.

Hildyard, V., and Valentine, M. Collapse of the ear canal during audiometry. *Arch. Otolaryngol.* 75:422, 1962.

Lupin, A. J. External auditory canal stenosis. *Arch. Otolaryngol.* 102:458, 1976.

Riedner, E., and Hiroshi, S. Collapsing ears and acoustic reflex measurement with circumaural ear cushions. *Arch. Otolaryngol.* 102:358, 1976.

Ventry, I., Chaiklin, J., and Boyle, W. Collapse of the ear canal during audiometry. *Arch. Otolaryngol.* 73:125, 1961.

Work, W. P. Lesions of the external auditory canal. *Ann. Otol. Rhinol. Laryngol.* 59:1062, 1970.

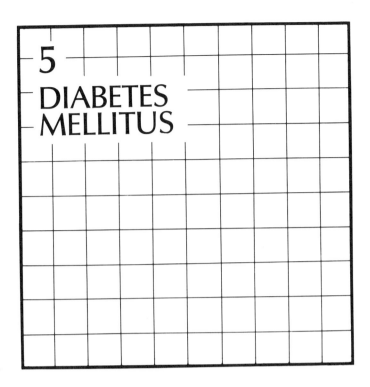

5 DIABETES MELLITUS

DESCRIPTION

1. The prefix "melli" means honey. The term *mellitus* refers to urine sweetened as with honey.

2. The prevalence of diabetes varies as a function of age, from about 0.1% of persons under 25 years of age to about 5.4% of individuals 65 to 74 years of age. An average prevalence is approximately 1.2% of individuals. However, in affluent societies, from 3% to 20% of persons may develop diabetes.
   Close relatives of diabetics develop diabetes 2½ times more frequently than the general population.
   On histologic examination, inner ear lesions are found in 50% of persons with diabetes (Jorgensen and Buch, 1961).

3. The age of symptom onset is one distinction between the maturity vs juvenile types of

Diabetes mellitus is a chronic systemic disease related to a relative or absolute deficiency of insulin.[1] Systemic abnormalities in diabetes may involve metabolic and vascular alterations. Metabolic disorders characteristically consist of abnormally elevated blood glucose levels with associated lipid and protein changes. Vascular disorders typically consist of defects in the structure or function of small blood vessels (microangiopathy) and atherosclerosis.

Complications of diabetes mellitus may include disorders of the eye, kidney, cranial nerves, and ear. Abnormalities of the auditory system may include atrophy of the spiral ganglion, degeneration of the myelin sheath of the eighth nerve, decrease in the number of nerve fibers in the spiral lamina, and thickening or narrowing of capillary walls of the stria vascularis and of the small arteries within the internal auditory canal.[2]

PATIENT CHARACTERISTICS

Onset of diabetes is after 40 years of age in approximately 80% of individuals.[3] In older individuals, diabetes is more prevalent in females than in males. For example, between 65 years and 74 years of age, diabetes occurs in about 4.5% of males and 6% of females. In diabetics under 40 years of age, the female-to-male ratio is approximately

diabetes. For further distinguishing characteristics, see Steinke and Soeldner, 1974.

4. The reported incidence of hearing loss in patients with diabetes ranges from about 10% to 55%.

5. Cerebrovascular disease is more common in diabetics than in the general population. For a description of auditory findings in cerebrovascular disease, see Chapter 2, Cerebrovascular Disorders.
   Estimates of the incidence of cranial nerve neuropathy in diabetes range from 5% to 15%. Usually, the incidence of neuropathy increases with the duration of the diabetes and the age of the patient.

equal. A hearing loss, if present, is characteristically bilateral.

CLINICAL COURSE

Progressive, bilateral sensorineural loss. The onset of hearing loss is characteristically insidious, but may be instantaneous in a few patients.[4] Approximately 20% of patients will also complain of dizziness.

SITE OF DISORDER

Cochlea and/or eighth nerve.[5]

GENERAL AUDIOLOGIC PATTERN

Pure tone sensitivity results characteristically show bilateral sensorineural hearing loss. However, on occasion, a unilateral sensorineural loss may occur. The degree of loss may vary from mild to profound. The audiometric configuration usually shows greater loss in the high frequency region than in low or mid frequency regions.

Maximum speech intelligibility scores vary depending on the site of the sensorineural disorder. In patients with cochlear site, maximum speech intelligibility performance is usually consistent with the degree of sensitivity loss. In patients with eighth nerve site, maximum speech intelligibility scores may be proportionate or disproportionate to the degree of pure tone sensitivity loss. However, in eighth nerve patients with normal or reduced maximum speech intelligibility performance, the shape of the PI function for speech materials generally shows abnormal rollover.

Impedance results characteristically show normal, type A, tympanograms and normal static compliance measures. Acoustic reflex results vary, however, depending on the site of disorder and the degree of sensitivity loss. As a general rule, reflexes are present in ears with cochlear disorder and absent in ears with eighth nerve disorder. Absent reflexes in patients with eighth nerve abnormality yield a diagonal crossed vs uncrossed reflex pattern. In addition to the above findings, acoustic reflex results in patients with diabetes mellitus may also reflect a disorder of the seventh cranial nerve. In these latter patients, the crossed vs uncrossed reflex pattern may vary depending on whether the seventh nerve is affected in isolation or in

6. For further information on audiometric findings in cochlear, eighth nerve, and seventh nerve sites, see Chapter 1, Acoustic Schwannoma; Chapter 7, Facial Nerve Disorders; and Chapter 14, Meniere's Disease.

combination with the eighth nerve. In isolated seventh nerve disorders, a vertical reflex pattern is characteristically observed; in combined seventh and eighth nerve disorders, an inverted L-shaped configuration typically occurs.[6]

Illustrative Patients

In general, patients with hearing loss directly attributable to diabetes mellitus are rare. A major difficulty in delineating hearing patterns in diabetes involves the many other possible causes of hearing loss that cannot always be adequately ruled out. For example, before a hearing loss can be associated with the presence of diabetes, other causal factors, such as aging and noise exposure, must be carefully evaluated. One approach to controlling the possibility that a hearing loss is reflecting factors other than diabetes is to select patients with unilateral hearing disorders. In this manner, auditory results on the uninvolved ear provide control data against which to compare performance on the involved ear. This "control ear" approach was used in selecting the following patient. In this individual, the diabetes apparently affected hearing ability on the left ear, but did not influence auditory findings on the right ear.

CASE 1. A 73-YEAR-OLD FEMALE WITH ADULT-ONSET DIABETES MELLITUS AND CRANIAL NERVE NEUROPATHY.

History

The patient was hospitalized for evaluation of double vision, increased salivation, severe shaking, sensations of coldness and nausea, inability to chew and to drink without a straw, episodic retroauricular pain, and left-sided facial weakness with inability to close the left eye. The double vision began 4 weeks prior to admission. The other difficulties began within the last 7 days. The patient was diagnosed as having diabetes mellitus approximately 10 years ago. However, she has not experienced significant complaints until the present episodes.

At hospitalization, neurologic examination noted involvement of cranial nerves five through ten on the left side and cranial nerves three and twelve on the right side. Diagnostic tests of facial nerve function indicated a lesion at or proximal to the facial

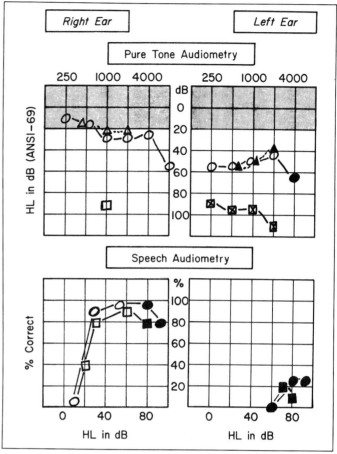

Case 5-1A

nerve nucleus on the left side. Results of computerized axial tomography (CT scan) were within normal limits. X-rays of the internal auditory canals and skull were normal.

The patient reports difficulty hearing and a constant roaring tinnitus in her left ear for about 10 years. The hearing loss and the tinnitus have become worse within the last 2 days. The patient has no hearing complaints about her right ear.

Results

The audiogram (Case 5-1A) shows a mild sensorineural loss on the right ear and a moderate sensorineural loss through 4000 Hz on the left ear. Sensitivity at 8000 Hz on the left ear shows profound impairment. The PTA scores (Case 5-1B) are 25 dB HL on the right ear and 47 dB HL on the left ear. On both ears bone conduction scores (Case 5-1A) at 500 Hz through 2000 Hz are superimposed on air conduction measures. The Weber test (Case 5-1B) at 500 Hz lateralizes to the right ear.

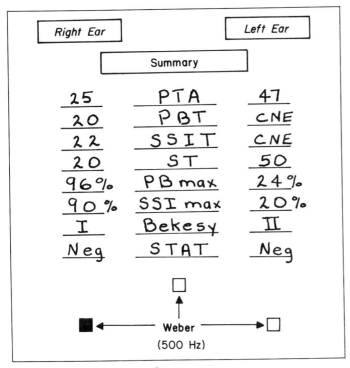

Right Ear		Left Ear
	Summary	
25	PTA	47
20	PBT	CNE
22	SSIT	CNE
20	ST	50
96%	PB max	24%
90%	SSI max	20%
I	Bekesy	II
Neg	STAT	Neg

Weber
(500 Hz)

Case 5-1B

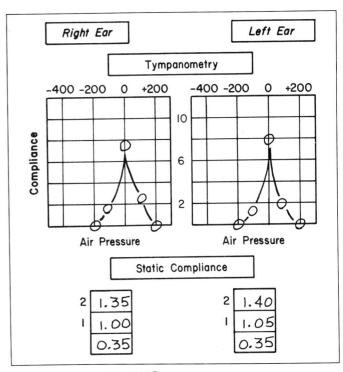

Case 5-1C

7. Remember, unusually poor speech understanding ability may characterize both patients with presbyacusis and patients with other retrocochlear lesions. In the present patient (73 years of age), results on the right ear may be viewed as a control for the effects of age on both pure tone and speech intelligibility measures. On both procedures, the large performance difference between ears votes against a "pure" presbyacusis effect and for a localized disorder affecting the left ear only.

Speech audiometry (Case 5-1A) on the right ear shows normal PI functions for both PB words and SSI materials. The PB max score (Case 5-1B) is 96%; the SSI max score is 90%. Speech thresholds on the right ear agree with average pure tone sensitivity results. The PBT and ST are 20 dB HL; the SSIT is 22 dB HL. On the left ear, the PI-PB and PI-SSI functions (Case 5-1A) show unusual deficits in the ability to understand speech materials. The PB max and SSI max scores (Case 5-1B) are only 24% and 20%, respectively.[7] On the left ear, speech thresholds for PB and SSI materials cannot be established. However, an ST of 50 dB HL agrees with average pure tone sensitivity.

Impedance audiometry (Case 5-1C) shows normal, type A, tympanograms and normal static compliance measures bilaterally. Crossed acoustic reflexes (Case 5-1A) with sound to the right ear are absent at all frequencies. In contrast, the uncrossed reflex at 1000 Hz on the right ear is within normal limits. On the left ear, crossed reflexes are present at normal HLs for 250 Hz through 1000 Hz. However, crossed reflex thresholds are elevated at 2000 Hz and absent at 4000 Hz. An uncrossed reflex at 1000 Hz on the left ear is absent at equipment limits.

The crossed vs uncrossed reflex pattern

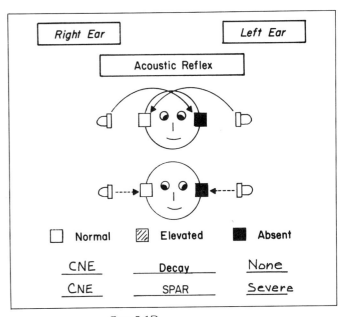

Case 5-1D

8. Remember, a vertical reflex pattern may be consistent with either middle ear or seventh nerve disorder. In this patient, a middle ear abnormality is rendered unlikely by bone conduction measures (Case 5-1A) and the Weber test

(Case 5-1D) is characterized by a vertical configuration on the left ear. Results are consistent with a seventh nerve disorder on the left side.[8] On the right ear the absence of crossed reflexes precludes measurement of reflex decay and SPAR. On the left ear, no reflex decay was observed at either 500 Hz or 1000 Hz. SPAR results predict a severe sensitivity loss in the 1000 to 4000 Hz region.

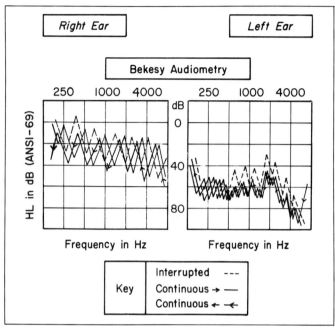

Case 5-1E

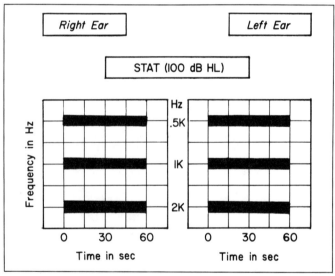

Case 5-1F

interwave latencies of all components at HLs from 60 to 100 dB on both ears.

Impression

RIGHT EAR: Mild sensorineural loss consistent with the patient's age.

LEFT EAR: Moderate sensorineural loss through 4000 Hz; profound sensorineural loss at 8000 Hz. Diagnostic test results are consistent with cochlear and seventh nerve disorders.

SELECTED READINGS

Axelsson, A., and Fagerber, S. Auditory function in diabetes. *Acta Otolaryngol.* 66:49, 1968.

Coats, A., and Martin, J. Human auditory nerve action potentials and brain stem evoked responses. *Arch. Otolaryngol.* 103:605, 1977.

Friedman, S., Schulman, R., and Weiss, S. Hearing and diabetic neuropathy. *Arch. Intern. Med.* 135:573, 1975.

Jackson, W. Diabetes mellitus in different countries and different races. *Acta Diabetol. Lat.* 7:361, 1970.

Jorgensen, M. The inner ear in diabetes mellitus. *Arch. Otolaryngol.* 74:373, 1961.

Jorgensen, M., and Buch, N. Studies on inner ear function and cranial nerves in diabetics. *Acta Otolaryngol.* 53:350, 1961.

Makishima, K., and Tanaka, K. Pathological changes of the inner ear and central auditory pathway in diabetes. *Ann. Otol. Rhinol. Laryngol.* 80:218, 1971.

Minami, Y., Minami, Y., and Hori, A. Hearing impairment in diabetics. *J. Otolaryngol. Jap.* 80:354, 1977.

Page, M., Asmal, A., and Edwards, C. Recessive inheritance of diabetes: The syndrome of diabetes insipidus, diabetes mellitus, optic atrophy and deafness. *Q. J. Med.* 45:505, 1976.

Steinke, J., and Soeldner, J. Diabetes Mellitus. In M. Wintrobe, G. Thorn, R. Adams, E. Braunwald, K. Isselbacher, and R. Petersdorf (eds.), *Principles of Internal Medicine* (7th ed.). New York: McGraw-Hill, 1974. Pp. 563–583.

Taylor, I., and Irwin, J. Some audiological aspects of diabetes mellitus. *J. Laryngol. Otol.* 92:99, 1978.

West, K. Epidemiology of Diabetes. In S. Fajans and K. Sussman (eds.), *Diabetes Mellitus: Diagnosis and Treatment.* New York: American Diabetes Association, 1974. Pp. 121–126.

(Case 5-1B). Further, a seventh nerve disorder on the left side is consistent with the patient's complaints of left-sided facial weakness.

Conventional Bekesy audiometry (Case 5-1E) yields a type I tracing on the right ear and a type II pattern on the left ear. No forward-backward discrepancy between continuous tracings was observed on either ear.

The STAT test (Case 5-1F) is negative on both ears at all frequencies. ABR audiometry (not shown) showed normal absolute and

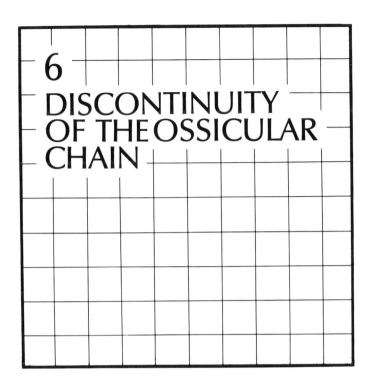

6

DISCONTINUITY OF THE OSSICULAR CHAIN

1. The vulnerability of the incus to disruption may be related to the more tenuous suspension of the incus between the firmly anchored malleus and stapes.

In 31 patients with ossicular chain derangement following skull injury, about 90% had incudostapedial joint separation. In contrast, only about 10% had malleolar fractures (Hough and Stuart, 1968) (see Chapter 24, Trauma).

2. The incidence of ossicular chain discontinuity is not reported.

Congenital ossicular chain discontinuity may be associated with branchial arch and facial anomalies; i.e., Pierre Robin and Treacher Collins syndromes and atresia/microtia.

DESCRIPTION

Discontinuity of the ossicular chain refers to a disruption of normal articulation between the malleus, incus, and stapes. Ossicular chain discontinuity may occur as a consequence of congenital defects, skull trauma, and middle ear disease. Traumatic severing of the ossicular chain may result from blows to the head, unusual changes in barometric pressure, and penetrating objects, such as gunshot wounds. A common site of ossicular chain disruption is the incus and/or the incudostapedial joint.[1] On occasion, in patients with ossicular chain discontinuity, the ossicles may become rejoined by fibrous tissue or fixed by a mass of new bony growth.[2]

PATIENT CHARACTERISTICS

The general characteristics of patients with ossicular chain discontinuity are variable. Of patients with middle ear injury due to head trauma, 50% are below 13 years of age and 70% are less than 22 years old. About 75% of patients with traumatic middle ear disorder are male. In approximately 80% of patients with middle ear disorder from head injury, the lesion is unilateral.

CLINICAL COURSE

Stable, usually unilateral, conductive loss. If the ossicular chain discontinuity is associ-

3. Type A_D tympanograms may also be found in isolated tympanic membrane abnormalities. In the differentiation of ossicular chain discontinuity and tympanic membrane disease, the degree of conductive loss is an important consideration. The combination of an A_D tympanogram and substantial conductive loss points to ossicular chain discontinuity. Tympanic membrane disease that produces an A_D shape seldom produces concomitant substantial conductive loss (see patient 1, Chapter 7, Facial Nerve Disorders).

If the probe tone frequency is 600 to 800 Hz, instead of 220 Hz, a W-shaped tympanogram may occur instead of the type A_D shape.

4. Static compliance measures may be particularly helpful in distinguishing between ossicular chain discontinuity and otosclerosis. In discontinuity, static compliance is generally above or within the high side of the normal range; in stapes fixation, static compliance is typically below or within the low side of the normal range.

ated with a longitudinal skull fracture, it may be accompanied by external ear canal lacerations or collapse, tympanic membrane rupture, mucous membrane hemorrhage, and seventh nerve disorder. Treatment may involve reconstructive surgery of the middle ear system.

SITE OF DISORDER

Middle ear.

GENERAL AUDIOLOGIC PATTERN

Pure tone sensitivity results characteristically show a conductive hearing loss of 40 to 60 dB HL. The audiometric configuration is generally flat. Maximum speech intelligibility scores are typically within normal limits.

Impedance results characteristically show an abnormally deep, type A (A_D), tympanogram, static compliance well above the normal range, and absent acoustic reflexes.[3] The reflex pattern is usually characterized by an inverted L-shaped configuration. Reflexes are normal only for uncrossed stimulation (sound and probe to the same ear) on the uninvolved ear. A qualification to this expected pattern of results is that static compliance measures may be in the high region of the normal range (1.0 to 1.6 cc) instead of outside normal limits.[4]

In contrast to the pattern presented above, totally different auditory findings may be found in patients with ossicular chain discontinuities characterized by a functional connection (i.e., the ossicles may be rejoined by adhesions, etc.). In these patients, hearing sensitivity may be surprisingly good. The air-bone gap may be minimal. The tympanogram may be rounded instead of a type A_D shape. Acoustic reflexes may be elevated or absent with sound to the conductive ear; but with probe to the conductive ear, reflexes may be observed at normal HLs. An abnormal sound effect and normal probe effect (diagonal pattern) in ears with ossicular chain discontinuity indicate a functional connection between the stapedial tendon and the tympanic membrane.

Illustrative Patients

CASE 1. A 15-YEAR-OLD FEMALE WITH OSSICULAR CHAIN DISCONTINUITY ON THE LEFT EAR.

Surgical Findings

Two years prior to audiologic evaluation, middle ear surgery on the left ear revealed interruption of the ossicular chain at the incudostapedial joint. Continuity of the chain was reestablished with incus interposition. Hearing sensitivity did not improve postoperatively, however.

At the time of the audiologic evaluation presented below, surgical findings on the left ear noted ossicular chain discontinuity between the interposed incus and the malleus. Adhesions pulled the interposed incus posteriorly. The apposition of the interposed incus and stapes appeared normal. The mobility of the stapes seemed adequate. There was no evidence of cholesteatoma or inflammation of middle ear structures.

History

The patient reports a hearing loss in the left ear for approximately 12 years. The hearing loss apparently occurred at the age of 3 years when she fell from a highchair. The patient notices a constant high-pitched ringing sound in her left ear. She has no hearing complaints about the right ear.

Results

The audiogram (Case 6-1A) shows normal sensitivity on the right ear and a mild conductive loss on the left ear. The PTA scores (Case 6-1B) are −2 dB HL on the right ear and 35 dB HL on the left ear. Bone conduction and SAL results (Case 6-1A) on the right ear are superimposed on air conduction. On the left ear, bone conduction and SAL measures show a conductive component of approximately 35 dB.

PI-PB and PI-SSI functions (Case 6-1A) on both ears show normal maximum intelligibility scores and no rollover. PB max and SSI max results (Case 6-1B) are 100% for the right and left ears. Speech thresholds (Case 6-1B) on each ear agree with average pure tone sensitivity. On the right ear, the PBT score is 0 dB HL; the SSIT score is 4 dB HL. On the left ear, the PBT is 40 dB HL; the SSIT is 37 dB HL.

Weber results at 500 Hz (Case 6-1B) are referred to the left ear. The Bing test at 500 Hz (not shown) shows an occlusion effect of 15 dB on the right ear. On the left ear, there is no difference between occluded and unoccluded results.

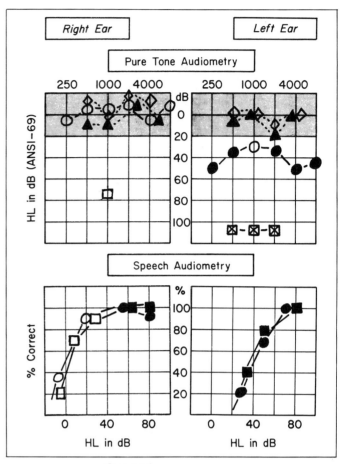

Case 6-1A

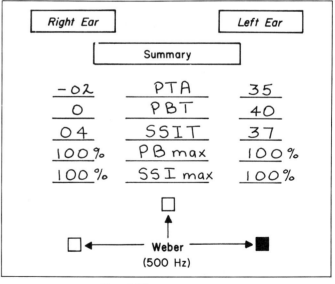

Case 6-1B

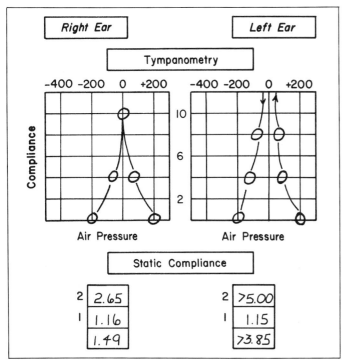

Case 6-1C

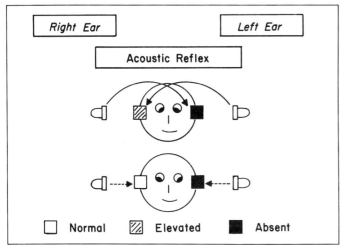

Case 6-1D

5. Notice how reflex thresholds on the left ear reflect the degree of conductive component. For example, assume that the reflex threshold at 1000 Hz on the normal, right ear represents the norm for this patient. The reflex norm then is 75 dB HL. The conductive component at 1000 Hz on the left ear is 30 dB. To determine

an expected reflex threshold HL at 1000 Hz in the left ear, we add the conductive component to the norm: 75 dB + 30 dB. The expected value is 105 dB HL; the observed value is 110 dB HL.

Impedance audiometry (Case 6-1C) on the right ear shows a normal, type A, tympanogram and normal static compliance. On the left ear, however, the tympanogram is a type A_D shape and static compliance is well above normal limits. Crossed acoustic reflexes (Case 6-1A) with sound to the right ear are absent at all frequencies. The uncrossed reflex at 1000 Hz on the right ear, however, is within normal limits. With sound to the left ear, crossed and uncrossed reflexes are elevated or absent at all frequencies.[5]

The reflex pattern at 1000 Hz (Case 6-1D) is characterized by an inverted L-shaped configuration. Only uncrossed reflexes on the right ear are normal; all other crossed and uncrossed reflexes are elevated or absent. An inverted L-shaped pattern indicates a combined probe effect (vertical pattern) and sound effect (diagonal pattern) on the left ear.

Impression

RIGHT EAR: Normal pure tone sensitivity.

LEFT EAR: Mild conductive loss. The overall pattern of results (abnormally deep, type A, tympanogram; unusually large static compliance measure; absent or elevated acoustic reflexes; and substantial air-bone gap) is consistent with ossicular chain discontinuity. Reflex absence with probe to the left ear suggests that there is no functional connection between the stapedial tendon and the tympanic membrane.

CASE 2. A 46-YEAR-OLD MALE WITH OSSICULAR CHAIN DISCONTINUITY ON THE LEFT EAR.

Surgical Findings

Surgical exploration of the left ear revealed fracture of the stapedial crura. Middle ear adhesions were noted.

History

The patient complains of decreased hearing and a constant ringing tinnitus in the left ear for approximately 1 year. The hearing loss occurred suddenly during a scuba diving excursion. The patient has no hearing complaints about the right ear. He has a 20-year history of noise exposure from industrial equipment.

Results

The audiogram (Case 6-2A) on the right ear shows normal pure tone sensitivity through 2000 Hz, then a profound high frequency sensorineural loss. On the left ear, the audiogram shows a mild mixed loss through 2000 Hz. Above 2000 Hz, there is no measurable hearing by air conduction or bone conduction. The PTA scores (Case 6-2B) are 5 dB HL on the right ear and 30 dB HL on the left ear.

SAL audiometry and bone conduction (Case 6-2A) on the right ear do not show a

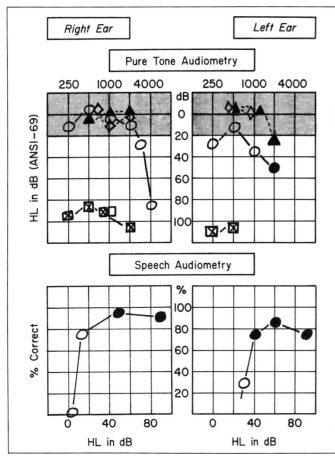

Case 6-2A

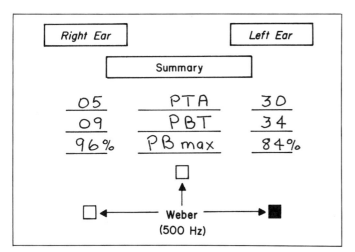

Case 6-2B

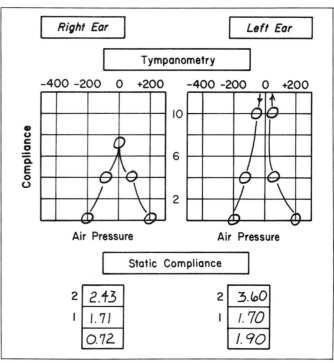

Case 6-2C

conductive component at any frequency. On the left ear, SAL and bone conduction measures show a conductive component of 20 dB to 35 dB at low and mid frequencies.

The Weber test at 500 Hz (Case 6-2B) lateralizes to the left ear. The Bing test at 500 Hz (not shown) shows an occlusion effect of 10 dB on the right ear. On the left ear, there

6. Remember, in conductive hearing loss, an abnormal sound condition and normal probe condition may occur in two types of disorder: ossicular discontinuity

is no difference between occluded and un-occluded measures.

The shape of the PI-PB functions (Case 6-2A) on both ears is normal. PB max scores (Case 6-2B) are 96% on the right ear and 84% on the left ear. Speech thresholds (Case 6-2B) agree with pure tone sensitivity results on both ears. The PBT is 9 dB HL on the right ear and 34 dB HL on the left ear.

Tympanometry and static compliance measures (Case 6-2C) on the right ear are within normal limits. On the left ear, however, a type A_D tympanogram and abnormally high static compliance are observed. Crossed and uncrossed acoustic reflexes (Case 6-2A) with sound to the right ear are present at normal HLs at 250 Hz through 1000 Hz. Crossed reflexes are elevated at 2000 Hz and absent at 4000 Hz, however. On the left ear, crossed and uncrossed reflexes are elevated or absent at all frequencies.

The reflex pattern at 1000 Hz (Case 6-2D) is characterized by a diagonal configuration. Reflexes are abnormal with sound to the left ear for both crossed and uncrossed conditions. However, with probe to the left ear and sound to the right ear, reflexes are present at normal HLs.[6]

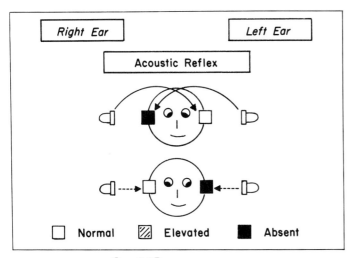

Case 6-2D

COMMENT

Results in these patients illustrate the audiometric signature of ossicular chain discontinuity. Audiometric results revolve around a triad of symptoms: substantial air-bone gap; abnormally deep, type A, tympanogram; and unusually large static compliance measure.

In the triad of audiometric results summarized above, notice that we did not include acoustic reflexes. In patients with ossicular chain discontinuity, acoustic reflex results usually show an inverted L-shaped pattern (Case 6-1D). However, a diagonal reflex configuration may occur, as shown in patient 2 (Case 6-2D). A diagonal reflex pattern indicates a residual connection between the tympanic membrane and the stapedial tendon in spite of the ossicular chain disruption.

SELECTED READINGS

Alberti, P., and Jerger, J. Probe tone frequency and the diagnostic value of tympanometry. *Arch. Otolaryngol.* 99:206, 1974.

Ballantyne, J. Traumatic Conductive Deafness. In W. Scott-Brown, J. Ballantyne, and J. Groves (eds.), *Diseases of the Ear, Nose, and Throat* (2nd ed.). Washington: Butterworth, 1965. Pp. 397–405.

Hough, J. Otologic Trauma. In M. Paparella and D. Shumrick (eds.), *Otolaryngology* (vol. 2). Philadelphia: Saunders, 1973. Pp. 241–262.

Hough, J., and Stuart, W. Middle ear injuries in skull trauma. *Laryngoscope* 78:899, 1968.

with a functional connection and collapsing ear canal (see patient 2, Chapter 4, Collapsing Ear Canal).

A diagonal (sensorineural) reflex pattern is not diagnostically misleading in this patient because of the abnormal tympanogram and static compliance. Remember the working rule: If any one impedance measure is abnormal, the possibility of a conductive component must be evaluated.

Impression

RIGHT EAR: Normal pure tone sensitivity through 2000 Hz; profound sensorineural loss above 2000 Hz. Results are consistent with patient's history of noise exposure.

LEFT EAR: Mild mixed loss through 2000 Hz; no measurable hearing above 2000 Hz. The combination of an abnormally deep, type A, tympanogram; unusually large static compliance measure; and significant air-bone gap is consistent with discontinuity of the ossicular chain. The presence of acoustic reflexes with sound in the right ear and probe in the left ear suggests a functional connection between the stapedial tendon and the tympanic membrane.

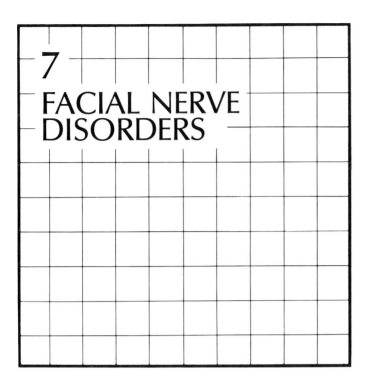

7
FACIAL NERVE DISORDERS

DESCRIPTION

1. Central and peripheral facial nerve disorders may be termed *upper motor neuron* and *lower motor neuron* lesions, respectively.

On rare occasions, facial nerve disorders do not produce concomitant facial paralysis (see patient 3, this chapter).

A primary characteristic of facial nerve disorders is partial or complete paralysis of the facial musculature on the affected side. Manifestations of the resulting facial paralysis vary, however, depending on whether the lesion is proximal or distal to the facial nerve nucleus in the brain stem. Facial nerve lesions proximal to the facial nerve nucleus (supranuclear or central) are characterized by paralysis of the lower two-thirds of the face on the affected side. The upper facial muscles of the forehead and eyebrow are unaffected, however. Facial nerve lesions at or distal to the facial nerve nucleus (termed *nuclear* and *peripheral* lesions, respectively) are characterized by paralysis of the entire face on the involved side.[1]

In peripheral facial nerve lesions, the site of disorder can be identified more precisely by testing separately the function of the branches of the facial nerve. These branches are concerned with tear secretion, the acoustic reflex, salivation, and taste sensation. For example, if acoustic reflexes are absent in patients with facial paralysis, the seventh nerve lesion may be placed above or proximal to the branch innervating the stapedial muscle. In contrast, if acoustic reflexes are present in persons with facial paralysis, then the lesion may be placed below or distal to the insertion of the branch

2. The prevalence of facial nerve disorder is not available. Bell's palsy occurs in about 22 per 100,000 persons annually. The incidence of Bell's palsy varies with age, however, from about 6 per 100,000 persons per year for individuals less than 10 years of age to approximately 27 per 100,000 persons per year for individuals 60 to 69 years of age.

Of 850 patients with facial paralysis, about 63% had Bell's palsy, about 13% had traumatic injury, and about 8% had herpes zoster oticus; about 5% resulted from otitis media, and about 5% were associated with neoplasms (Cawthorne, 1969).

3. Bilateral facial paralysis may be called *facial diplegia.*

to the stapedial muscle. Disorders of the facial nerve may result from (1) trauma, such as temporal bone fractures; (2) neoplasms, such as neuromas of the seventh or eighth nerve, parotid tumors, or pontine gliomas; (3) infections, such as herpes zoster or otitis media; (4) toxic or metabolic defects, such as diabetes; (5) congenital abnormalities, such as cholesteatoma; and (6) an idiopathic origin, such as Bell's palsy.[2]

PATIENT CHARACTERISTICS

Initial onset of symptoms in idiopathic facial paralysis is usually between 20 and 50 years of age. The initial attack occurs before 30 years of age in more than 50% of individuals, however. The female-to-male ratio is approximately 1.2 : 1. In facial nerve disorders, either or both sides of the face may be affected. In a series of 35 patients with peripheral facial nerve sites (Powers, 1974), 48% had right-sided involvement, 51% had left-sided lesions, and 1% had bilateral disorders. In the latter circumstance, the face may present a "masked" appearance.[3]

CLINICAL COURSE

The onset of facial paralysis may be acute or slowly progressive. It may be accompanied by complaints of tinnitus and/or otalgia. The facial paralysis may occur in varying degrees of completeness and severity. The symptoms of facial paralysis may be chronic or may show complete recovery. In idiopathic facial paralysis, about 80% of patients show spontaneous recovery with little or no residual weakness. However, idiopathic facial nerve disorder may recur in 3% to 10% of individuals. Treatment may include drug therapy, surgery, and physical therapy.

SITE OF DISORDER

Seventh cranial nerve.

GENERAL AUDIOLOGIC PATTERN

The distinguishing audiologic characteristics of patients with facial paralysis are related to the stapedial muscle reflex. In general, reflexes are absent in lesions proximal to the innervation of the stapedial muscle and present at normal HLs in lesions distal to the stapedial muscle innervation. Absent re-

4. Remember, before a vertical pattern may be attributed to facial nerve disorder, the possibility of a middle ear site must be ruled out.

5. Increased sensitivity to loud sounds is reported in about 30% of patients with Bell's palsy.

Abnormal performance on auditory tests at high intensity levels may be related to the observation that the acoustic reflex, when normal, extends the dynamic range of the ear about 20 dB (Borg and Zakrisson, 1973).

6. See patient 1, Chapter 5, Diabetes Mellitus.

flexes result in a vertical pattern. Both crossed and uncrossed reflexes are absent with probe to the affected side.[4] In patients with systematic recovery of facial muscle function, serial reflex testing may show concurrent systematic recovery of acoustic reflexes. The vertical reflex pattern may change to a normal configuration with all threshold HLs returning to within the normal range. However, in contrast to the normal threshold values, reflex amplitude growth functions may continue to be abnormal relative to the uninvolved ear.

In some patients with facial nerve disorder and consequent abnormal acoustic reflexes, audiologic test results at loud intensity levels may show unusual abnormalities on the involved side. For example, rollover of the performance-intensity function for speech materials may occur. Further, the loudness discomfort level, or the intensity level where sounds are first reported as annoying, may occur at a reduced HL relative to the normal ear.[5]

In contrast to these findings, other audiologic results are generally within normal limits. Tympanograms and static compliance measures are usually normal. Maximum speech intelligibility scores are typically within the normal range. Pure tone sensitivity results are generally normal on both ears. One exception to the above generalities is that a hearing loss may predate and/or accompany the seventh nerve disorder in some patients. For example, a conductive loss may be present if the facial paralysis is a consequence of middle ear disease or a longitudinal skull fracture. A sensorineural hearing loss may be present if the facial paralysis is related to an eighth nerve Schwannoma or a metabolic-vascular disorder such as diabetes.[6]

If the PI function for speech materials shows rollover and/or acoustic reflexes are abnormal in the presence of normal middle ear function, further tests to evaluate the possibility of eighth nerve disorder are indicated. Appropriate tests may include Bekesy and BCL audiometry, STAT, TDT, and ABR testing.

Illustrative Patients

CASE 1. A 19-YEAR-OLD MALE WITH FACIAL PARALYSIS OF UNKNOWN ETIOLOGY (BELL'S PALSY) ON THE RIGHT SIDE.

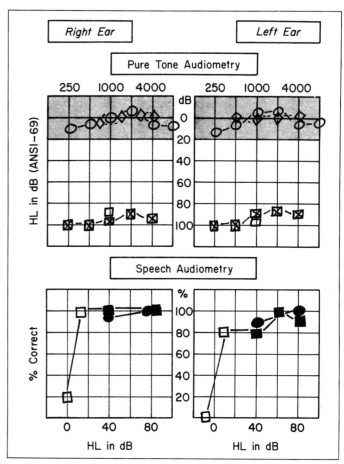

Case 7-1A

History

One week ago the patient awoke with partial paralysis of the right side of his face. Over the next 3 days, the right-sided paralysis became complete. The patient complains of a right-sided twitching sensation and a change in taste. He does not notice any change in his hearing ability.

Results

The audiogram (Case 7-1A) shows bilaterally normal pure tone sensitivity. The PTA scores (Case 7-1B) are 0 dB HL on the right ear and −3 dB HL on the left ear. SAL audiometry (Case 7-1A) does not show a conductive component in either ear. The Weber test (Case 7-1B) at 500 Hz is referred to the middle of the head.

PI-SSI functions (Case 7-1A) are normal on both ears. SSI max scores (Case 7-1B) are 100% bilaterally. SSIT scores, 5 dB HL on the right ear and 4 dB HL on the left ear, agree with pure tone sensitivity levels. PB testing at high intensity levels (Case 7-1A) shows normal intelligibility scores and no

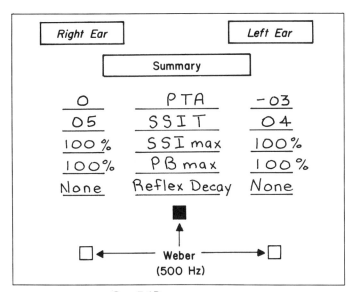

Case 7-1B

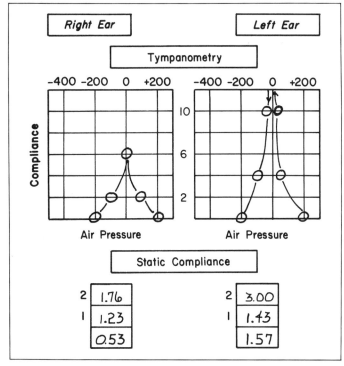

Case 7-1C

7. Notice that the tympanogram on the left ear mimics results in ossicular discontinuity. Remember, however, the combination of an abnormally deep type A tympanogram without concomitant conductive

loss points to tympanic membrane disease, not discontinuity. Contrast results in this patient to results on patient 2, Chapter 6, Discontinuity of the Ossicular Chain.

rollover. PB max scores (Case 7-1B) are 100% in each ear.

Impedance audiometry (Case 7-1C) shows a type A tympanogram on the right ear and a type A$_D$ tympanogram on the left ear.[7] Static compliance measures are within normal limits on both ears. Crossed and uncrossed acoustic reflexes (Case 7-1A) are present at normal HLs at all frequencies on both ears. Reflex decay testing at 1000 Hz (Case 7-1B) does not show any change in reflex amplitude during the 10-sec test period on either ear.

Impression

Normal pure tone sensitivity on both ears. Impedance audiometry indicates essentially normal middle ear function bilaterally. However, the left middle ear system is unusually compliant relative to the right middle ear. Crossed and uncrossed acoustic reflexes with probe to the right side are present at normal HLs at all frequencies suggesting that the facial nerve is intact proximal to the innervation of the stapedial muscle.

CASE 2. A 25-YEAR-OLD FEMALE WITH FACIAL PARALYSIS OF UNKNOWN ETIOLOGY (BELL'S PALSY) ON THE RIGHT SIDE.

History

The patient reports complete facial paralysis on the right side for the past 11 days. During this time, she also complains of headaches and pain around the right ear. Neurologic examination is within normal limits except for the right facial paralysis. Skull x-rays and routine laboratory studies are normal. The patient does not notice any hearing difficulties. However, since the facial paralysis, loud sounds bother her in the right ear.

Results

The audiogram (Case 7-2A) shows normal pure tone sensitivity bilaterally. The PTA scores (Case 7-2B) are 0 dB HL on the right ear and 2 dB HL on the left ear. SAL audiometry (Case 7-2A) does not show a conductive component on either ear.

Speech audiometry (Case 7-2A) shows maximum intelligibility scores of 100% for both PB and SSI materials on the right and left ears. On the right ear, however, the PI-PB and PI-SSI functions show mild rollover. Speech thresholds (Case 7-2B) on both ears agree with pure tone sensitivity results. The SSIT scores are 2 dB HL on both ears. The PBT scores are 0 dB HL on the right ear and 6 dB HL on the left ear.

Impedance audiometry (Case 7-2C) shows normal, type A, tympanograms and normal static compliance measures bilaterally. Crossed acoustic reflexes (Case 7-2A) on the right ear are present at normal HLs at all frequencies. However, uncrossed reflexes on the right ear could not be elicited at equipment limits. With sound to the left ear, crossed reflexes are absent at all fre-

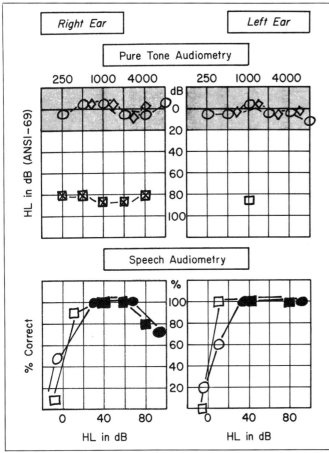

Case 7-2A

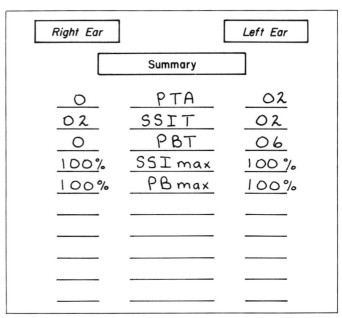

Case 7-2B

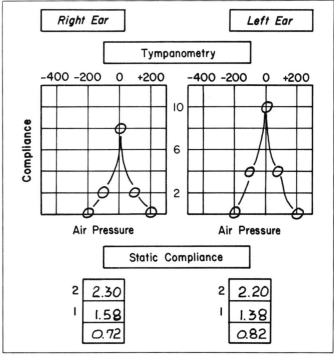

Case 7-2C

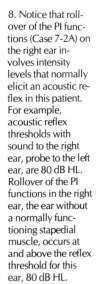

8. Notice that rollover of the PI functions (Case 7-2A) on the right ear involves intensity levels that normally elicit an acoustic reflex in this patient. For example, acoustic reflex thresholds with sound to the right ear, probe to the left ear, are 80 dB HL. Rollover of the PI functions in the right ear, the ear without a normally functioning stapedial muscle, occurs at and above the reflex threshold for this ear, 80 dB HL.

9. Remember, the vertical reflex pattern, in and of itself, is diagnostically nonspecific. A vertical configuration may reflect either a right middle ear disorder or a right

quencies. The uncrossed reflex threshold at 1000 Hz in the left ear, however, is within normal limits. The reflex pattern at 1000 Hz (Case 7-2D) is characterized by a vertical configuration. Reflex thresholds are normal with probe to the left ear and abnormal with probe to the right ear.[8] The vertical pattern is consistent with a seventh nerve disorder on the right side.[9] Reflex decay testing at 1000 Hz was measured in the crossed condition on the right ear and in the uncrossed condition on the left ear. Results do not show any decline in reflex amplitude during the 10-sec test period on either ear.

Impression

Normal pure tone sensitivity on both ears. Absent acoustic reflexes with probe to the right ear and mild rollover of PI functions for speech materials on the right ear are consistent with a seventh nerve disorder on the right side.

CASE 3. A 10-YEAR-OLD MALE WITH A 1-CM MESENCHYMAL TUMOR OF THE LEFT SEVENTH NERVE.

seventh nerve site. In this patient, a right middle ear site is ruled out by SAL audiometry and the normal, symmetric pure tone sensitivity.

Surgical Findings

Surgery revealed a 1-cm mesenchymal tumor attached by a fibrous, pedunculated strand to the mastoid segment of the left facial nerve proximal to the origin of the chorda tympani nerve. An arachnoid layer was noted to be occluding the left internal auditory canal. The cochlear and vestibular divisions of the eighth cranial nerve were

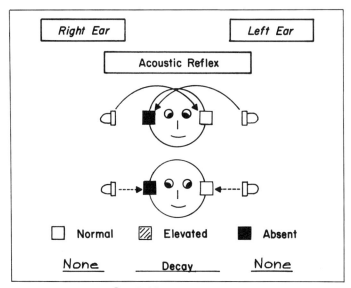

Case 7-2D

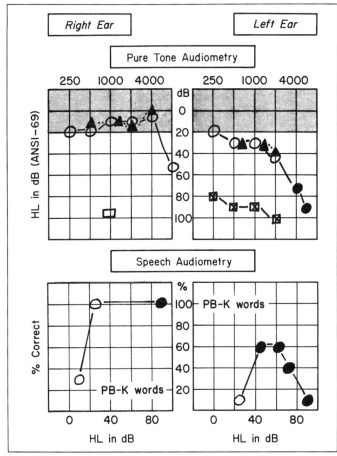

Case 7-3A

10. Notice that facial paralysis is not always present in patients with facial nerve disorders. In fact, as many as one-third of patients with facial nerve neoplasms may not have detectable facial paralysis.

matted together. There was a marked flattening of the left eighth nerve.

History

The child's parents report a progressive hearing loss in the left ear for approximately 2 years. The loss was initially noted on a school hearing screening examination. The child does not notice any tinnitus or dizziness. Neurologic examination is essentially within normal limits except for a possible left eighth nerve disorder. No evidence of facial paralysis is observed on either side. The child is enrolled in a special education class for the mentally retarded. He is receiving individual therapy for speech and language problems.[10]

Results

The audiogram (Case 7-3A) on the right ear shows normal pure tone sensitivity with the exception of a moderate sensorineural loss at 8000 Hz. Pure tone sensitivity results on the left ear show a moderate, sloping sensorineural loss with greater impairment in the high frequency region than in the low frequency region. The PTA scores (Case 7-3B) are 15 dB HL on the right ear and 37 dB HL on the left ear. Bone conduction thresholds (Case 7-3A) are superimposed on air conduction thresholds bilaterally.

11. Normal speech intelligibility performance on the right ear provides a valuable control condition for this

The PI function for PB-kindergarten (PB-K) words (Case 7-3A) is normal on the right ear, but shows a reduced maximum intelligibility score and substantial rollover on the left ear. The PB-K max scores (Case 7-3B) are

child's speech and language problems. Results on the right ear allow us to say that depressed speech intelligibility scores on the left ear are due to a specific auditory disorder, rather than generalized speech and language problems.

On the left ear, a speech threshold may not be determined by the 50% intelligibility level due to the depressed PB-K max score. In this circumstance, a PBT is determined by the 25% intelligibility level.

12. Notice how reflex thresholds on the left ear reflect the sloping audiometric contour. For each dB change in air conduction threshold HLs, there

100% on the right ear and 60% on the left ear. The PBT scores, 13 dB HL on the right ear and 32 dB HL on the left ear (Case 7-3B), agree with average pure tone sensitivity.[11]

Impedance audiometry (Case 7-3C) shows normal, type A, tympanograms and normal static compliance measures on both ears. Crossed acoustic reflexes (Case 7-3A) with sound to the right ear are absent at all frequencies. The uncrossed reflex at 1000 Hz, however, is present at a normal HL. With sound to the left ear, crossed acoustic reflexes are present at normal HLs from 250 through 2000 Hz. A crossed acoustic reflex could not be elicited at 4000 Hz, however. Uncrossed reflexes on the left ear are absent at equipment limits.[12]

The reflex pattern (Case 7-3D) is characterized by a vertical configuration. Reflexes are absent with probe to the left ear and present with probe to the right ear. A vertical pattern, in the presence of normal middle ear function, is consistent with a seventh nerve disorder on the left side. The SPAR test (Case 7-3D) could not be carried out on the

48

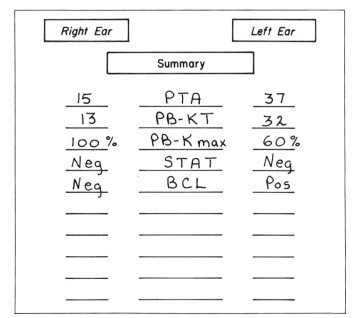

Case 7-3B

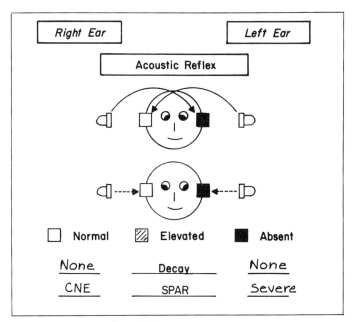

Case 7-3D

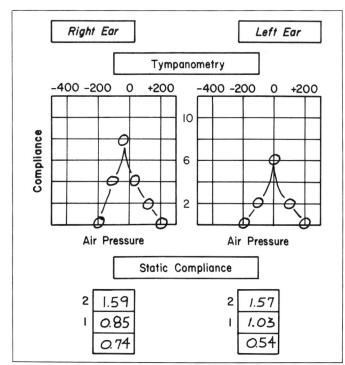

Case 7-3C

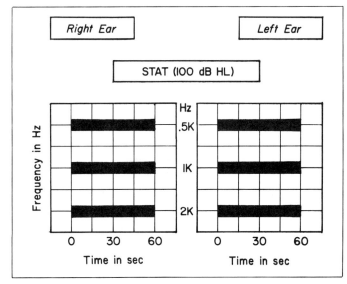

Case 7-3E

13. Notice on the right ear that the continuous tracings run above the interrupted tracing. Remember, in contrast to the conventional threshold Bekesy procedure, this result is a normal behavior pattern for suprathreshold BCL audiometry.

14. The interpretation of the delayed

is a corresponding dB shift in acoustic reflex threshold HLs. Consequently, the sensation level of acoustic reflexes remains at 55 dB to 60 dB.

right ear. On the left ear, SPAR measures predict severe sensitivity loss in the high frequency region. Reflex decay measures at 1000 Hz (Case 7-3D) were obtained in the uncrossed condition on the right ear and in the crossed condition on the left ear. Results on both ears show a normal reflex time course with no reflex amplitude decay.

The STAT (Case 7-3E) does not show abnormal adaptation at any frequency on either ear. BCL audiometry (Case 7-3F) yields negative results on the right ear and positive results on the left ear.[13] The positive pattern on the left ear is characterized by a substantial discrepancy for continuous forward vs backward tracings between 250 and 1000 Hz. ABR audiometry, based on the latency of wave V (Case 7-3G), is within normal limits on the right ear, but is substantially delayed at 60 and 70 dB HL on the left ear.[14]

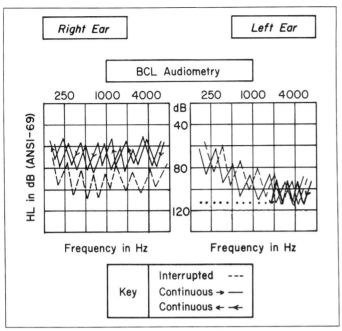

Case 7-3F

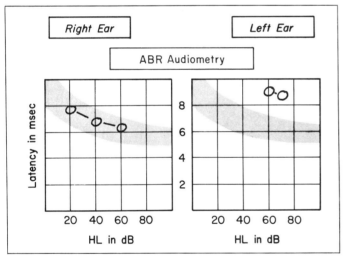

Case 7-3G

15. Note the difference in the degree of rollover observed in patient 3 with combined seventh and eighth nerve sites (Case 7-3A) and in patient 2 with an isolated seventh nerve disorder (Case 7-2A).

response latency on the left ear must be tempered by the sloping audiometric contour and the severe hearing loss above 2000 Hz. If response latencies are adjusted by 1 msec to compensate for the severe high frequency loss, adjusted latencies on the left ear continue to fall outside the normal range.

Impression

RIGHT EAR: Normal pure tone sensitivity with the exception of a moderate sensorineural loss at 8000 Hz.

LEFT EAR: Moderate sensorineural loss. Diagnostic test results are most consistent with a combined seventh and eighth nerve disorder. A seventh nerve abnormality is indicated by absent acoustic reflexes with probe to the left ear. An eighth nerve site is suggested by the presence of delayed wave V latencies on ABR audiometry, abnormal adaptation on BCL testing, and abnormal

rollover and reduced maximum intelligibility scores on speech audiometry.[15]

COMMENT

These results illustrate the three substantially different audiometric patterns that may characterize findings in patients with facial nerve disorder. The first patient illustrates auditory findings in a facial nerve lesion presumed to be distal to the innervation of the stapedial muscle. Results on pure tone audiometry (Case 7-1A), speech audiometry (Case 7-1A), and impedance testing (Cases 7-1A and 7-1C) are consistently within normal limits.

The second patient represents results characteristic of a facial nerve lesion presumed to be proximal to the innervation of the stapedial muscle. In this patient, pure tone sensitivity (Case 7-2A), maximum speech intelligibility scores (Case 7-2A), tympanometry and static compliance measures (Case 7-2C) are within the normal range. However, acoustic reflexes are absent with probe to the affected side (Cases 7-2A and 7-2D). Further, PI functions for speech materials show mild rollover on the affected side. The rollover effect becomes apparent at intensity levels that would trigger an acoustic reflex in a normally functioning ear.

Results in the third patient represent findings in a facial nerve lesion that is producing secondary eighth nerve involvement in addition to the primary seventh nerve site. The seventh nerve site is proximal to the chorda tympani nerve and the innervation of the stapedial muscle. The presence of a combined seventh and eighth nerve disorder dramatically changes the audiometric picture. Pure tone sensitivity (Case 7-3A) and maximum speech intelligibility performance (Case 7-3A) are no longer normal. Rollover of the PI function for PB words (Case 7-3A) becomes more pronounced.

In the third patient, with combined seventh and eighth nerve sites, evidence of abnormal adaptation (Case 7-3F) and abnormal ABR responses (Case 7-3G) are observed. However, the overall pattern of audiometric results is not as clearcut as that usually seen in pure eighth nerve disorders (see Chapter 1, Acoustic Schwannoma). In particular, acoustic reflex results in patient 3 do not reflect the secondary eighth nerve in-

16. A more common reflex pattern in combined seventh and eighth nerve disorders is the inverted L-shaped configuration. An inverted L-shaped pattern indicates an abnormal sound effect and probe effect on the involved ear (see patient 1, Chapter 1, Acoustic Schwannoma).

volvement. With sound to the affected ear, acoustic reflex threshold HLs are normal and no reflex decay is apparent (Case 7-3D). The reflex pattern, a vertical configuration (Case 7-3D), indicates only the peripheral seventh nerve site of disorder.[16]

SELECTED READINGS

Alford, B., Jerger, J., Coats, A., Peterson, C., and Weber, S. Diagnostic tests of facial nerve function. *Otolaryngol. Clin. North Am.* 7:331, 1974.

Alford, B., Weber, S., and Sessions, R. Neurodiagnostic studies in facial paralysis. *Ann. Otol. Rhinol. Laryngol.* 79:227, 1970.

Antoli-Candela, F., and Stewart, T. The pathophysiology of otologic facial paralysis. *Otolaryngol. Clin. North Am.* 7:309, 1974.

Borg, E., and Zakrisson, J. Stapedius reflex and speech features. *J. Acoust. Soc. Am.* 54:525, 1973.

Cawthorne, T. Intratemporal facial palsy. *Arch. Otolaryngol.* 90:137, 1969.

Citron, D., and Adour, K. Acoustic reflex and loudness discomfort in acute facial paralysis. *Arch. Otolaryngol.* 104:303, 1978.

Hauser, W., Karnes, W., Annis, J., and Kurland, L. Incidence and prognosis of Bell's palsy in the population of Rochester. *Mayo Clin. Proc.* 46:258, 1971.

Neely, J. Neoplastic involvement of the facial nerve. *Otolaryngol. Clin. North Am.* 7:385, 1974.

Neely, J., and Alford, B. Facial nerve neuromas. *Arch. Otolaryngol.* 100:298, 1974.

Powers, W. Peripheral facial paralysis and systemic disease. *Otolaryngol. Clin. North Am.* 7:397, 1974.

Shambaugh, G., and Clemis, J. Facial Nerve Paralysis. In M. Paparella and D. Shumrick (eds.), *Otolaryngology* (vol. 2). Philadelphia: Saunders, 1973. Pp. 263–282.

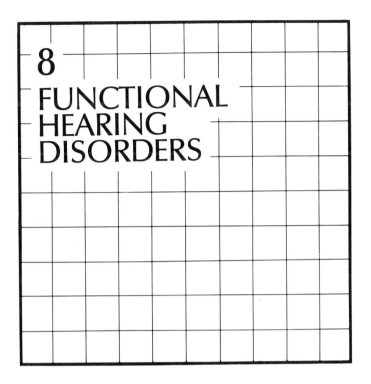

8 FUNCTIONAL HEARING DISORDERS

DESCRIPTION

1. Other terms used to describe functional hearing loss *are nonorganic psychogenic, pseudohypoacusis, malingering,* and *conversion hysteria disorder.* To some clinicians, the above terms may have substantially different implications about the possibility of unknown organic etiologies and conscious vs unconscious motivations. For a discussion of these terms see Hopkinson, 1973.

2. The prevalence of functional hearing loss is estimated as . . . less than 2% in the general population . . . about 7% in children between 6 and 17 years of age . . . between about 10% to 50% in persons tested for compensation purposes or in military-related audiology services.

Functional hearing disorders are apparent losses that cannot be attributed to an organic etiology or a structural change.[1] In adults, functional hearing loss may be related to monetary gains, to emotional stresses, and/or to a desire to avoid specific situations, such as military service. In children, functional hearing disorders may be used to attract attention or to shift parental concerns toward hearing, rather than other behaviors, such as academic failure. On occasion, functional hearing loss in both adults and children may reflect genuine emotional problems. The motivations for functional hearing loss may range over a continuum from wholly conscious to wholly unconscious. In numerous individuals, a functional hearing loss may be superimposed on a true organic deficit. In these persons, the functional component is referred to as a *functional overlay.*[2]

PATIENT CHARACTERISTICS

Functional hearing loss may occur in patients of any age. However, children with functional hearing disorders are usually at least 8 years old. On psychological testing, patients with functional loss may appear to have a greater degree of emotional immaturity, instability, neurotic anxiety, and/or feelings of inferiority than the general

3. An unusually calm attitude in patients with functional disorders has been termed *la belle indifférence* by some investigators.

population. During the initial formal interview, the psychosocial behavior of functional patients may be characterized by excessive nervousness; an unusually loud voice; frequent, unsolicited comments about his hearing problems; an extremely passive, anxious effect; or exaggerated attempts to hear or to lipread. In contrast to the exaggerated descriptions of his hearing problems, the patient may have a rather casual emotional reaction to his hearing loss.[3] His manner toward the clinician may be amiable and/or ingratiating. In subsequent informal conversational situations, functional patients, especially children, may appear to understand without difficulty.

Functional hearing loss may be unilateral or bilateral. A sex prevalence is not reported. However, in adults, a review of the literature suggests a larger prevalence of functional hearing loss in males than in females. The preponderance of male patients, however, may reflect a disproportionate number of studies conducted in military-related settings. An exception to the above observation is that hearing disorders due to conversion hysteria (not under conscious control) are more prevalent in females than in males. In children, functional hearing loss is three times more common in females than in males.

CLINICAL COURSE

4. Of patients with functional hearing loss in a military setting, 86% had underlying medically diagnosed organic hearing loss (Gleason, 1958).

Remember, an erroneous air conduction hearing loss may be caused by stenosis of the external ear canal, rather than a functional hearing disorder (see Chapter 4, Collapsing Ear Canal).

In patients with functional hearing loss, an apparent, erroneous sensitivity loss may be superimposed on normal hearing or any type of hearing disorder.[4] The onset of the functional loss may be vague and uncertain or may be sudden and referred to a specific incident. In general, functional hearing disorders occur at a time or in a manner that provides a "solution" to a perceived problem. The reported hearing loss may be accompanied by tinnitus. In fact, a patient may report that the tinnitus confuses him and interferes with his hearing or his ability to perform the hearing test. Treatment of functional hearing disorders may involve psychological or psychiatric counseling.

GENERAL AUDIOLOGIC PATTERN

Pure tone results characteristically show a moderate to severe air conduction and bone conduction sensitivity loss. The audiometric

5. In a series of 64 patients with functional hearing loss, 66% had a pure tone test-retest difference of more than 10 dB. On pure tone testing, functional patients may adopt an unusually strict listening criterion. For example, "false alarm" responses may be observed in about 85% of hearing loss patients, but only about 20% of functional individuals (Ventry and Chaiklin, 1965).

6. About 70% to 85% of functional patients have a difference of more than 10 dB between pure tone and speech thresholds (Ventry and Chaiklin, 1965; Jerger and Jerger, 1976).
In a series of children with functional hearing loss, 39 of 40 individuals scored at least 90% correct on traditional speech intelligibility testing (Dixon and Hayes, 1959).

7. In adults with functional hearing loss, type V Bekesy tracings occur in 60% to 75% of patients (Stein, 1963; Rintelmann and Harford, 1967; Jerger et al., 1972).
In a series of adults with functional hearing loss, 10 of 11 individuals had significant discrepancy between forward vs backward continuous tracings (Jerger et al., 1972).

contour is generally relatively flat. An exception involves patients with functional overlay on a true hearing loss. In these individuals, any configuration may result. However, isolated high frequency sensitivity loss rarely, if ever, occurs. A primary characteristic of pure tone threshold results in patients with functional hearing disorders may be unusual threshold variability (a difference of 15 dB or more), particularly for ascending vs descending threshold-seeking procedures.[5]

Impedance results characteristically show normal tympanograms, normal static compliance, and normal acoustic reflexes. Sensitivity prediction from acoustic reflex (SPAR) measures may be particularly helpful in estimating whether the functional hearing disorder is superimposed on normal hearing or a sensorineural hearing loss. On occasion, especially in children, impedance results may be consistent with the presence of middle ear disorder.

Speech audiometry may show maximum intelligibility scores and speech threshold results that are disproportionately good relative to the apparent pure tone sensitivity loss. In fact, a discrepancy between average pure tone sensitivity and speech threshold results is a hallmark of functional loss.[6]

In patients with functional hearing disorders, special tests may be administered to document the presence of a functional component to the hearing problem and to estimate the probable organic hearing status of the involved ear(s). In unilateral functional disorders, appropriate tests may include the SPAR technique, the Stenger procedure, ABR audiometry, and threshold Bekesy audiograms with forward vs backward tracings for continuous signals. In addition to these procedures, another indication of functional disorder is the absence of crossover responses, or a shadow curve for pure tone and speech signals presented to the reportedly bad ear without adequate masking noise to the uninvolved, good ear. In bilateral functional hearing disorders, appropriate tests may include the SPAR technique, ABR audiometry, and threshold Bekesy audiometry with continuous forward vs backward tracings.[7]

It is important to note that diagnostic procedures for the differentiation of middle ear, cochlear, and retrocochlear sites of disorder

are *contraindicated* by the presence of functional hearing problems. In particular, BCL audiometry, the tone decay test, the suprathreshold adaptation test, SAL measures, and sensitized speech tests may yield erroneous and misleading results in patients with functional hearing problems.

CLINICAL MANAGEMENT OF FUNCTIONAL HEARING LOSS

It is the clinician's responsibility to identify functional hearing loss and to quantify, if possible, the true underlying organic hearing status. Toward this goal, experienced clinicians maintain a calm, objective attitude toward the patient. A thoughtful clinician's manner does not convey surprise or annoyance when the hearing loss appears spurious. Importantly, during the hearing testing session, a patient is not confronted or accused of feigning his hearing difficulties. Usually, the presence and degree of functional impairment may be sufficiently documented with the battery of tests specified above. In addition, more reliable voluntary threshold sensitivity measures may result from simply restructuring the listening tasks. To do this, a patient's response may be changed (i.e., he may be instructed to count the number of sounds he hears during a specified listen interval) or the pure tone and speech signals may be modified (pulsed tones vs continuous tones vs warble tones; quiet vs background noise, etc.).

Illustrative Patients

CASE 1. A 42-YEAR-OLD FEMALE WITH FUNCTIONAL HEARING LOSS ON THE LEFT EAR.

History

Approximately 1 month ago the patient was hospitalized for elective surgery. During her hospitalization, she was struck on the left side of the head by an x-ray machine. Since the accident, the patient complains of severe head and neck pain, weakness of the lower extremities, and a hearing loss in her left ear. She is unable to return to work.

Neurologic examination is within normal limits. There is no evidence of spinal cord compression or radiculopathy. Skull films, CT scan, electromyographic studies, and otorhinolaryngologic findings are normal. The patient does not have any hearing com-

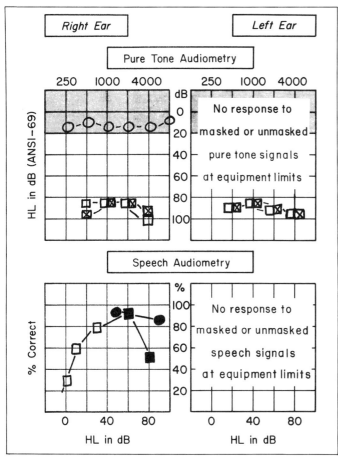

Case 8-1A

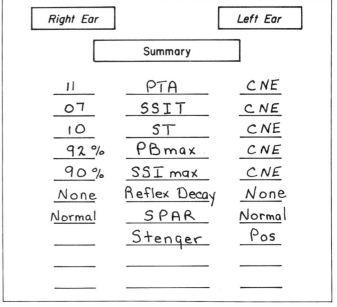

Case 8-1B

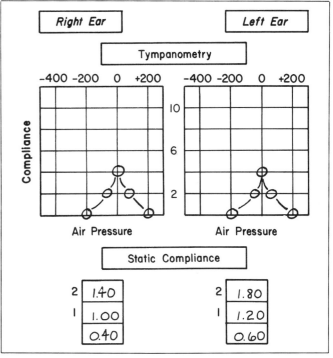

Case 8-1C

8. Notice the lack of crossover responses (a shadow curve) with sound at maximum intensity to the left ear and no masking noise to the right ear. Absence of crossover is a strong suggestion of functional loss in the left ear (for an example of an appropriate shadow curve, see patient 2, Chapter 24, Trauma).

9. In this patient, presence of SSI rollover coupled with absence of PB rollover is not interpreted as a strong indication of retrocochlear site, but is interpreted much more cautiously. Remember, tests with a high correct identification rate for retrocochlear site (such as PI-SSI roll-

plaints about her right ear. She thinks the hearing in her left ear was normal before the accident.

Results

The audiogram (Case 8-1A) shows normal pure tone sensitivity on the right ear. On the left ear, there is no response to masked or unmasked pure tone signals at equipment limits.[8] The PTA score (Case 8-1B) on the right ear is 11 dB HL. A PTA score on the left ear could not be established.

Speech audiometry (Case 8-1A) on the right ear shows normal maximum speech intelligibility scores for both PB and SSI materials. The PB max score (Case 8-1B) is 92%; the SSI max score is 90%. On the right ear, the PI-SSI function shows a rollover effect of approximately 40%. However, PB testing at high intensity levels does not show the rollover phenomenon.[9] The SSIT score on the right ear, 7 dB HL, agrees with average pure tone sensitivity. On the left ear, there is no response to masked or unmasked speech signals at equipment limits.

over) are inevitably coupled with a high false alarm rate in normal and cochlear ears. Correct identification rates and false alarm rates provide useful information to the clinician for interpreting test results.

Impedance audiometry (Case 8-1C) shows normal, type A, tympanograms and normal static compliance measures bilaterally. Crossed and uncrossed acoustic reflexes (Case 8-1A) on both ears are present at normal HLs at all frequencies. Reflex decay testing (Case 8-1B) at 1000 Hz does not show any decline in reflex amplitude during the 10-sec test period on either ear.

54

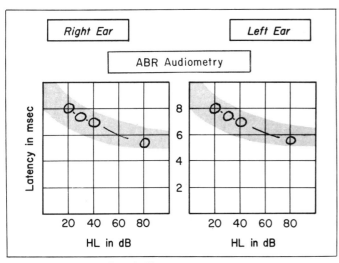

Case 8-1D

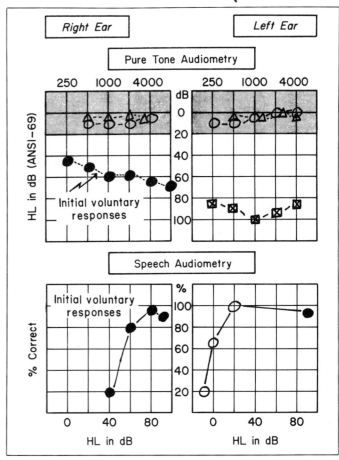

Case 8-2A

10. Remember, the likelihood of a normal SPAR prediction in the presence of even a mild hearing loss is relatively low, less than 20%.

11. Notice that Stenger results suggest relatively normal sensitivity on the left ear at least for the speech frequencies.

12. Functional patients with normal hearing in the good ear and a total absence of voluntary responses in the bad ear are relatively infrequent, about 2% of individuals in a series of 64 subjects (Ventry and Chaiklin, 1965).

In this patient, notice how results on the normal, right ear provide a valuable control condition for results on the left ear. In particular, symmetric findings on the two

The SPAR measure predicts normal pure tone sensitivity on both ears.[10]

The voluntary speech threshold for spondee words (ST) (Case 8-1B) on the right ear is 10 dB HL. On the left ear, there is no response to spondee words at equipment limits with or without masking to the right ear. The speech Stenger test (Case 8-1B) is positive. The patient ceased responding when spondee words were presented to both ears at 14 dB HL.[11]

ABR audiometry (Case 8-1D) on both ears shows a normal latency-intensity function for wave V. The amplitude of ABR responses is symmetric on the two ears. The lowest click intensity eliciting a repeatable wave V response is 20 dB HL on both ears.

Impressions

RIGHT EAR: Normal pure tone sensitivity.

LEFT EAR: No voluntary responses to pure tone or speech signals are observed at equipment limits with or without masking.[12] SPAR results predict normal pure tone sensitivity. ABR audiometry yields a normal latency-intensity function with well-formed, repeatable wave V responses at 20 dB HL. The Stenger test for functional hearing loss is positive. The Stenger speech interference level on the left ear is 14 dB HL. SPAR results, ABR findings, and the Stenger test suggest symmetric hearing sensitivity on the two ears.

CASE 2. A 22-YEAR-OLD BLIND FEMALE WITH FUNCTIONAL HEARING LOSS ON THE RIGHT EAR.

ears for SPAR measures (Case 8-1B) and ABR audiometry (Case 8-1D) are a strong indication of symmetric hearing sensitivity.

13. Remember, a functional patient may seem unconcerned about his hearing loss if it is solving a problem for him. This young blind girl had been saving her money for years for a trip to Europe alone. She was to leave in a few weeks. The present hospitalization depleted her trip funds. She could no longer afford to go.

History

The patient was admitted to the hospital with complaints of dizziness, nausea, vomiting, and hearing loss accompanied by severe pain in the right ear. The symptoms began 10 days ago accompanied by rash and edema of the right external auditory canal. The patient has a history of external otitis in both ears.

At admission, neurologic examination, physical findings, and routine laboratory studies are essentially normal, except for decreased hearing in the right ear and blindness in both eyes secondary to retrolental fibroplasia. Otorhinolaryngologic examination is within normal limits. The patient has no hearing complaints about her left ear. In fact she seems unconcerned about the hearing loss in her right ear.[13] Psychiatric evaluation at this admission yielded a final diagnosis of conversion hysteria.

Results

Initial voluntary threshold hearing levels (Case 8-2A) show a moderate sensitivity loss

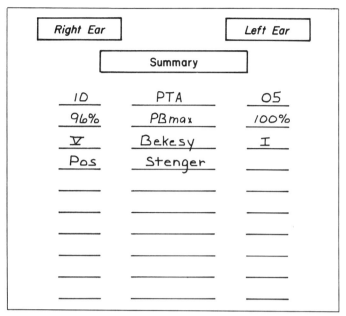

Case 8-2B

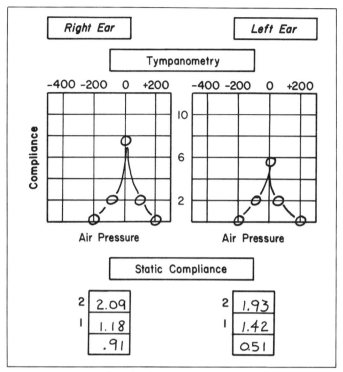

Case 8-2C

14. Agreement between PBT vs PTA scores (false-negative results) may occur in about 15% of patients with functional loss (Jerger and Jerger, 1976).

15. Notice how helpful uncrossed reflexes would have been in this patient. More specifically, absent crossed reflexes with sound to the right ear may be reflecting either a sound effect on the right ear or a probe effect on the left ear. Uncrossed reflexes would have allowed us to differentiate between the possibility of a middle ear-muscle site on the normal, left ear, vs a "retrocochlear" pattern on the affected, right, ear.

16. Agreement between voluntary spondee thresholds and pure tone thresholds (false-negative results) may occur in about 30% of functional hearing loss

on the right ear and normal pure tone sensitivity on the left ear. PI-PB functions (Case 8-2A) show normal maximum speech intelligibility scores on both ears. The PB max scores (Case 8-2B) are 96% on the right ear and 100% on the left ear. Speech thresholds on both ears agree with initial voluntary pure tone sensitivity results. The PBT scores (not shown) are 51 dB HL on the right ear and −5 dB HL on the left ear.[14]

Impedance audiometry (Case 8-2C) shows normal, type A, tympanograms and normal static compliance measures bilaterally. Crossed acoustic reflexes on the left ear are present at normal HLs between 250 and 4000 Hz. Crossed acoustic reflexes (Case 8-2A) on the right ear are absent at all frequencies. Uncrossed reflexes are not available due to equipment limitations. Unanswered, therefore, is the interesting question of whether the right ear reflexes are absent on a purely psychogenic basis.[15]

Conventional threshold Bekesy audiometry (Case 8-2D) shows a type V tracing on the right ear and type I tracing on the left ear.

Voluntary speech thresholds for spondee words (ST) (not shown) are 6 dB HL on the left ear and 60 dB HL on the right ear.[16] The speech Stenger test (Case 8-2B) is positive. With speech signals at 20 dB HL in the left ear and 10 dB HL in the right ear, the patient ceased responding.

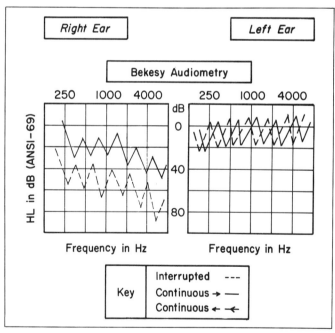

Case 8-2D

patients (Ventry and Chaiklin, 1965).

Results in this patient stress that neither the PTA vs PBT nor PTA vs ST relation is a perfect clinical tool for distinguishing patients with functional problems.

ABR audiometry on both ears (Case 8-2E) shows a normal latency-intensity function for wave V. The lowest click intensity yielding repeatable wave V responses was 10 dB HL on both ears.

At this time, voluntary pure tone threshold results were repeated on the right ear. However, for this test, the patient was instructed

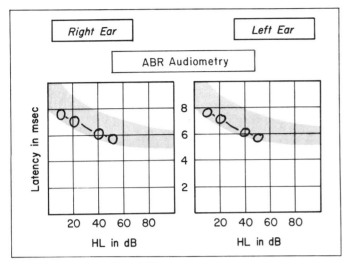

Case 8-2E

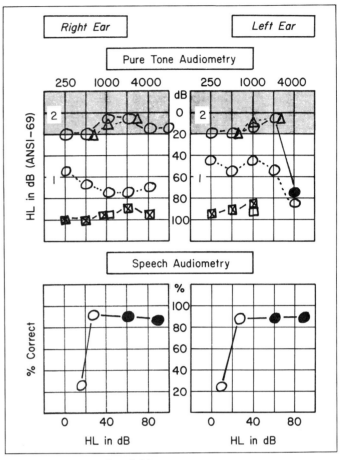

Case 8-3A

to count the number of sounds that she heard during designated listening intervals. With this technique, voluntary threshold HLs on the right ear (Case 8-2A) are within normal limits at 500 Hz through 4000 Hz. Unmasked bone conduction threshold HLs do not show a conductive component on either ear. The PTA scores (Case 8-2B) are 10 dB HL on the right ear and 5 dB HL on the left ear.

Impression

Normal pure tone sensitivity on both ears.

CASE 3. A 14-YEAR-OLD FEMALE WITH BILATERAL FUNCTIONAL HEARING LOSS.

History

The patient was brought to the audiology service by a child welfare social worker. Approximately 1 month ago, she failed a school hearing screening examination. The child thinks she has a hearing loss in both ears. She reports earaches in each ear for the past year. Otorhinolaryngologic examination at this time is within normal limits. The patient is having academic problems at school.

Results

Initial voluntary pure tone sensitivity results ("1," Case 8-3A) show a severe hearing loss in the right ear and a moderate hearing loss in the left ear. PI-PB functions are normal on both ears with maximum intelligibility scores of 92% bilaterally. PBT scores (Case 8-3B) are 20 dB HL on the right ear and 17 dB HL on the left ear. Spondee thresholds

17. Notice that speech thresholds in this child contradict the obtained pure tone sensitivity results.

18. Remember, for SPAR measures, normal hearing is predicted with considerably greater accuracy than degree of sensorineural hearing loss. The predictive accuracy for mild to moderate hearing impairment is about 40% to 60% (Jerger et al., 1978).

19. Notice how helpful Bekesy audiometry is in documenting the presence of functional disorder in this patient. However, a type II Bekesy pattern on the right ear is considered non-

(ST) (Case 8-3B) are 21 dB HL on the right ear and 13 dB HL on the left ear.[17]

Tympanometry and static compliance measures (Case 8-3C) are normal on both ears. Crossed and uncrossed acoustic reflexes (Case 8-3A) with sound to the right ear are present at normal HLs at all frequencies. Crossed and uncrossed acoustic reflexes with sound to the left ear are present at normal HLs from 250 Hz through 1000 Hz. However, crossed acoustic reflexes are absent at 2000 Hz and 4000 Hz. Reflex decay testing (Case 8-3B) does not show amplitude decay on either ear. SPAR results (Case 8-3B) predict a mild to moderate sensitivity loss on each ear.[18]

Conventional threshold Bekesy audiometry (Case 8-3D) shows a type II tracing on the right ear and a type V tracing on the left ear. A significant forward-backward discrepancy is observed on both ears.[19]

Voluntary pure tone thresholds were repeated at this time. The child was instructed to count the number of sounds that she

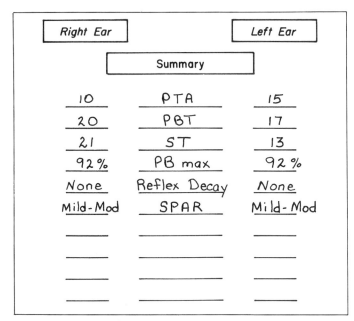

Right Ear	Summary	Left Ear
10	PTA	15
20	PBT	17
21	ST	13
92%	PB max	92%
None	Reflex Decay	None
Mild-Mod	SPAR	Mild-Mod

Case 8-3B

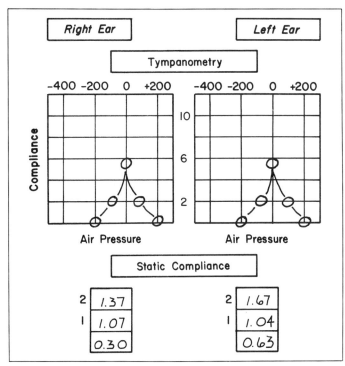

Case 8-3C

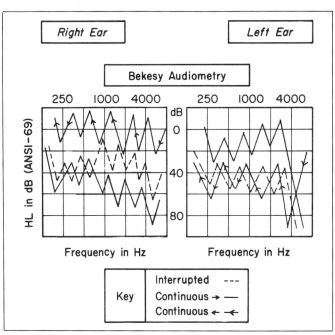

Case 8-3D

diagnostic. Remember, results of behavioral site of lesion tests are generally unreliable in patients with functional disorder.

heard during specified listening intervals. The final audiogram ("2," Case 8-3A) shows normal pure tone sensitivity on the right ear. On the left ear, the audiogram shows normal pure tone sensitivity through 2000 Hz, then a severe high frequency sensitivity loss. Unmasked bone conduction thesholds at 500, 1000, and 2000 Hz do not show an air-bone gap on either ear. The PTA scores

20. Notice, however, that estimates of sensitivity obtained from the Bekesy tracing for continuous backward signals yield better threshold HLs than the final voluntary threshold HLs plotted on the audiogram.

21. Notice that estimates of sensitivity from the Bekesy continuous forward tracings agree with the final voluntary threshold HLs plotted on the audiogram. Acoustic reflex thresholds with sound to the left ear also support the presence of a valid high frequency sensitivity loss.

(Case 8-3B) are 10 dB HL on the right ear and 15 dB HL on the left ear.

Impression

RIGHT EAR: Pure tone sensitivity within normal limits.[20]

LEFT EAR: Pure tone sensitivity within normal limits through 2000 Hz, then a severe high frequency sensorineural loss.[21]

Recommendation

Reevaluation of hearing sensitivity in 1 year.

COMMENT

Notice in these three patients that there was no individual audiologic test procedure or result that consistently and reliably alerted the clinician to the presence of a functional hearing disorder. For example, in one patient (Case 8-1A) the presence of a functional hearing loss was initially suggested by the lack of appropriate crossover responses (a shadow curve) for pure tone and speech signals to the affected, bad, ear and no masking noise in the uninvolved, good, ear. Another strong indication of functional loss in this patient was the presence of acoustic reflexes at HLs the patient denied hearing (Case 8-1A) and a SPAR prediction of normal hearing sensitivity (Case 8-1B). However, crossover responses and acoustic reflex measures were not particularly helpful in another of the patients (Case 8-3A). In this patient, testing for a shadow curve was inappropriate because of the relatively mild sensitivity difference between ears. The SPAR test, instead of predicting normal sensitivity, suggested mild to moderate sensitivity loss at some audiometric frequency on both ears. Further, the relation between acoustic reflex threshold HLs and initial voluntary behavioral pure tone threshold HLs was not sufficiently reduced to suggest functional impairment. In this patient, the presence of functional loss was first indicated by a discrepancy between voluntary speech thresholds and initial voluntary pure tone sensitivity levels (Cases 8-3A and 8-3B). The PBT vs initial PTA discrepancy was about 50 dB on the right ear and 30 dB on the left ear, striking evidence of a functional hearing disorder on both ears.

In contrast to results on this patient, the relation between the PTA and speech thresholds yielded false agreement in another patient (Case 8-2A). This latter patient had good agreement between initial voluntary pure tone threshold HLs and both speech threshold measures, the PBT and ST. Further, acoustic reflex measures were not helpful in suggesting the presence of functional loss. Instead, acoustic reflexes were absent with sound to the affected ear. The first indication of a functional hearing loss in this patient was her unusually amiable affect. She was a young blind girl who seemed unconcerned about losing her normal hearing ability in one ear. In addition, conventional threshold Bekesy audiometry (Case 8-2D) was helpful in documenting the reality of functional impairment in this patient.

In short, there was no individual clinical test procedure or relation between test procedures that consistently indicated the presence of a functional hearing loss in these three patients.

SELECTED READINGS

Dixon, R., and Hayes, N. Children with non-organic hearing problems. *Arch. Otolaryngol.* 70:619, 1959.

Gleason, W. Psychological characteristics of the audiologically inconsistent patient. *Arch. Otolaryngol.* 68:42, 1958.

Hopkinson, N. Functional Hearing Loss. In J. Jerger (ed.), *Modern Developments in Audiol-ogy* (2nd ed.). New York: Academic Press, 1973. Pp. 175–210.

Jerger, J., Hayes, D., Anthony, L., and Mauldin, L. Factors Influencing Prediction of Hearing Level from the Acoustic Reflex. In *Monographs in Contemporary Audiology* (vol. 1). Minneapolis: Maico, 1978. Pp. 1–20.

Jerger, J., and Jerger, S. Estimated speech threshold from the PI-PB function. *Arch. Otolaryngol.* 102:487, 1976.

Jerger, J., Jerger, S., and Mauldin, L. The forward-backward discrepancy in Bekesy audiometry. *Arch. Otolaryngol.* 96:400, 1972.

Martin, F. Differential Diagnostic Evaluation: Nonorganic Loss and Other Special Procedures. In J. Katz (ed.), *Handbook of Clinical Audiology*. Baltimore: Williams & Wilkins, 1972. Pp. 357–373.

Reich, P., and Kelly, M. The Neuroses. In M. Wintrobe, G. Thorn, R. Adams, E. Braunwald, K. Isselbacher, and R. Petersdorf (eds.), *Harrison's Principles of Internal Medicine* (7th ed.). New York: McGraw-Hill, 1974. Pp. 1875–1882.

Rintelmann, W., and Harford, E. The detection and assessment of pseudohypoacusis among school-age children. *J. Speech Hear. Disord.* 28:141, 1963.

Rintelmann, W., and Harford, E. Type V Bekesy pattern: Interpretation and clinical utility. *J. Speech Hear. Res.* 10:733, 1967.

Stein, L. Some observations on type V Bekesy tracings. *J. Speech Hear. Res.* 6:339, 1963.

Ventry, I., and Chaiklin, J. Multidiscipline study of functional hearing loss. *J. Aud. Res.* 5:179, 1965.

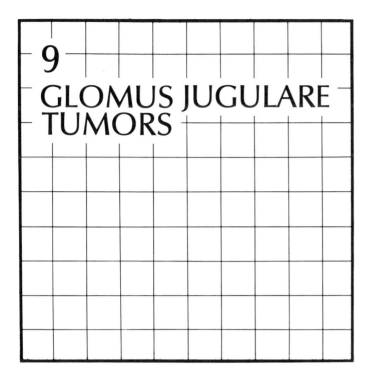

9
GLOMUS JUGULARE TUMORS

DESCRIPTION

Glomera jugularae are tiny, neural bodies that may occur normally in man. Within the temporal bone, glomus jugulare bodies have been found on the top of the jugular bulb just below the floor of the middle ear, along the course of the glossopharyngeal and vagus nerves, and in the mucosa and tympanic plexus on the cochlear promontory. The purpose of glomus jugulare bodies is unknown. One function may be to act as chemoreceptors, regulating the physical and chemical composition of blood (Ballenger, 1977).

From an otologic viewpoint, neoplasms of glomus jugulare formations may be thought of as arising from one of two general areas: the middle ear cavity or the jugular bulb region. However, glomus jugulare tumors originating in the jugular bulb area may erode the bony floor of the middle ear and spread into the middle ear space. Other sites that may be affected by pressure or invasion as glomus jugulare tumors increase in size include the mastoid process, the cochlea, the facial nerve, the posterior fossa, and/or the external auditory canal.[1]

1. Glomus jugulare tumors . . . may be termed *chemodectomas* or *nonchromaffin paragangliomas* . . . may be called *glomus tympanicum tumors* if arising from and contained within the middle ear cavity . . . are the most common type of middle ear tumor (Shapiro and Neues, 1964).

PATIENT CHARACTERISTICS

Glomus jugulare tumors are most frequently diagnosed in patients between 40 and 60 years of age. The average time interval be-

tween initial onset of symptoms and diagnosis is about 6 years (Alford and Guilford, 1962). Approximately 80% of patients are female. The tumor is unilateral in about 99% of patients.

CLINICAL COURSE

2. In a series of 277 patients, 90% had hearing loss, 52% had pulsating tinnitus, 56% had a polypoid mass in the external ear canal, and 44% had facial paralysis (Alford and Guilford, 1962).

Insidious increase in symptoms. Specific symptomatology may vary, however, depending on whether the tumor arises from glomus jugulare formations within the middle ear cavity or within the region of the jugular bulb. Neoplasms originating in the middle ear may be initially characterized by pulsatile tinnitus and conductive hearing loss. Facial nerve paralysis may be present. Neoplasms arising from the jugular bulb region may be initially characterized by involvement of cranial nerves nine through twelve. The eighth nerve may be affected.[2] Treatment of glomus jugulare tumors may involve surgery and/or radiotherapy. In some patients, however, glomus jugulare tumors may recur after treatment.

SITE OF DISORDER

Middle ear. Secondary sites may be the cochlea and/or eighth nerve. On rare occasions, auditory function may be completely normal.

GENERAL AUDIOLOGIC PATTERN

3. Of 170 patients with hearing loss on audiologic testing, 65% had sensorineural loss, 32% had conductive loss, and 4% had mixed loss (Alford and Guilford, 1962).

Pure tone sensitivity results may show a sensorineural, conductive, or mixed hearing loss. The degree of loss varies.[3] On occasion, normal pure tone sensitivity may occur. Speech intelligibility results may be normal or abnormal depending on the extent of middle ear, cochlea, and eighth nerve involvement. Impedance results may vary depending on the nature and extent of ossicular chain involvement. A unique finding on impedance testing may be a periodic pulsating baseline measure. The pulsations are synchronous with the patient's heartbeat and reflect the increased vascularity of the tumor mass.[4]

4. Pulsating fluctuations superimposed on baseline impedance measures may be observed not only in patients with glomus jugulare tumors, but also in individuals with active chronic otitis media or objective tinnitus.

Illustrative Patients

CASE 1. A 53-YEAR-OLD MALE WITH A GLOMUS JUGULARE TUMOR AFFECTING THE LEFT EAR.

Radiographic and Surgical Findings

A left common carotid angiogram shows a highly vascular neoplasm at the base of the left petrous bone in the area of the jugular fossa. Polytomography shows a destructive lesion of the left jugular vault with extension into the inferior aspect of the left petrous bone and middle ear space. At surgery a glomus jugulare tumor was noted to involve the middle ear space, the mastoid portion of the facial nerve, and the temporal bone in the area of the jugular foramen and jugular bulb. The tumor was totally removed from the middle ear space. A portion of the facial nerve was decompressed. Remaining tumor segments were treated with radiotherapy.

History

The patient is admitted to the hospital for a 1-year postoperative evaluation of coronary artery bypass surgery. In response to routine questioning, however, he reported hearing loss and pulsatile tinnitus in his left ear. Otorhinolaryngologic examination reveals a red mass in the left middle ear space. Cranial nerves two through twelve appear intact. The patient is essentially asymptomatic except for hearing complaints about his left ear. He has no hearing complaints about his right ear.

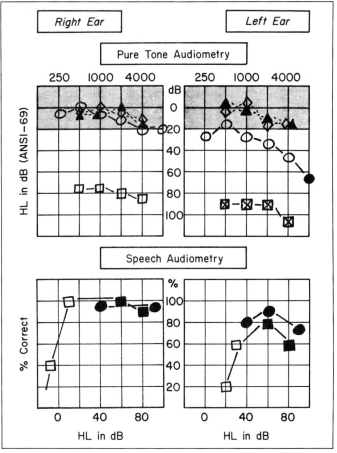

Case 9-1A

Results

5. In patients with conductive loss, a sloping audiometric contour may be referred to as a *mass tilt*. Contrast the audiometric configuration in this patient with the "stiffness tilt" of patient 2 in Chapter 18, Otosclerosis.

The audiogram (Case 9-1A) shows normal sensitivity on the right ear and a mild conductive loss on the left ear. PTA scores (Case 9-1B) are 5 dB HL on the right ear and 24 dB HL on the left ear.[5] Bone conduction and SAL audiometry (Case 9-1A) on the right ear are superimposed on air conduction. On the left ear, bone conduction and SAL results show a conductive component of approximately 15 to 25 dB.

The Weber test (Case 9-1B) at 500 Hz lateralizes to the left ear. The Bing test (not shown) at 500 Hz on the right ear shows an occlusion effect of 15 dB. On the left ear, however, threshold sensitivity in occluded vs unoccluded conditions does not show improvement (5 dB).

The PI-SSI function and PB testing at high intensity levels (Case 9-1A) on the right ear show normal maximum intelligibility scores and no rollover. The SSI max (Case 9-1B) is 100%; the PB max is 96%. Relative to performance on the right ear, the PI-SSI func-

6. In patients with questionable rollover effects, a rollover index may be computed to aid in differentiation of site of disorder. To do this, the PB minimum (76%) is subtracted from the PB max (88%). The difference is divided by the PB max (88% − 76%) ÷ (88%). In this patient, the rollover index is 0.14, a level well below the smallest rollover index (0.45) usually found in eighth nerve site.

tion and PB testing at high intensity levels (Case 9-1A) on the left ear show mildly reduced maximum intelligibility scores and mild rollover.[6] The SSI max (Case 9-1B) is 80%; the PB max is 88%. The SSIT scores (Case 9-1B) agree with average pure tone sensitivity bilaterally. The SSIT score is −5 dB HL on the right ear and 30 dB HL on the left ear.

Tympanometry and static compliance measures (Case 9-1C) are within normal limits on both ears. With both sound and probe to the right ear (uncrossed condition), acoustic reflexes (Case 9-1A) are present at normal HLs from 500 through 4000 Hz. With sound to the left ear and probe to the right ear (crossed condition), reflexes are present at normal HLs at 500 through 2000 Hz. The crossed reflex at 4000 Hz on the left ear, however, is elevated. Acoustic reflexes with probe to the left ear could not be accurately measured due to unusually large periodic pulsations superimposed on the baseline impedance. Case 9-1D shows

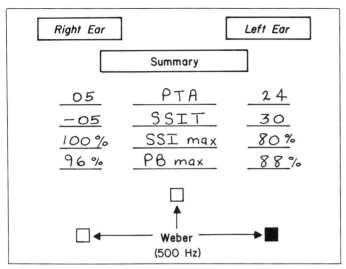

Case 9-1B

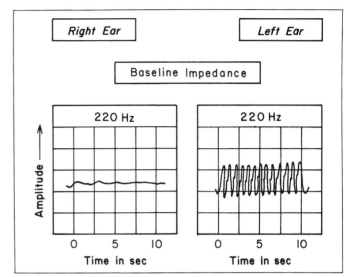

Case 9-1D

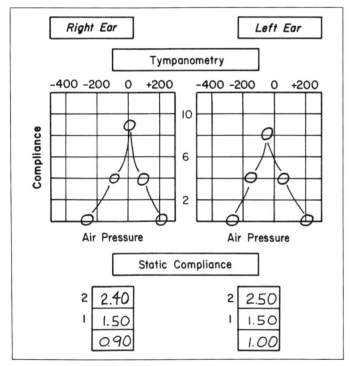

Case 9-1C

baseline impedance recordings at atmospheric pressure on both ears during a 10-sec test interval. Notice the difference between baseline measures on the right and left ears. With probe to the right ear, the baseline is relatively flat with minimal random fluctuations. With probe to the left ear, however, strong periodic pulsations are superimposed upon the baseline measure. The pulsation rate is 78 pulses per minute. The rhythmic fluctuations are synchronous with the patient's heartbeat (radial pulse).

7. Remember, in glomus jugulare tumors, the pulsations are reflecting the unusual vascularity of the tumor mass. The pulsations may be decreased or increased by partially occluding, on the affected side, the carotid artery (to decrease) or the venous outflow of the internal jugular vein (to increase).

With an application of +200 mm H_2O, the pulsations were damped.[7]

Impression

RIGHT EAR: Normal.

LEFT EAR: Mild conductive loss. Impedance audiometry is characterized by a type A tympanogram, normal static compliance measure, and a periodic pulsating resting impedance at a rate of 78 pulses per minute.

CASE 2. A 50-YEAR-OLD FEMALE WITH A GLOMUS JUGULARE TUMOR AFFECTING THE LEFT EAR.

Radiographic and Biopsy Findings

Lumbar pneumoencephalography and left vertebral and left carotid angiography show a highly vascular mass in the region of the left jugular bulb and jugular foramen. The neoplasm appears to extend into the left posterior fossa, the left middle ear space, the retronasopharyngeal soft tissue adjacent to the left jugular foramen, and the soft tissue caudal to the base of the skull. Displacement and distortion of the lateral aspect of the fourth ventricle, the caudal aspect of the pons, and the medulla is noted. Plane skull films document bone destruction at the region of the left jugular foramen. Tympanotomy reveals a pulsating red mass occupying the lower half of the middle ear and hypotympanic area. Diagnosis from pathologic report is glomus jugulare tumor. The patient was treated with radiation therapy.

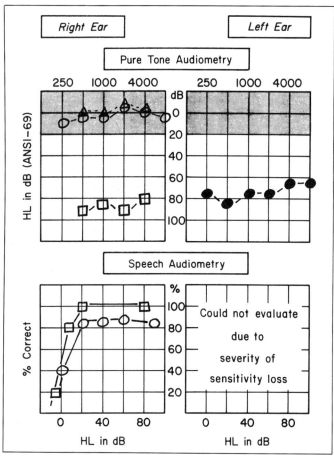

Right Ear | Left Ear

Pure Tone Audiometry

250 1000 4000   250 1000 4000

HL in dB (ANSI-69)

Speech Audiometry

% Correct

Could not evaluate due to severity of sensitivity loss

HL in dB   HL in dB

Case 9-2A

Right Ear | Left Ear

Summary

02	PTA	78
O	SSIT	CNE
05	PBT	CNE
-05	SAT	70
100%	SSI max	CNE
88%	PB max	CNE
I	Bekesy	III

Case 9-2B

History

For the past 10 years the patient has noticed hoarseness and occasional difficulty in swallowing. During the past 5 years she reports a gradually increasing hearing loss on the left ear accompanied by a roaring tinnitus. She has no hearing complaints about her right ear. Physical examination reveals left vocal cord paralysis, reduced hearing in the left ear, decreased sensation in the left cheek, and mild cerebellar ataxia. The Romberg test is negative. No pathologic reflexes are noted. Corneal and forehead sensations are within normal limits. Otorhinolaryngologic examination reveals a mass at the inferior aspect of the left tympanic membrane.

Results

The audiogram (Case 9-2A) shows normal sensitivity on the right ear and a severe sensorineural loss on the left ear. The PTA scores (Case 9-2B) are 2 dB HL on the right ear and 78 dB HL on the left ear. Unmasked

8. Notice that the presence of a middle ear disorder would have been missed in this patient without tympanometry and static compliance measures. More specifically, a conductive component was not observed on conventional bone conduction testing due to the severity of the sensorineural loss. However, tympanometry and static compliance clearly show extreme restriction of middle ear mobility.

bone conduction thresholds (Case 9-2A) on the right ear are superimposed on air conduction thresholds. On the left ear, there is no response to bone conducted signals at the limits of the equipment with masking to the right ear.

PI-SSI and PI-PB functions (Case 9-2A) on the right ear are within normal limits. The SSI max score (Case 9-2B) is 100%; the PB max score is 88%. On the right ear, speech threshold measures agree with average pure tone sensitivity. The SSIT is 0 dB HL; the PBT is 5 dB HL; the SAT is −5 dB HL. On the left ear, SSI and PB speech intelligibility tests could not be administered due to the severity of the pure tone sensitivity loss. However, an SAT of 70 dB HL on the left ear agrees with average pure tone sensitivity.

Impedance audiometry (Case 9-2C) on the right ear shows a normal, type A, tympanogram and normal static compliance. On the left ear, the tympanogram is an unusually shallow, type B, shape and static compliance is reduced below normal limits.[8] Acoustic reflexes (Case 9-2A) with both sound and probe to the right ear (uncrossed condition) are present at normal HLs at all frequencies. With sound to the left ear and probe to the right ear (crossed condition), acoustic reflexes are absent at all frequencies. Acoustic reflexes with probe to the left ear could not be accurately mea-

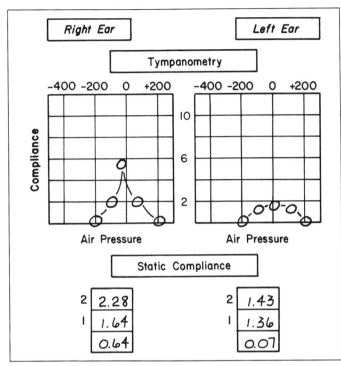

Case 9-2C

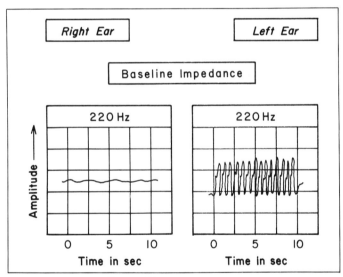

Case 9-2D

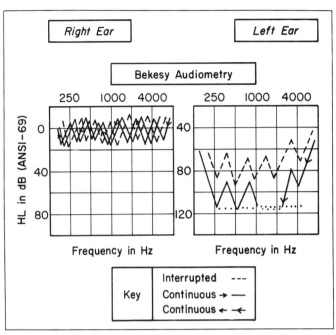

Case 9-2E

sured due to unusual pulsations superimposed on the baseline impedance (Case 9-2D). The rhythmic fluctuations on the left ear are synchronous with the patient's heartbeat (radial pulse) at a rate of 88 beats per minute.

Conventional threshold Bekesy audiometry (Case 9-2E) on the right ear yields a normal, type I, tracing with no forward-backward discrepancy. On the left ear, the Bekesy audiogram is a type III pattern with a

9. Notice the valuable contribution to diagnostic audiometry that conventional Bekesy audiometry provides in this patient. Without threshold Bekesy results, the possibility of eighth nerve site is unusually difficult to evaluate in this patient due to the severity of the pure tone sensitivity loss. For example, threshold HLs on the left ear preclude the administration of some test procedures, i.e., speech audiometry (Case 9-2A); and limit the interpretation of test results, i.e., absent ABR response or absent acoustic reflexes with sound to the left ear (Case 9-2A). In contrast, the administration and interpretation of conventional Bekesy audiometry is not adversely influenced by pure tone sensitivity levels.

significant difference between continuous forward vs backward tracings.[9]

Impression

RIGHT EAR: Normal pure tone sensitivity.

LEFT EAR: Severe sensorineural loss. Impedance audiometry is consistent with a middle ear disorder characterized by a flat, type B, tympanogram, reduced static compliance, and a periodic pulsating resting impedance at a rate of 88 beats per minute. Administration of diagnostic test procedures for site of disorder is limited by the severity of the pure tone sensitivity loss. However, results of conventional Bekesy audiometry are consistent with the presence of eighth nerve disorder. A type III Bekesy audiogram with significant discrepancy between continuous forward vs backward tracings was observed.

SELECTED READINGS

Alford, B., and Guilford, F. A comprehensive study of tumors of the glomus jugulare. *Laryngoscope* 72:765, 1962.

Balkany, T. Pulsatile impedance tympanometry. *Impedance Newsletters* 4:25, 1975.

Ballenger, J. J. *Diseases of the Nose, Throat, and Ear.* Philadelphia: Lea & Febiger, 1977. Pp. 791–805.

Bratt, G., Bess, F., Miller, G., and Glasscock, M. Glomus tumor of the middle ear: Origin, symptomatology, and treatment. *J. Speech Hear. Disord.* 44:121, 1979.

Friedmann, I. *Pathology of the Ear.* Oxford: Blackwell, 1974. Pp. 167–182.

Guild, S. The glomus jugulare, a nonchromaffin paraganglioma, in man. *Ann. Otol. Rhinol. Laryngol.* 62:1045, 1953.

Rock, E. The glomus jugulare tumor. *Impedance Newsletters* 3:10, 1974.

Rosenwasser, H. Glomus jugulare tumors. *Arch. Otolaryngol.* 88:29, 1968.

Shapiro, M., and Neues, D. Technique for removal of glomus jugulare tumors. *Arch. Otolaryngol.* 79:219, 1964.

Taylor, D., Alford, B., and Greenberg, D. Metastases of glomus jugulare tumors. *Arch. Otolaryngol.* 82:5, 1965.

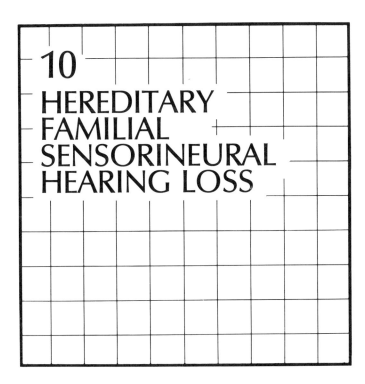

10

HEREDITARY FAMILIAL SENSORINEURAL HEARING LOSS

DESCRIPTION

Hereditary hearing loss may occur when one gene or a pair of genes is abnormal for hearing. If one abnormal gene is sufficient to produce a hearing defect, the hereditary loss is termed a *dominant* trait. If a pair of abnormal genes (one from each parent) is necessary to produce the disorder, the hereditary defect is termed a *recessive* trait.

In dominantly transmitted hereditary hearing loss, one parent is affected (hearing impaired) and passes the abnormality to about one-half of his children. In recessively transmitted loss, both parents are usually unaffected (normal hearing) carriers and pass the hearing defect to approximately one-fourth of their children. On occasion, the abnormal gene may be located on the X (sex) chromosome. This condition is termed a *sex-linked* (X-linked) hereditary characteristic. X-linked traits may be dominant or recessive.[1]

Classification of hereditary sensorineural hearing loss is based on either etiologic, genetic, or histopathologic features. Presently, there is no clinical pattern that consistently identifies the different types of hereditary sensorineural hearing disorders (Ibrahim and Linthicum, 1979). Temporal bone studies in patients with inherited sensorineural hearing loss may show absence of the organ of Corti in the basal turn, spiral ganglion degeneration of the basal turn, and irregular degeneration of the stria vascularis (Paparella and Capps, 1973).

PATIENT CHARACTERISTICS

Hereditary sensorineural hearing loss usually becomes manifest during childhood or early adulthood (Paparella and Capps, 1973). However, the onset of hearing loss may occur at any age. A sex ratio for hereditary familial sensorineural hearing loss is unavailable. In children, however, hearing disorders due to genetic or environmental factors are more prevalent in males than in females. The male-to-female ratio is about 1.2 : 1 (Schein, 1979).

Genetic differences between the sexes provide the basis for two striking characteristics of X-linked hearing disorders. First, a cardinal feature of X-linked traits is a lack of father-to-son transmission, since sons receive only Y chromosomes from the father. Second, females with an abnormal gene for hearing loss on the X chromosome may not manifest any abnormality. Instead, a female may be an asymptomatic, normal hearing, carrier of the disorder. In contrast, unaffected carrier males do not exist. Males with an abnormal gene on the X chromosome always manifest a hearing loss. Theoretically, females may be unaffected due to the presence of a normal gene on the additional X chromosome. Males are consistently affected due to the presence of a single, abnormal X chromosome that is genetically unopposed.[2] Hereditary sensorineural hearing loss is characteristically bilateral.[3]

CLINICAL COURSE

Hereditary sensorineural hearing loss may be present at birth or of delayed onset. If the hearing loss is congenital, the degree of loss is usually stable. If, however, the hearing loss develops subsequent to birth, the degree of loss may progress in severity over time. In persons with delayed hereditary sensorineural hearing disorders, the onset of loss is characteristically insidious. The observation of unstable pure tone sensitivity in some patients stresses the importance of serial audiometric evaluations of all individuals with hereditary sensorineural hearing loss.

1. Hereditary hearing loss occurs in about 1 per 2000 to 1 per 6000 live births (Proctor and Proctor, 1967). In consanguineous marriages, the prevalence of hereditary hearing loss is increased.

Of hereditary hearing loss with no associated abnormalities, about 80% to 90% is through recessive transmission and about 10% to 20% occurs through dominant transmission of the trait. Of recessive type inherited hearing loss, about 6% of persons show X-linked defects (Schein and Delk, 1974, cited in Catlin, 1978).

In the United States, the prevalence of childhood hearing disorders due to genetic or environmental factors is higher in the West and the South than in the north central and northeastern states (Schein, 1979).

2. Normal hearing carriers of genes for deafness may exhibit subtle audiologic abnormalities, such as peculiar "dips" on sweep frequency Bekesy audiometry and elevated acoustic reflex thresholds at isolated frequencies (Anderson and Wedenberg, 1976; Parving, 1978).

3. In a series of schoolchildren with unilateral hearing loss, the loss was attributable to hereditary factors in only 10% of persons (Everberg, 1960).

Hereditary hearing loss occurs in isolation with no associated abnormalities in about two-thirds of individuals. In the remaining one-third of patients, the loss is part of an identifiable syndrome of abnormalities (Paparella and Capps, 1973).

The management of persons with hereditary sensorineural hearing loss usually involves medical, educational, and counseling specialties. In particular, genetic counseling of high-risk individuals is considered a primary avenue toward the control and/or prevention of hereditary abnormalities. The treatment of persons with hereditary sensorineural hearing loss generally involves amplification.

SITE OF DISORDER

Cochlea.[4]

GENERAL AUDIOLOGIC PATTERN

Pure tone sensitivity results characteristically show a bilateral sensorineural loss. The hearing loss is generally symmetric on the two ears. On rare occasions, a unilateral loss may be observed. The degree of loss varies from mild to severe impairment. The audiometric contour may be sloping, flat, rising, or basin-shaped. In persons with an unstable loss that progresses in severity over time, the audiometric contour may also change over time. For example, the loss may be initially restricted to a narrow range of frequencies and may progress to involve all frequencies.

Maximum speech intelligibility scores are usually consistent with the degree of sensitivity loss. The shape of the PI function is usually normal.

Impedance results characteristically show normal, type A, tympanograms and normal static compliance measures. Acoustic reflexes are generally present at normal HLs and reduced sensation levels. In patients with severe hearing loss, reflex thresholds cannot be measured because signals cannot be presented at sufficiently high intensity levels.

Illustrative Patients

In general, patients with sensorineural hearing loss attributable to hereditary factors are difficult to isolate. A major difficulty involves the many other possible causes of hearing loss that cannot always be adequately ruled out. In the following patients, a clinical diagnosis of hereditary familial sensorineural hearing loss was based on (1) a careful history of the problem in relation to its occurrence in other members of the family, and (2) a careful ruling out of other possible etiologies. No cause other than heredity could be found in any person.

CASE 1. A 41-YEAR-OLD FEMALE WITH HEREDITARY SENSORINEURAL HEARING LOSS ON BOTH EARS.

History

The patient's chief complaint is hearing loss in both ears. She has noticed hearing problems for "as long as I can remember." She has a mother, an aunt, and a cousin with hearing loss.

Physical examination and otorhinolaryngologic examination are within normal limits except for a hearing loss on both ears. The patient denies any previous serious illnesses, accidents, exposure to loud noises, atypical or unusual drug use, and head trauma. This is the patient's first audiologic evaluation. She is interested in obtaining a hearing aid.

Results

The audiogram (Case 10-1A) shows a moderate sensorineural hearing loss on both ears. The PTA scores (Case 10-1B) are 52 dB HL on the right ear and 48 dB HL on the left ear. Unmasked bone conduction thresholds (Case 10-1A) are superimposed on air conduction thresholds bilaterally.

Speech audiometry (Case 10-1A) shows reduced maximum intelligibility scores for both word and sentence materials. PB max scores (Case 10-1B) are 56% on the right ear and 76% on the left ear. SSI max scores are 50% on the right ear and 60% on the left ear. No rollover is observed on either ear.

Speech thresholds on both ears agree with average pure tone sensitivity. On the right ear, the PBT is 55 dB HL; the SSIT is 60 dB HL. On the left ear, the PBT is 50 dB HL; the SSIT is 55 dB HL.[5]

Impedance audiometry (Case 10-1C) shows type A tympanograms on both ears. Static compliance measures are within normal limits bilaterally. Crossed and uncrossed acoustic reflexes (Case 10-1A) are

4. In addition to hereditary familial sensorineural hearing loss, other types of hereditary hearing loss occur and may be associated with other sites within the auditory system. See Chapter 1, Acoustic Schwannoma (von Recklinghausen's disease); Chapter 5, Diabetes Mellitus; Chapter 18, Otosclerosis; and Chapter 20, Paget's Disease.

5. Notice that the PB max score in the right ear is 20% poorer than PB max performance in the left ear. In view of the relatively symmetric pure tone sensitivity on both ears, asymmetric PB max performance is unusual.

Remember, if

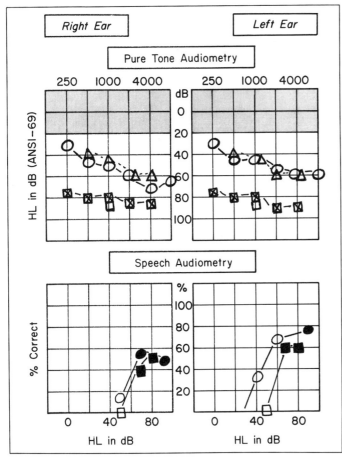

Case 10-1A

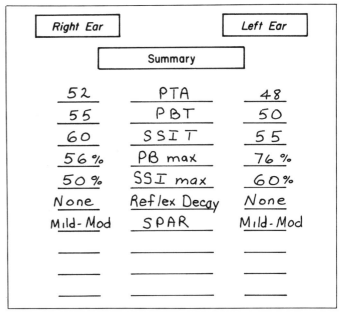

Case 10-1B

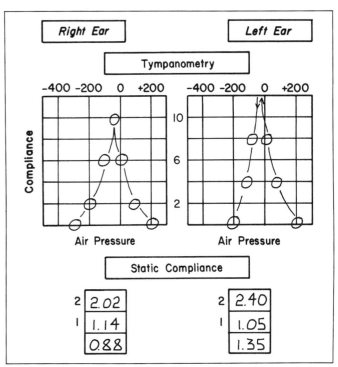

Case 10-1C

maximum speech intelligibility performance is at or near the 50% intelligibility level, speech thresholds are determined on a steeper part of the function. For example, in the left ear, the PBT was determined from the 50% intelligibility level, but the SSIT was based on the 25% intelligibility score.

present at normal HLs and reduced sensation levels at all frequencies. No reflex decay (Case 10-1B) at 500 Hz or 1000 Hz is observed on either ear. The SPAR measure predicts a mild to moderate sensitivity loss on both ears.

Impression

Moderate sensorineural hearing loss on both ears. Impedance audiometry is consistent with normal middle ear function on the right ear and essentially normal, although unusually compliant, middle ear function on the left ear.

Recommendations

1. Hearing aid evaluation pending otologic consultation.
2. Monitoring of pure tone sensitivity at regular intervals.

Comment

The above patient has been married three times. She has 11 children. Of the 11 children, 9 have a hearing loss. The following

audiograms present results on three of the children: one from the first husband, one from the second husband, and one from the third husband.

CASES 2, 3, AND 4. A 13-YEAR-OLD FEMALE, A 12-YEAR-OLD FEMALE, AND A 7-YEAR-OLD MALE WITH BILATERAL HEREDITARY SENSORINEURAL HEARING LOSS.

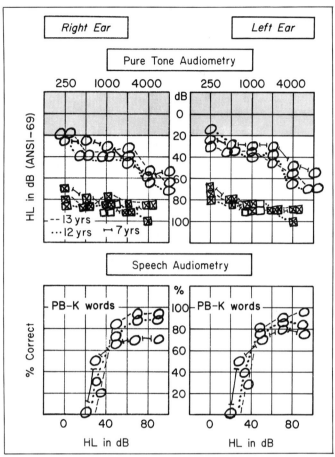

Case 10-2A

History

All three children became aware of a hearing loss after failing a hearing screening test at school. The children primarily notice trouble hearing at school. They do not notice hearing difficulties at home. The 13-year-old wears a hearing aid during school hours. She has worn the aid for 4 years.

The children do not remember any serious illnesses, noise exposure, atypical or unusual drug use, or head trauma. Physical examination and otorhinolaryngologic examination are within normal limits except for decreased hearing on both ears of all three individuals.

Results

6. Notice the marked similarity of the audiograms in the children (Case 10-2A) and the mother (Case 10-1A). Similar audiometric contours are a primary feature

Case 10-2A shows audiometric results for the three children. The audiogram shows a mild to moderate sensorineural loss on both ears of all children. The PTA scores (not shown) range from 33 to 40 dB HL on the right ear and from 30 to 38 dB HL on the left ear.[6]

of some types of hereditary sensorineural hearing loss (Konigsmark and Gorlin, 1976).

Notice the slight increase in the degree of loss as age increases from 7 years (a PTA of about 30 dB, Case 10-2A) to 41 years (a PTA of about 50 dB, Case 10-1A). Remember, hereditary sensorineural hearing loss may progress in severity over time in many individuals (Konigsmark, 1972).

Speech audiometry (Case 10-2A) shows slightly more variability among the three children than pure tone sensitivity results. PB-K max scores range from 72% to 96% on the right ear and from 80% to 96% on the left ear. The shape of the PI function is normal in all three children. Speech thresholds agree with pure tone sensitivity results on both ears of all children. The PBT scores range from 30 dB to 40 dB HL on each ear.

Tympanometry and static compliance measures (not shown) are normal on both ears of all three children. Crossed and uncrossed acoustic reflexes (Case 10-2A) are present at normal HLs and reduced sensation levels at all frequencies.

Impression

Mild to moderate sensorineural hearing loss on both ears of each child. Impedance audiometry is consistent with normal middle ear function.

Recommendations

1. Hearing aid evaluation pending otologic consultation.
2. Monitoring of pure tone sensitivity at regular intervals, preferably by the public school audiologist.
3. Preferential classroom seating.

Comment

The above patients illustrate a critical feature of hereditary familial sensorineural hearing loss. A hearing loss may occur at a very young age. In this circumstance, the audiologist's role must shift toward the considerations and implications of hearing loss in children. Social, emotional, and educational issues become vital concerns. This particular situation requires close cooperation between the audiologist, otologist, educator, and educational psychologist/ counselor.

SELECTED READINGS

Anderson, H., and Wedenberg, E. Identification of normal hearing carriers of genes for deafness. *Acta Otolaryngol.* 82:245, 1976.

Catlin, F. Etiology and Pathology of Hearing Loss in Children. In F. Martin (ed.), *Pediatric Audiology.* Englewood Cliffs, N.J.: Prentice-Hall, 1978. Pp. 3–34.

Everberg, G. Further studies on hereditary unilateral deafness. *Acta Otolaryngol.* 51:615, 1960.

Gacek, R. The pathology of hereditary sensori-neural hearing loss. *Ann. Otol. Rhinol. Laryngol.* 80:289, 1971.

Ibrahim, R., and Linthicum, F. Clinical records. Hereditary deafness in children. Diagnosis and a family report. *J. Laryngol. Otol.* 93:495, 1979.

Konigsmark, B. Genetic hearing loss with no associated abnormalities: A review. *J. Speech Hear. Disord.* 37:89, 1972.

Konigsmark, B., and Gorlin, R. *Genetic and Metabolic Deafness.* Philadelphia: Saunders, 1976. Pp. 1–44.

Paparella, M., and Capps, M. Sensori-neural Deafness in Children—Genetic. In M. Paparella and D. Shumrick (eds.), *Otolaryngology* (vol. 2). Philadelphia: Saunders, 1973. Pp. 320–337.

Parving, A. Reliability of Bekesy threshold tracing in identification of carriers of genes for an X-linked disease with deafness. *Acta Otolaryngol.* 85:40, 1978.

Proctor, C. Diagnosis, prevention, and treatment of hereditary sensori-neural hearing loss. *Laryngoscope* Suppl. 7:1, 1977.

Proctor, C., and Proctor, B. Understanding hereditary nerve deafness. *Arch. Otolaryngol.* 85:45, 1967.

Ruben, R., and Rozycki, D. Clinical aspects of genetic deafness. *Ann. Otol. Rhinol. Laryngol.* 80:255, 1971.

Schein, J. Symposium on environmental and genetic hearing loss: Epidemiology of childhood hearing loss. *Hearing Aid J.* 32:8, 1979.

Schuknecht, H. Pathology of Sensori-neural Deafness of Genetic Origin. In F. McConnell and P. Ward (eds.), *Deafness in Childhood.* Nashville: Vanderbilt University Press, 1967. Pp. 69–90.

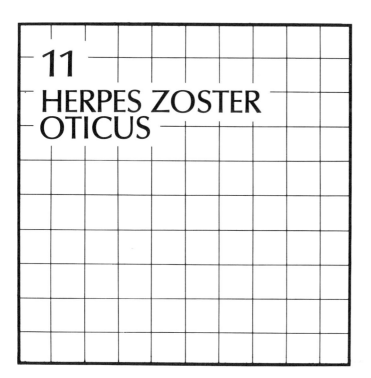

11

HERPES ZOSTER OTICUS

DESCRIPTION

Herpes zoster oticus is a temporary inflammatory viral infection that is usually characterized by herpetic eruptions on the skin. The skin rash typically occurs within the external auditory canal and/or portions of the auricle. On occasion, however, the skin lesions may appear on other areas of the head, such as the face, mouth, throat, and palate. Otalgia, hearing loss, or facial paralysis may precede or follow the eruption of the rash.

In a 69-year-old woman with herpes zoster oticus (Friedmann, 1974), histologic temporal bone studies showed extensive round cell infiltration of the seventh nerve, the eighth nerve, the cochlea, and the mastoid process. The organ of Corti near the apical turn appeared destroyed.[1]

PATIENT CHARACTERISTICS

Herpes zoster usually occurs in persons over 45 years of age; the disease is more common in males than in females (Adams et al., 1978). The hearing loss and accompanying symptoms are characteristically unilateral. Many affected persons report a previous history of chickenpox.[2]

CLINICAL COURSE

Unstable, unilateral sensorineural hearing loss. The onset of the hearing loss may be

1. Herpes zoster oticus may be called *Ramsay Hunt syndrome.*

The prevalence of herpes zoster oticus is not reported.

In patients with neoplasms (particularly lymphomas such as Hodgkin's disease), the prevalence of herpes zoster is increased.

Of patients with facial paralysis, 2% to 7% have herpes zoster oticus.

2. Chickenpox and herpes zoster may be different manifestations of infection with a common viral agent. In fact, patients with herpes zoster may be the source of an outbreak of chickenpox among susceptible contacts, such as children (Ribble, 1974).

3. Factors favorable for recovery of auditory function include mild initial hearing loss, cochlear site of disorder, absence of vertigo, and age of less than 65 years (Byl and Adour, 1977).

relatively sudden. The hearing loss may be accompanied by complaints of tinnitus, nausea, vomiting, facial paralysis, and dizziness. Cranial nerves five through twelve may be affected. As the herpes zoster infection subsides, recovery of the hearing loss may occur.[3]

SITE OF DISORDER

Cochlea and/or eighth nerve.

GENERAL AUDIOLOGIC PATTERN

Pure tone sensitivity results characteristically show unilateral sensorineural hearing loss. The initial degree of loss may vary from mild to profound impairment. The audiometric configuration usually shows greater loss in the high frequency region than in the low and mid frequency regions.

As the herpes zoster infection diminishes, the hearing loss may show complete recovery. However, individuals with an initially severe degree of sensitivity loss rarely recover to within normal limits. Further, in spite of substantial improvement in hearing sensitivity, a high frequency sensorineural loss may persist in some patients, particularly elderly individuals.

Maximum speech intelligibility scores vary depending upon the severity and site of the sensorineural disorder. In patients with cochlear site, maximum speech intelligibility performance is usually consistent with the degree of sensitivity loss. An exception to this observation, however, is patients with mild to moderate cochlear sensitivity loss and completely normal speech intelligibility scores. In patients with eighth nerve site, maximum speech intelligibility scores may be proportionate or disproportionate to the degree of pure tone sensitivity loss. However, in patients with eighth nerve disorder, the PI function for speech materials generally shows abnormal rollover.

Impedance results characteristically show normal, type A, tympanograms and normal static compliance measures. Acoustic reflex results vary, however, depending on the degree of sensitivity loss and the site of disorder. The possible sites of disorder affecting acoustic reflex results are the cochlea, the eighth nerve, and/or the seventh nerve. As a general rule, in patients with cochlear disorder, reflexes are present at normal HLs and

4. In a series of 172 patients with facial paralysis and herpes zoster oticus, 37% reported tinnitus, hearing loss, and/or increased sensitivity to loud sounds on the involved side (Byl and Adour, 1977).

For a discussion of audiologic findings in persons with facial paralysis, see Chapter 7, Facial Nerve Disorders.

reduced sensation levels for all frequencies. In patients with eighth nerve disorder, however, reflexes are usually absent for both crossed and uncrossed conditions with sound to the affected ear. The reflex abnormality in individuals with eighth nerve site yields a diagonal reflex pattern. In patients with seventh nerve disorder, reflexes are usually absent for both crossed and uncrossed conditions with probe to the affected side. The reflex pattern in patients with seventh nerve abnormality is characterized by a vertical configuration.[4]

If the PI function for speech materials shows substantial rollover and/or acoustic reflexes show the diagonal reflex pattern in the absence of severe pure tone sensitivity loss, further tests to evaluate the possibility of eighth nerve disorder are indicated. Appropriate tests may include Bekesy and BCL audiometry, STAT, TDT, and ABR testing.

Illustrative Patients

CASE 1. AN 18-YEAR-OLD FEMALE WITH HERPES ZOSTER OTICUS ON THE LEFT SIDE.

History

About 5 days ago the patient began to experience double vision, dizziness, and nausea. At approximately the same time, she noticed tinnitus, hearing loss, and severe pain in the left ear. Subsequently, a skin rash appeared on the concha of the left auricle. She denies noticing any facial weakness. She does not have any hearing complaints about her right ear.

Neurologic examination indicates involvement of cranial nerves six and eight on the left side. There is no evidence of seventh nerve disorder, however. Skull x-rays and computerized axial tomographic (CT) scanning are within normal limits. Otorhinolaryngologic examination reveals a slightly injected left tympanic membrane. The walls of the external auditory canal appear edematous with desquamation of canal wall skin and tympanic membrane. On the pinna, a hemorrhagic-appearing area is noted on the concha. However, no herpetic eruptions are seen. There is no otoscopic indication of middle ear infection.

Results

The audiogram (Case 11-1A) shows normal pure tone sensitivity on the right ear and a

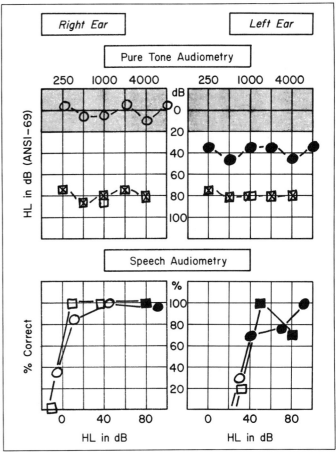

Case 11-1A

5. On the left ear, notice the relatively normal speech intelligibility performance in the presence of a 40 dB sensorineural loss (see General Audiologic Pattern, p. 71).

6. The PI-SSI function is more sensitive to the presence of retrocochlear disorder than the PI-PB function (Jerger and Hayes, 1977; e.g., see patient 1, Chapter 2, Cerebrovascular Disorders). The price one pays for this increased sensitivity to retrocochlear site, however, is a higher false alarm rate in normal and cochlear ears. As a consequence, the presence of SSI rollover coupled with

mild sensorineural loss on the left ear. The PTA scores (Case 11-1B) are 0 dB HL on the right ear and 40 dB HL on the left ear. The Weber test (Case 11-1B) at 500 Hz is referred to the right ear.

PI-PB and PI-SSI functions (Case 11-1A) on both ears show normal maximum intelligibility scores of 100% correct.[5] On the left ear, however, the PI-SSI function shows a rollover effect of 30%.[6]

Speech thresholds (Case 11-1B) on each ear agree with average pure tone sensitivity. On the right ear, the PBT is 0 dB HL; the SSIT is −2 dB HL. On the left ear, the PBT is 36 dB HL; the SSIT is 39 dB HL.

Impedance audiometry (Case 11-1C) shows normal, type A, tympanograms and normal static compliance measures bilaterally. Crossed and uncrossed acoustic reflexes (Case 11-1A) on both ears are present at normal HLs at all frequencies. Reflex decay testing at 1000 Hz (Case 11-1B) is normal on both ears. Results do not show any decline in reflex amplitude during a

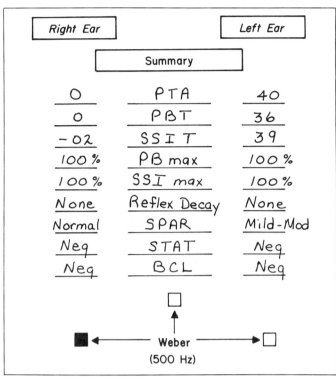

Right Ear		Left Ear
	Summary	
0	P T A	40
0	P B T	36
- 02	S S I T	39
100 %	P B max	100 %
100 %	S S I max	100 %
None	Reflex Decay	None
Normal	S P A R	Mild-Mod
Neg	S T A T	Neg
Neg	B C L	Neg

Weber
(500 Hz)

Case 11-1B

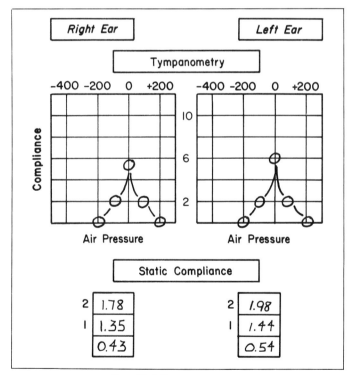

Case 11-1C

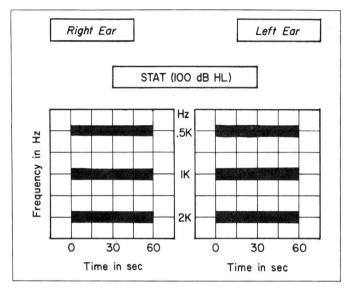

Case 11-1D

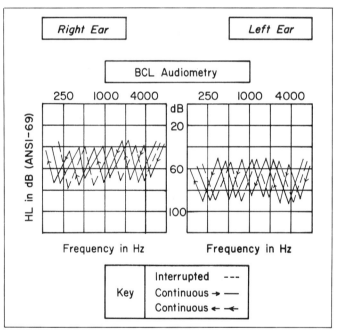

Case 11-1E

the absence of PB rollover is not interpreted as a strong indication of retrocochlear site, but is interpreted much more cautiously (see patient 1, Chapter 8, Functional Hearing Disorders).

7. Notice that bone conduction testing is unnecessary in this patient. Remember

10-sec test period. The SPAR measure predicts normal pure tone sensitivity on the right ear and a mild-to-moderate sensitivity loss on the left ear.[7]

The STAT (Case 11-1D) does not show abnormal adaptation at any frequency on either ear. BCL audiometry (Case 11-1E) yields negative results on the right and left ears. The tracings for interrupted, continuous-forward, and continuous-backward pure tone signals are superimposed on both ears.

the working rule: If all three impedance measures are normal, the loss is sensorineural.

Impression

RIGHT EAR: Normal.

LEFT EAR: Mild sensorineural loss. Diagnostic test results are consistent with cochlear site. Acoustic reflexes are present at normal HLs and reduced sensation levels at all frequencies. There is no evidence of eighth nerve disorder on reflex decay testing, STAT, or BCL audiometry.

Audiologic Reevaluation

Approximately 1 month after dismissal from the hospital, the patient returned for audiologic reevaluation. She reports that her hearing in the left ear has returned to normal. Otorhinolaryngologic examination at this date is within normal limits. Neurologic testing is consistently normal.

Results

The audiogram (Case 11-1F) shows normal pure tone sensitivity on the right ear and a mild sensorineural loss on the left ear. The PTA scores (Case 11-1G) are 1 dB HL on the right ear and 12 dB HL on the left ear. Speech audiometry (Case 11-1F) shows maximum intelligibility scores of 100% for both PB and SSI materials on the right and left ears. On the right ear, however, the PI-SSI function shows mild rollover. The SSIT (Case 11-1G) measures on both ears agree with pure tone sensitivity results. The SSIT scores are −2 dB HL on the right ear and 6 dB HL on the left ear.

Tympanometry, static compliance, and acoustic reflex (Case 11-1F) results are the same as those previously obtained (Cases 11-1A and 11-1C).

Impression

Pure tone sensitivity on the left ear has improved approximately 30 dB since results of approximately 1 month ago. Maximum speech intelligibility scores and impedance audiometry remain within normal limits.

CASE 2. A 26-YEAR-OLD MALE WITH HERPES ZOSTER OTICUS ON THE RIGHT SIDE.

History

The patient reports pain in the right ear for the past 6 days. One day after the pain started, he began to experience unsteadiness and a high-pitched ringing sound, a feeling of pressure, and "muffled" hearing in the

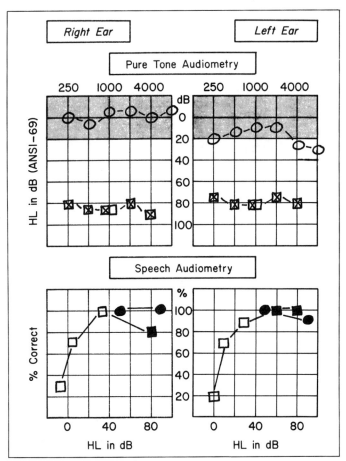

Case 11-1F

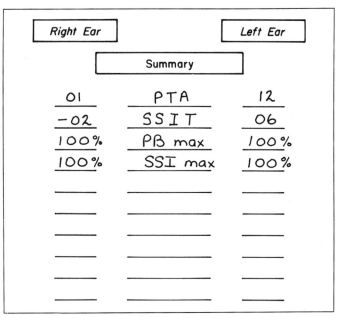

Case 11-1G

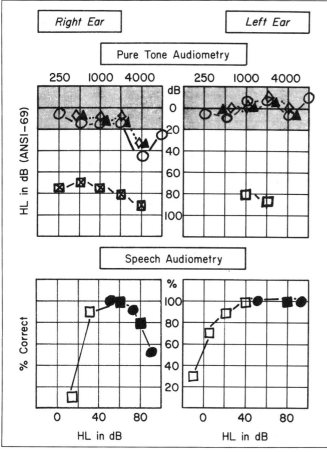

Case 11-2A

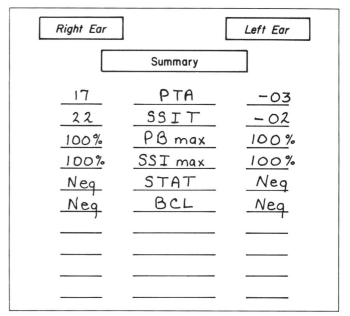

Case 11-2B

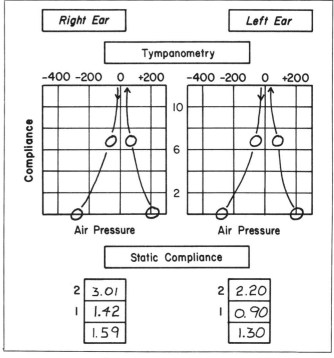

Case 11-2C

8. Notice that pure tone thresholds at 250 Hz through 2000 Hz on the right ear are within the lower limits of the normal range. However, in this patient, a more sensitive interpretation of threshold measures may be gained by comparing results on the right ear to thresholds on the

right ear. Three days ago the right side of his face became weak. He cannot close his right eye.

Physical examination is within normal limits except for right facial paralysis. Results of facial nerve studies are consistent with right neuropraxia. Skull x-rays and computerized axial tomographic (CT) scanning are normal. Otorhinolaryngologic examination reveals a scabbing lesion in the right inferior concha, just above the earlobe. The right tympanic membrane appears injected superiorly. The patient's neck shows an enlarged node inferior to the right ear, just behind the angle of the mandible.

Results

The audiogram (Case 11-2A) shows a mild sensorineural loss on the right ear and normal pure tone sensitivity on the left ear. The PTA scores (Case 11-2B) are 17 dB HL on the right ear and −3 dB HL on the left ear.[8] Bone conduction testing and SAL audi-

left, normal, ear. In comparison to thresholds on the normal control ear, pure tone sensitivity results on the right ear represent a sensorineural loss of about 20 dB.

9. Recall that rollover of the PI func-

ometry (Case 11-2A) do not show a conductive component on either ear.

Speech audiometry (Case 11-2A) shows maximum intelligibility scores of 100% for both PB and SSI materials on the right and left ears. On the right ear, however, the PI-PB and PI-SSI functions show rollover.[9] SSIT measures (Case 11-2B) agree with average pure tone sensitivity bilaterally. The

76

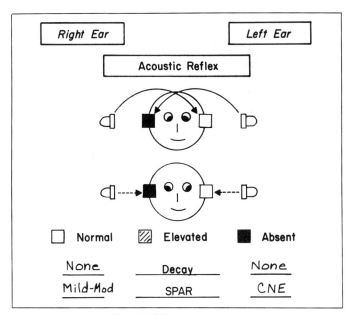

Case 11-2D

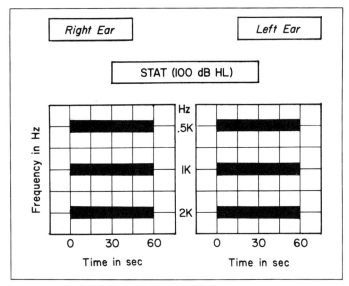

Case 11-2E

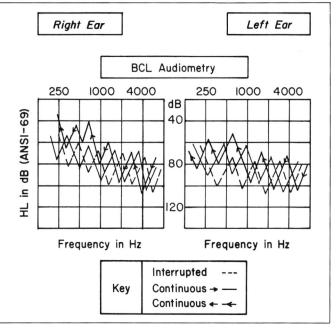

Case 11-2F

tion may occur in patients with seventh nerve disorder. Abnormal performance at high intensity levels may be related to the observation that the acoustic reflex, when normal, extends the dynamic range of the ear about 20 dB (Borg and Zakrisson, 1973).

10. The presence of an abnormally deep type A tympanogram without a concomitant air-bone gap (Case 11-2A) is consistent with unusual tympanic membrane compliance, rather than ossicular chain discontinuity (see comments on patient 1, Chapter 7, Facial Nerve Disorders).

SSIT is 22 dB HL on the right ear and −2 dB HL on the left ear.

Impedance audiometry (Case 11-2C) shows type A_D tympanograms and normal static compliance measures on both ears.[10] Crossed acoustic reflexes (Case 11-2A) on the right ear are present at normal HLs at all frequencies. However, uncrossed reflexes on the right ear could not be elicited at equipment limits. With sound to the left ear, crossed reflexes are absent at all frequencies. Uncrossed reflex thresholds at 1000 and 2000 Hz on the left ear, however, are within normal limits. The reflex pattern at 1000 Hz (Case 11-2D) is characterized by a vertical configuration. Reflex thresholds are normal with probe to the left ear and abnormal with probe to the right ear. The vertical pattern is consistent with a seventh nerve disorder on the right side. Reflex decay testing at 1000 Hz was measured in the crossed condition on the right ear and in the uncrossed condition on the left ear. Results did not show any decline in reflex amplitude during the 10-sec test period on either ear. The SPAR measure on the right ear predicts mild to moderate sensitivity loss. SPAR results on the left ear could not be obtained.

The STAT (Case 11-2E) does not show abnormal adaptation at any frequency on either ear. BCL audiometry (Case 11-2F) is negative on the right and left ears. ABR audiometry (not shown) shows normal abso-

lute and interwave latencies of all components on both ears.

Impression

RIGHT EAR: Mild sensorineural loss. Diagnostic test results are most consistent with a cochlear site. Crossed acoustic reflexes are present at normal HLs at all frequencies. ABR latency measures are within normal limits. There is no evidence of eighth nerve disorder on reflex decay testing, STAT, or BCL audiometry. Impedance audiometry is consistent with an essentially normal, although unusually compliant, middle ear system and a facial nerve disorder proximal to the innervation of the stapedial muscle.

LEFT EAR: Normal.

SELECTED READINGS

Adams, G., Boies, L., and Paparella, M. *Boies' Fundamentals of Otolaryngology* (5th ed.). Philadelphia: Saunders, 1978. Pp. 478–479.

Borg, E., and Zakrisson, J. Stapedius reflex and speech features. *J. Acoust. Soc. Am.* 54:525, 1973.

Byl, F., and Adour, K. Auditory symptoms associated with herpes zoster oticus or idiopathic facial paralysis. *Laryngoscope* 87:372, 1977.

Friedmann, I. *Pathology of the Ear.* Oxford: Blackwell, 1974. Pp. 442–448.

Harbert, F., and Young, I. Audiologic findings in Ramsay Hunt syndrome. *Arch. Otolaryngol.* 85:632, 1967.

Hunt, J. R. The symptom-complex of the acute posterior poliomyelitis of the geniculate, auditory, glossopharyngeal and pneumogastric ganglia. *Arch. Intern. Med.* 5:631, 1910.

Jerger, J., and Hayes, D. Diagnostic speech audiometry. *Arch. Otolaryngol.* 85:632, 1977.

Ribble, J. Chickenpox (Varicella) and Herpes Zoster. In M. Wintrobe, G. Thorn, R. Adams, E. Braunwald, K. Isselbacher, and R. Petersdorf (eds.), *Harrison's Principles of Internal Medicine* (7th ed.). New York: McGraw-Hill, 1974. Pp. 969–972.

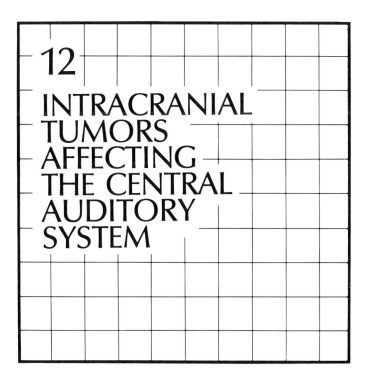

12

INTRACRANIAL TUMORS AFFECTING THE CENTRAL AUDITORY SYSTEM

DESCRIPTION

1. In large series of necropsies, the prevalence of intracranial tumors is about 1% to 2% of individuals.

The annual incidence of cerebral tumors in Rochester, Minnesota, between 1935 and 1968 was 12.6 per 100,000 inhabitants (Percy et al., 1972).

Cerebral tumors are more common in whites than in blacks (Behrend, 1974).

This chapter focuses on neoplasms affecting the auditory pathways within the brain stem (intraaxial) or at the level of the temporal lobe. For information on auditory findings in patients with neoplasms at other sites within the auditory system, see Chapter 1, Acoustic Schwannoma; Chapter 3, Cholesteatoma; Chapter 7, Facial Nerve Disorders (patient 3); and Chapter 9, Glomus Jugulare Tumors.

Intracranial tumors may arise from the skull, the meninges, the blood vessels, the choroid plexus, the pituitary gland, the pineal body, the cranial nerves, and the neurons and neuroglia of the brain (Northfield, 1973). Neoplasms appear to develop from alterations of normal cells with subsequent uncontrolled growth (Slager, 1970). The pathologic mechanisms producing neoplastic growth are not clearly defined.[1]

The classification of intracranial tumors may be based upon the cell type of the tumor tissue. For example, tumors originating from astrocytic cells may be termed *astrocytomas.* Classification of tumor type may be used for predicting a neoplasm's biologic behavior, growth pattern, response to therapy, and the patient's prognosis. Intracranial tumors may also be classified depending on whether they are situated above or below the tentorium. The former are called *supratentorial;* the latter are called *infratentorial.* Infratentorial tumors are also called *posterior fossa tumors.*

The signs and symptoms of intracranial neoplasms may arise from cellular invasion and destruction, increased intracranial pressure, interference with the blood supply to an area, edema, obstruction of cerebrospinal fluid, and displacement or compression of brain tissue.

2. In contrast to a variable sex ratio for all brain tumors in general, certain types of brain tumors appear to show a unique sex and age predilection (Slager, 1970):

Meningioma
1. More common in females; 2. occurs in middle and later decades of life.

Astrocytoma
1. More common in males; 2. occurs at all ages; incidence decreases after 40 years of age.

Glioblastoma
1. More common in males; 2. peak incidence is around 50 years of age.

Ependymoma
1. More common in males; 2. peak incidence is in children and young adults.

Medulloblastoma
1. More common in males; 2. peak incidence is between 7 and 12 years of age.

Pinealoma
1. More common in males; 2. peak incidence is in second and third decades of life.

3. Remember, although the auditory

PATIENT CHARACTERISTICS

Brain tumors may occur at any age. However, of patients with symptomatic primary brain neoplasms, only about 10% to 20% are less than 17 years old. About 2% are less than 3 years old.

The age prevalence for various types and sites of disorder shows striking differences between children and adults. For example, most intraaxial brain stem tumors occur in childhood or adolescence (Lassman, 1974). In fact, of all brain tumors occurring in children, about 65% are located in the posterior fossa (Green et al., 1976). In contrast, posterior fossa tumors account for no more than about 25% of all brain neoplasms in adults (Koos and Miller, 1971).

In children, about 75% of brain tumors are gliomas (Green et al., 1976). In adults, however, gliomas are much less common than extraaxial neoplasms, such as meningiomas and neuromas (Stein, 1976).

The sex ratio for intracranial tumors is unsettled. Some studies (Zulch, 1965) report that brain tumors are more prevalent in males than in females. The ratio of male to female is approximately 11:9. A male sex predilection may be most pronounced in the first six years of life (Koos and Miller, 1971). In contrast to these studies, other studies (Kurland et al., 1962) report that the prevalence of primary brain tumors is higher in females than in males. Still other, more recent, studies (Behrend, 1974), however, do not show any sex preponderance of primary neoplasms of the central nervous system.[2]

In patients with intracranial tumors affecting the central auditory system, the laterality of the auditory disorder varies depending upon the site of involvement. In patients with temporal lobe site, the auditory disorder is characteristically unilateral. The ear presenting the abnormal symptomatology is generally the ear opposite the affected side of the brain. In contrast to this observation, in patients with brain stem site the auditory disorder is characteristically bilateral. However, in these latter patients, the severity of the auditory abnormality is rarely symmetric. Brain stem tumors generally grow eccentrically larger on one side. The abnormal auditory symptomatology is usually greater on the ear opposite the most severely involved side of the brain stem.[3]

system receives bilateral input at all levels higher than the cochlear nuclei, the crossed ascending auditory pathways are functionally dominant. Consequently, primary auditory deficits are usually observed on the ear opposite the affected side of the brain.

4. Klüver and Bucy (1939) produced bilateral ablations of the temporal lobes in monkeys and observed abnormal behavior in four areas (the 4 Fs syndrome): fighting, feeding, fearing, and fornicating. Remember, temporal lobe structures associated with the limbic system are thought to play a part in a person's emotional responses, instinctual activities, and visceral reactions (Strobos, 1974).

CLINICAL COURSE

Clinical manifestations of intracranial tumors vary depending on the site of the tumor and its histologic nature. Some neoplasms grow slowly and may cause very few symptoms over a period of many years. Other neoplasms grow rapidly and may cause death within a few months.

In addition to different growth patterns, clinical symptoms may vary depending on whether the neoplasm occurs in a "silent" or "vocal" part of the brain. For example, in patients with temporal lobe tumors, a paucity of symptoms may be observed even in tumors of considerable size. In contrast, in patients with intraaxial brain stem tumors, clinical symptoms are typically pronounced. The brain stem is densely packed with important nuclei and neuronal pathways. Considerable neurologic abnormalities may be observed even in tumors of unusually small size.

Children may have fewer clinical symptoms than adults. A difference between children and adults may be related to the increased elasticity of a child's skull, the ability of the immature brain to compensate for functional impairment, and a child's limited ability to verbalize subtle symptomatology.

In patients with either temporal lobe or brain stem site, subjective auditory complaints are rare. In patients with temporal lobe site, specific clinical symptoms may include hemiparesis, seizures, memory impairment, emotional blunting or instability, gustatory and olfactory hallucinations, visual field defects, déjà vu phenomena, and personality changes. Vertigo and/or tinnitus may be reported by about 12% of patients. Lesions of the dominant temporal lobe may be associated with aphasia in about 60% of individuals (Strobos, 1974). Individuals with extensive deep destruction of the temporal lobe may show disturbances in behavior relating to basic drives. On occasion, a partial Klüver-Bucy syndrome may be seen in persons with temporal lobe disease.[4]

In patients with brain stem site, specific clinical symptomatology may include hemiparesis, sensory loss, visual abnormalities, ocular muscle weakness, involuntary movement or tremors, abnormal corneal reflex, hydrocephalus, nystagmus,

5. The audiologic evaluation of some patients may be complicated by other symptoms of brain damage; i.e., increased fatigability, inability to concentrate, increased distractibility, increased irritability, impaired intellectual function, and emotional instability.

6. Remember, central auditory tests may be difficult to interpret in patients with peripheral hearing loss. Results in these patients are equivocal. They may be reflecting either the peripheral or the central auditory problem.

7. Intraaxial brain stem lesions with exophytic extensions present special diagnostic problems because the exophytic component may masquerade as an independent extraaxial mass and may conceal the presence of the intraaxial disorder. Auditory findings may be uniquely helpful in resolving this diagnostic challenge.

dizziness, facial paralysis, ataxia, vomiting, inadequate gag and cough reflexes, defective swallowing, and hoarseness of the voice.[5]

Treatment of intracranial tumors may involve surgery, radiotherapy, or chemotherapy. In patients with intraaxial brain stem neoplasms, the majority of tumors are inoperable. The course of the disease in these patients is usually steadily downhill with minor periods of improvement or stability. Early detection of intracranial neoplasms is important for maximum recovery.

CLINICAL EVALUATION OF CENTRAL AUDITORY DISORDER

Clinical manifestations of auditory disorder increase in subtlety as the site of lesion progresses from the peripheral to the central auditory system. For example, patients with central auditory disorder usually have little or no difficulty with pure tone and PB word tests. In order to demonstrate the presence of central auditory abnormality, considerably more subtle auditory tasks are required. This fact places a unique responsibility on clinicians. A critical aspect of the clinical evaluation of patients with central auditory disorder is to be alert to the possibility of a central auditory problem.

One key to documenting the presence of central auditory abnormality is to screen all patients with relatively normal sensitivity for the possibility of a central auditory site.[6] The possibility of central auditory disorder may be screened for with the PI-PB function, the PI-SSI function, and the SSW test. Possible findings on these procedures are detailed below under General Audiologic Pattern.

SITE OF DISORDER

Brain stem or temporal lobe. In patients with an intraaxial brain stem disorder characterized by an exophytic growth into the cerebellopontine angle, an eighth nerve disorder may be observed.[7]

GENERAL AUDIOLOGIC PATTERN

Pure tone results characteristically show normal sensitivity on both ears. On occasion, however, a mild, bilateral, high frequency loss may be observed. In general, pure tone sensitivity results are symmetric on the two ears.[8]

Maximum speech intelligibility scores are generally within normal limits for monosyllabic (PB) words and generally disproportionately depressed for SSI materials. A discrepancy between PB max and SSI max scores is a hallmark of retrocochlear disorders. Although PB max performance is characteristically normal, if a PI-PB function is carefully constructed across many intensity levels, two abnormalities may be observed. First, the function may show a consistent performance difference between ears that cannot be accounted for by a peripheral sensitivity difference. This performance deficit usually appears on the ear contralateral to the affected side of the brain. Second, rollover of the PI-PB function may occur. The presence of rollover, in the absence of any sensitivity loss, is suggestive of central auditory disorder.

In addition to PI functions, the SSW test is a helpful screening procedure. If a performance difference occurs between the two ears for the simultaneous dichotic condition, results are consistent with a temporal lobe site.

If one or more of the screening procedures is positive, performance deficits can be further explored with the SSI materials. Performance is measured for both a contralateral competing message (CCM) and an ipsilateral competing message (ICM). The patient's relative performance on the two tasks (ICM and CCM) assists in differentiating intraaxial brain stem and temporal lobe sites. A relatively greater performance deficit for ICM than for CCM suggests a brain stem site, whereas a relatively greater deficit for CCM than for ICM suggests a temporal lobe site. The unique difference between brain stem and temporal lobe sites is that patients with intraaxial brain stem disorders have more difficulty with degraded monotic signals and patients with temporal lobe disorders have more difficulty with dichotic signals. In addition to the SSI and SSW procedures, unusual performance deficits may be observed for speech tasks degraded by filtering, temporal interruption, acceleration, or compression.[9]

Impedance audiometry characteristically shows normal tympanograms and normal static compliance measures. Acoustic reflex results vary, however, depending on the site of disorder. As a general rule, reflexes are normal in patients with temporal lobe site and abnormal in patients with intraaxial brain stem site. In the latter patients, reflex thresholds on both ears are characteristically elevated in the crossed condition and present at normal HLs in the uncrossed condition. The reflex pattern is characterized by a horizontal configuration of abnormality. A notable exception to the above observations involves patients with brain stem site who show normal acoustic reflexes for both crossed and uncrossed stimulation. The site of disorder in these patients is usually above the level of the acoustic reflex pathways in the brain stem.[10]

In occasional patients with intraaxial brain stem or temporal lobe disorders, striking exceptions to the above general audiologic pattern may be observed. For example, in patients with intraaxial brain stem neoplasms characterized by exophytic extensions that invade the cerebellopontine angle, auditory findings may be consistent with eighth nerve site. The overall pattern of results may show unilateral sensitivity loss, reduced PB max scores, significant rollover, abnormal crossed and uncrossed acoustic reflexes, and abnormal Bekesy audiograms. The above pattern may be observed on the ear ipsilateral to the radiographic site of disorder. However, as a general rule, auditory findings in patients with exophytic extensions that invade the cerebellopontine angle, as well as the intraaxial brain stem pathways, usually show abnormalities on both ears. Hearing deficits on both ears, particularly on the ear contralateral to the radiographic abnormality, strongly support the possibility of an intraaxial brain stem site.[11]

In patients with temporal lobe site, two unusual exceptions to the general pattern of results outlined above may occur. The first exception involves patients with deep, extensive lesions of the left temporal lobe. Auditory abnormalities in these patients may be observed on the left ear, the ear ipsilateral to the affected side of the brain. This ipsilateral ear effect is in direct contrast to the contralateral ear effect characterizing most temporal lobe patients. An ipsilateral ear effect has been explained on the basis of two conditions: (1) the greater efficiency of the

---

Marginal notes:

8. The symmetry of pure tone sensitivity on the two ears is frequently helpful in distinguishing between extraaxial (eighth nerve) and intraaxial brain stem disorders. For example, in a series of 16 patients with confirmed intraaxial brain stem disorders, the audiogram was symmetric on the two ears in about 80% of persons (Jerger and Jerger, 1974). In contrast, in a series of 25 patients with confirmed extraaxial (eighth nerve) brain stem disorders, the audiogram was asymmetric on the two ears in all patients (Neely et al., 1977).

9. In our experience, the combination of the SSI procedure and the SSW test offers an unusually effective diagnostic tool for differentiating temporal lobe and brain stem sites. More specifically, the SSW test offers unique assistance in differentiating temporal lobe disorders. It does not, however, consistently identify patients with brain stem disorders. Conversely, the SSI procedure provides unique assistance in distinguishing brain stem site. It does not, however, consistently identify patients with temporal lobe site.

10. In 6 patients with confirmed intraaxial brain stem disorders, the horizontal reflex pattern was observed in 4 of the 6 individuals (Jerger and Jerger, 1977).

11. In a series of 6 patients with intraaxial brain stem tumors with exophytic extensions critically invading the cerebellopontine angle, auditory findings were useful in distinguishing the presence of an intraaxial brain stem disorder in 4 of the 6 individuals (Jerger and Jerger, 1975).

contralateral pathways under difficult listening conditions, and (2) the specialization of the left hemisphere for language. The left ear deficit in a deep, extensive left temporal lobe lesion is attributed to the fact that the pathways from the left ear to the right temporal lobe are blocked from proceeding from the right temporal lobe to the left temporal lobe for processing (Sparks et al., 1970).

The other unusual exception involves patients with bilateral temporal lobe disease. In these rare patients, cortical "deafness" may be observed. The audiogram may show a severe hearing loss on both ears. Maximum intelligibility scores for monosyllabic (PB) words may be severely impaired bilaterally. Serial hearing tests over time may show some return of auditory function. However, demonstrable deficits usually remain and are characteristically more pronounced on one ear than the other.

Other deficits associated with the presence of central auditory disorder may include abnormalities on masking level difference (MLD) tasks, binaural fusion tests, intensity discrimination functions, threshold vs signal-duration functions, and temporal order tasks. "Decruitment" may be observed on the alternate binaural loudness balance (ABLB) procedure. The auditory brain stem response may be delayed and poorly formed. The MLD tests, binaural fusion tests, and brain stem evoked response audiometry are noted for their sensitivity to the presence of an intraaxial brain stem disorder at or below the level of the inferior colliculi. These three procedures are usually normal in patients with temporal lobe site.

Illustrative Patients

CASE 1. A 51-YEAR-OLD FEMALE WITH A RIGHT TEMPORAL LOBE DISORDER. SURGICAL FINDINGS REVEALED A GRADE IV TEMPORAL LOBE ASTROCYTOMA, 2½ CM IN DIAMETER.[12]

History

Approximately 6 months ago, in another state, the patient experienced a grand mal seizure. The family described the attack as consisting of generalized muscle convulsions (clonic movements) with the eyes rolling backward. The patient did not have any other neurologic problems. She was placed on drug therapy.[13]

12. Notice that a number (grade) may be added to the cytologic classification of a brain tumor. The number specifies the degree of malignancy and may range from I (benign) to IV (malignant).

13. Seizures are a frequent symptom of temporal lobe disease and may be observed in 40% to 60% of individuals

with temporal lobe disorder (Northfield, 1973).

Approximately 5 months ago, the patient experienced another seizure. She was admitted to the Neurosensory Center hospital for evaluation of the seizure disorder. EEG findings showed a focus of slow activity in the right temporal region. A computerized axial tomographic (CT) scan revealed a high density mass lesion at the medial aspect of the posterior right temporal lobe.

At the present hospitalization, the patient is admitted for evaluation of pain behind the eyes and a feeling of pressure over the suboccipital region. She reports that she has experienced no seizures since her last hospitalization. She denies any previous history of alcoholism, trauma to the head, hypertension, and unusual drug use except for the anticonvulsant medication. She reports occurrences of episodes of a drawing and burning sensation on the right side of the face. The episodes last about 1 minute and are accompanied by sensations of an unpleasant taste and odor. The patient denies any other symptomatology. However, the family reports that the patient seems to have unusual difficulty remembering things. They feel she has had a personality change. The patient is right-handed.

At the present time, physical examination is unremarkable. Neurologic evaluation reveals a loss of sight in the corresponding left lateral halves of the eyes (left homonymous hemianopia). Cerebellar function appears intact except for a slightly unsteady gait. The CT scan shows an increase in the size of the right temporal lobe mass since the previous scan. Lateral displacement of adjacent structures is noted for the first time.

The patient does not have any hearing complaints on either ear. The audiologic results presented below were obtained just prior to a right temporal craniotomy.

Results

The audiogram (Case 12-1A) shows normal pure tone sensitivity on both ears with the exception of a very mild high frequency sensitivity loss. The PTA scores (Case 12-1B) are 8 dB HL on both ears.

The PI-SSI functions (Case 12-1A) are normal on the right ear, but show slightly reduced maximum performance and substantial rollover on the left ear. The SSI max scores (Case 12-1B) are 100% on the right ear and 80% on the left ear. The SSIT scores,

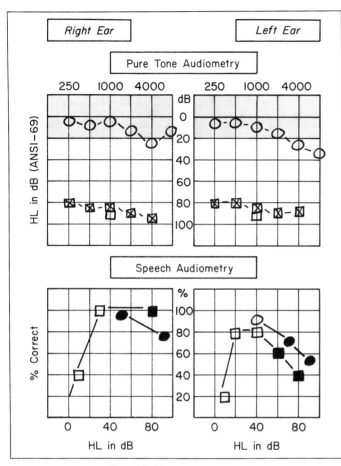

Case 12-1A

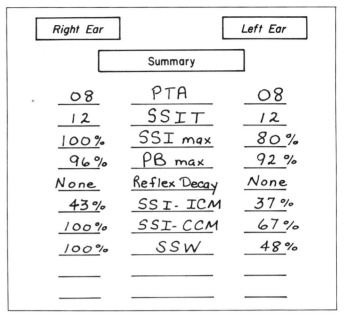

Case 12-1B

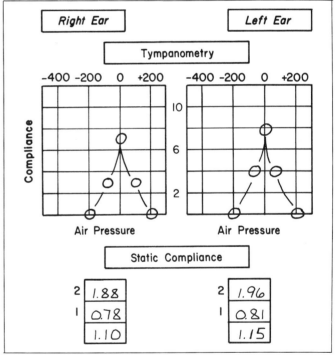

Case 12-1C

14. Notice that rollover of the PI functions on the left ear and the difference between ears on SSI maximum performance suggests the possibility of a retrocochlear disorder. The normal, symmetric, pure tone sensitivity suggests that any auditory disorder is above the level of the eighth nerve and cochlear nucleus. If acoustic reflex results support this hypothesis, we will proceed to the SSI central test battery to evaluate further the speech intelligibility performance deficits.

12 dB HL on both ears, agree with average pure tone sensitivity measures bilaterally.

PB testing at high intensity levels (Case 12-1A) shows normal maximum intelligibility scores on both ears. The PB max scores (Case 12-1B) are 96% on the right ear and 92% on the left ear. PB testing shows mild rollover on the right ear and pronounced rollover on the left ear.[14]

Tympanometry and static compliance measures (Case 12-1C) are normal on both ears. Crossed and uncrossed acoustic reflexes (Case 12-1A) are present at normal HLs at all frequencies on both ears. No reflex decay is observed at 500 Hz or 1000 Hz on either ear.

SSI-ICM performance (Case 12-1D) shows depressed scores on both ears. Average performance (Case 12-1B) is 43% on the right ear and 37% on the left ear. SSI-CCM performance (Case 12-1D) is normal on the right ear but shows an unusually large performance deficit on the left ear. Average CCM performance scores (Case

15. In patients with temporal lobe disorders, the SSI procedure may yield poor performance on both ICM and CCM tasks. ICM deficits may be observed on both ears or the contralateral ear only. The CCM

12-1B) are 100% on the right ear and 67% on the left ear.[15]

SSW results (Case 12-1B) show a large performance difference between ears. Average scores for the competing condition are 100% on the right ear, but only 48% on the left ear.

Auditory brain stem evoked response (ABR) audiometry (Case 12-1E) yields

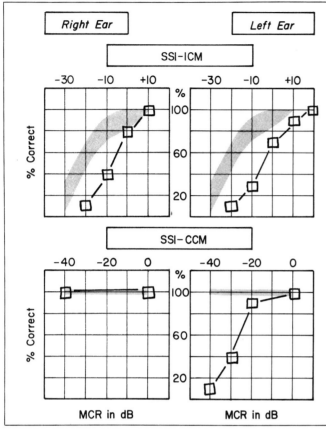

Case 12-1D

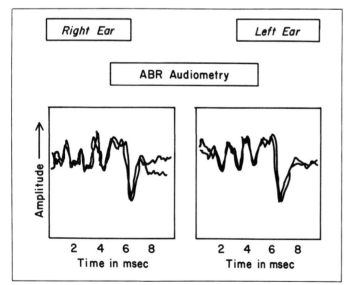

Case 12-1E

In some patients, ICM deficits may be related to secondary, indirect, involvement of the auditory pathways in the brain stem. For example, autopsy results in this patient revealed compression of the lateral ventricle, the third ventricle, and the midbrain.

16. Results in this patient illustrate the contralateral ear effect. We observe left ear deficits in association with a right temporal lobe disorder. Remember, however, determining the affected side of the brain in patients with temporal lobe site is not always as clearcut as it is in patients with disorders at other levels of the auditory system. For example, the next patient (case 2) illustrates an ipsilateral ear effect.

17. About 1 year after the audiologic evaluation, the patient was diagnosed as having receptive aphasia.

deficit is observed on the contralateral ear only. The overriding principle in these patients is the relatively greater deficit for CCM tasks than for ICM tasks.

well-formed responses with normal wave V latencies on both ears. The absolute and interwave latencies of all component waves are within normal limits. Repeatable wave V responses were elicited at intensity levels down to 40 dB HL on both ears.

Impression

Pure tone sensitivity within normal limits bilaterally except for a very slight high frequency sensitivity loss. Impedance audiometry is consistent with normal middle ear function on both ears. Diagnostic test results are consistent with a central auditory disorder at the level of the temporal lobe. A temporal lobe site is supported by a substantial SSI-CCM deficit in the presence of a relatively less severe SSI-ICM deficit and a large loss for the competing condition on the SSW test. Performance deficits on dichotic speech tasks are observed on the left ear only.[16]

CASE 2. A 25-YEAR-OLD FEMALE WITH A LEFT TEMPORAL LOBE DISORDER. SURGICAL FINDINGS REVEALED AN EXTENSIVE GRADE III ASTROCYTOMA IN THE DEEP LEFT POSTERIOR PARIETOTEMPORAL REGION. THE CORPUS CALLOSUM APPEARED MASSIVELY EXPANDED AND IRREGULAR.

History

The audiologic evaluation was carried out about 1½ years after temporal lobe surgery. Electroencephalography and brain scan results show evidence of tumor recurrence.

The patient is admitted to the hospital for evaluation of a right leg weakness during walking. Neurologic evaluation shows right hemiparesis, a loss of sight in the corresponding right lateral halves of the eyes (right homonymous hemianopia) and edema of the optic papilla (papilledema) in both eyes. The patient appears to have some difficulty in naming objects (anomia).[17] Cranial nerve function appears fairly intact. She denies head trauma, unusual drug use, and noise exposure. She does not have any hearing complaints about either ear.

Results

The audiogram (Case 12-2A) shows normal pure tone sensitivity bilaterally. The PTA scores (Case 12-2B) are 9 dB HL on the right ear and 11 dB HL on the left ear.

Speech audiometry (Case 12-2A) shows normal maximum intelligibility scores for both PB words and SSI materials on both ears. The PB max scores (Case 12-2B) are 92% on the right ear and 88% on the left ear. The SSI max scores are 100% on both

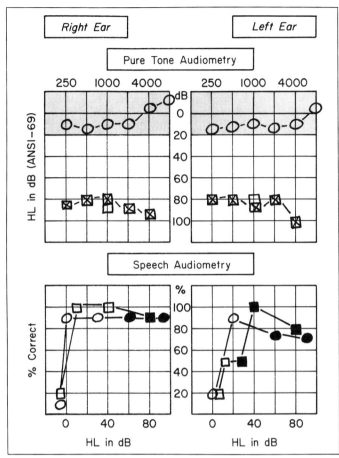

Case 12-2A

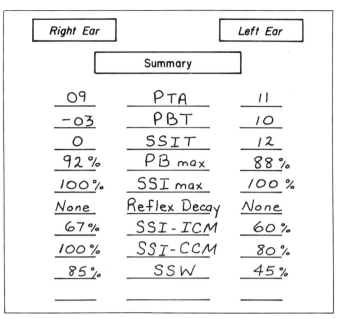

Case 12-2B

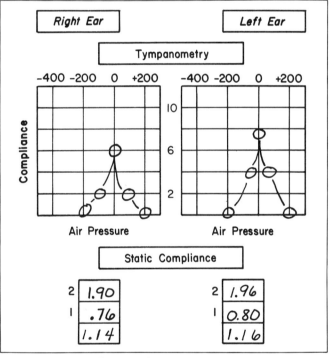

Case 12-2C

ears. The shape of the PI-PB and PI-SSI functions (Case 12-2A) is normal on the right ear but shows mild rollover on the left ear.

Speech thresholds (Case 12-2B) on both ears agree with average pure tone sensitivity. On the right ear, the PBT is −3 dB HL; the SSIT is 0 dB HL. On the left ear, the PBT is 10 dB HL; the SSIT is 12 dB HL.

Impedance audiometry (Case 12-2C) shows normal tympanograms and normal static compliance measures bilaterally. On both ears, crossed and uncrossed acoustic reflexes (Case 12-2A) are present at normal HLs. No reflex decay is observed at 500 Hz or 1000 Hz on either ear.

SSI-ICM performance (Case 12-2D) is normal on the right ear and shows a very mild performance deficit on the left ear. Average performance scores (Case 12-2B) are 67% on the right ear and 60% on the left ear.

The SSI-CCM task (Case 12-2D) is performed without difficulty on the right ear,

18. Notice that the performance deficit on the SSW test is more dramatic in this patient than the SSI-CCM perfor-

but shows a moderate performance deficit on the left ear. Average performance scores (Case 12-2B) are 100% on the right ear and 80% on the left ear.

The SSW test (Case 12-2B) shows a large performance difference between ears. Average scores for the competing condition are 85% on the right ear, but only 45% on the left ear.[18]

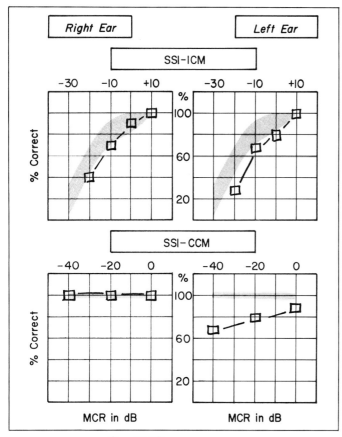

Case 12-2D

mance loss. In our experience, the SSW test is a more sensitive tool for distinguishing temporal lobe site than the SSI-CCM procedure. However, the observation of a relatively more severe SSI-CCM loss than SSI-ICM loss still holds true.

19. Notice that an ipsilateral ear effect in this patient is consistent with the history of a deep, extensive left temporal lobe disorder with involvement of the corpus callosum.

Impression

Pure tone sensitivity within normal limits bilaterally. Impedance audiometry is consistent with normal middle ear function on each ear. Diagnostic test results are consistent with a temporal lobe site. A temporal lobe disorder is supported by the observation of a large performance deficit for the competing condition on the SSW test and a relatively greater loss on the SSI-CCM procedure than on the SSI-ICM task. All abnormal auditory findings are observed on the left ear.[19]

CASE 3. A 25-YEAR-OLD FEMALE WITH A BRAIN STEM DISORDER ECCENTRIC TO THE RIGHT. SURGERY REVEALED A PINEALOBLASTOMA AND SECONDARY HYDROCEPHALUS.

History

The patient is admitted to the hospital with a 9-month history of headache, nausea, vomiting, visual problems, and poor motor control. Approximately 4 months ago, the patient developed hydrocephalus. She underwent a surgical shunt procedure in another

country. She had been well before the onset of these symptoms.

At the present time, neurologic examination reveals papilledema, a loss of upward eye gaze, and bilateral horizontal nystagmus. Cerebellar and motor function is within normal limits except for a resting tremor. Deep tendon reflexes appear to be more active on the right side than on the left side. Routine laboratory studies are within normal limits. A CT scan reveals an infiltrating mass lesion involving the pons, midbrain, and right subthalamic region with obliteration of the fourth ventricle chamber, moderately severe distention of the third and lateral ventricles in the midline, and hydrocephalus.

The patient does not have any hearing complaints on either ear. She denies unusual drug use, head trauma, and noise exposure. The patient's native language is Spanish. She appears to have only a limited understanding of English. The history information was obtained through an interpreter. The audiologic evaluation was obtained just prior to a right temporal craniotomy.

Results

The audiogram (Case 12-3A) shows normal pure tone sensitivity on both ears. The PTA scores (Case 12-3B) are 13 dB HL on the right ear and 15 dB HL on the left ear. Unmasked bone conduction thresholds (Case 12-3A) are superimposed on air conduction thresholds bilaterally. The Weber test (Case 12-3B) is heard in the midline.

20. Remember, when the performance plateau of a PI function is at or near the 50% intelligibility level, speech thresholds are more accurately obtained on a steeper part of the function, such as the 25% intelligibility level.

PI-SSI functions for Spanish materials (Case 12-3A) are abnormal on both ears. On the right ear, substantial rollover is observed even though maximum intelligibility performance is normal (100%). On the left ear, an unusually poor maximum intelligibility score (60%) is obtained. The SSIT scores agree with average pure tone sensitivity bilaterally. SSIT scores are 20 dB HL on the right ear and 22 dB HL on the left ear.[20]

Impedance audiometry (Case 12-3C) shows a type C tympanogram on the right ear and an unusually shallow, type A, tympanogram on the left ear. Static compliance measures are within normal limits on the right ear but slightly below the normal range on the left ear. Crossed and uncrossed acoustic reflexes (Case 12-3A) on both ears are present at normal HLs at all frequencies.

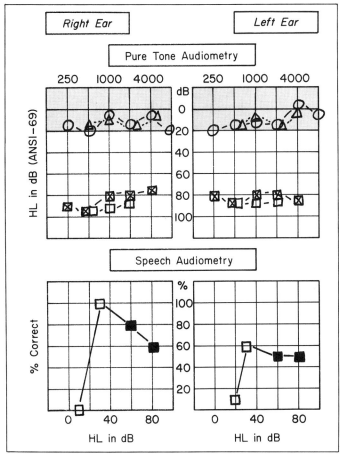

Case 12-3A

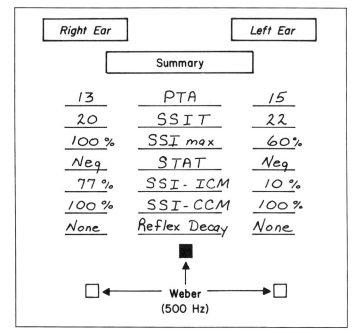

Case 12-3B

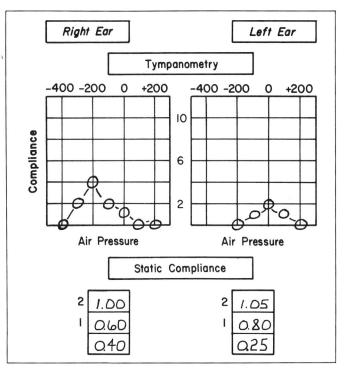

Case 12-3C

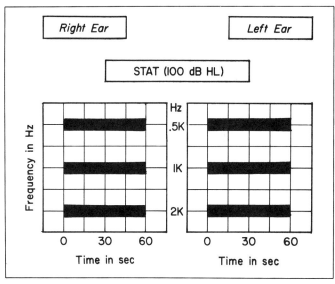

Case 12-3D

No reflex decay is observed at 500 Hz or 1000 Hz on either ear.

The STAT (Case 12-3D) does not show abnormal adaptation at any frequency on either ear. The SSI-ICM procedure (Case 12-3E) shows impaired performance on the left ear and normal performance on the right ear. Average SSI-ICM scores (Case 12-3B) are 10% on the left ear and 77% on the right ear. In contrast to SSI-ICM performance, SSI-CCM performance (Case 12-3E) is nor-

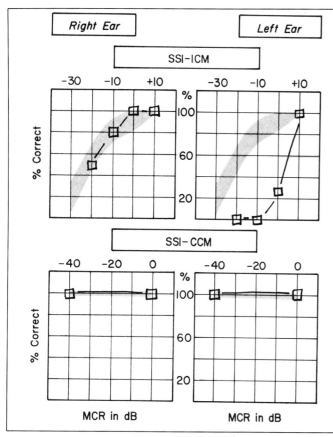

Case 12-3E

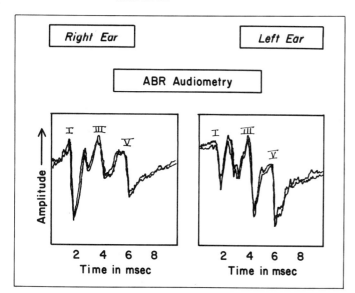

Case 12-3F

range, it is helpful to obtain the interwave latency between waves I and V. In some patients, particularly individuals with eighth nerve disorder, wave V latency may still be within the normal range, but the I to V interwave latency may be abnormal. In the present patient, wave I to V interwave latency was normal on both ears.

Note, however, that on the right ear the amplitude of wave V is less than the amplitude of wave I. The left ear shows a more normal I/V amplitude ratio. The abnormality of the amplitude ratio on the right ear may be considered a marginal positive finding for brain stem involvement.

22. Notice that the only abnormal findings in this patient are speech audiometric results. In other patients with brain stem site, however, speech audiometry may be only mildly abnormal in the presence of relatively more dramatic ABR and acoustic reflex abnormalities (see patient 3, Chapter 15, Multiple Sclerosis). Variable results on isolated test procedures emphasize the importance of a test battery approach for precise site prediction.

mal on both ears. SSI-CCM scores (Case 12-3B) are 100% at all test conditions.

ABR audiometry (Case 12-3F) shows normal latency measures for wave V on both ears. A well-formed response (waves I through V) is observed bilaterally.[21]

21. In patients with suspected retrocochlear site and wave V latencies within the normal

Impression

Pure tone sensitivity is within normal limits bilaterally. Impedance audiometry shows negative middle ear pressure on the right ear and slightly decreased mobility of the middle ear system on the left ear. However, bone conduction measures are superimposed on air conduction thresholds bilaterally. Diagnostic test results indicate a central auditory disorder involving the brain stem pathways on the right side. A brain stem site is supported by a substantial SSI-ICM (Spanish materials) performance deficit in the presence of normal SSI-CCM performance and by abnormal PI-SSI functions. SSI-ICM performance deficits are observed on the left ear only and indicate a disorder on the opposite, right, side of the brain stem. The possibility of eighth nerve involvement is rendered unlikely by the normal, relatively symmetric, pure tone sensitivity, normal acoustic reflex threshold HLs, no reflex decay, no abnormal adaptation on STAT, and normal ABR results. The observation of well-formed waves I through V on ABR audiometry and normal acoustic reflexes suggest involvement of the central auditory pathways at a relatively rostral level of the brain stem.[22]

CASE 4. A 7-YEAR-OLD MALE WITH A BRAIN STEM DISORDER GREATER ON THE LEFT SIDE. RADIOGRAPHIC STUDIES REVEALED A LARGE INTRAAXIAL PONTOMEDULLARY AND MIDBRAIN MASS ECCENTRICALLY LARGER ON THE LEFT SIDE OF THE BRAIN. TREATMENT INVOLVED RADIATION THERAPY FOR A PERIOD OF APPROXIMATELY 35 DAYS.

History

Approximately 3 months ago, the patient began to complain of double vision (diplopia) and blurred vision. His left eye appeared to deviate inward. He seemed well before the beginning of these symptoms. During the next 3 months, the symptoms became progressively worse.

Presently, the patient complains of difficulty with walking and weakness on his right side, difficulty with swallowing and occasional hoarseness. Cranial nerve examination shows a persistent medial deviation of the left eye, a bilaterally decreased corneal reflex, and a decreased gag reflex bilaterally. The patient has a mild to moder-

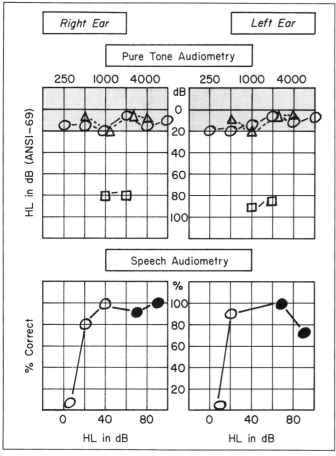

Case 12-4A

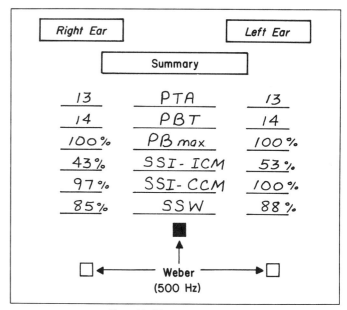

Case 12-4B

ate right-sided hemiparesis and a slightly dystaxic gait.

Tests of cerebellar function show dysmetria on the right side on finger to nose testing. Deep tendon reflexes are slightly hyperactive on the right side relative to the left side. An extensor plantar response on the left side is noted. Evaluation of sensory systems appears to be within normal limits. Vertebral and carotid angiograms reveal a large pontomedullary and midbrain mass eccentrically larger on the left. The floor of the fourth ventricle appears elevated.

The patient has no history of other serious illnesses, unusual drug use, or noise exposure. However, about 2 years ago, he fell and received a blow to the head. He has no hearing complaints on either ear.

Results

The audiogram (Case 12-4A) shows normal pure tone sensitivity on both ears. The PTA scores (Case 12-4B) are 13 dB HL on both ears. Unmasked bone conduction scores

23. In patients with a horizontal reflex pattern, it is important to rule out the possibility of a collapsing ear canal on each ear. Remember, any occlusion of the ear canal will elevate crossed reflexes, but not uncrossed reflexes. This patient did not have a collapsing ear canal on either ear.

(Case 12-4A) are superimposed on air conduction thresholds bilaterally. The Weber test is referred to the midline.

The PI-PB functions (Case 12-4A) show normal maximum intelligibility scores (100%) on both ears. The shape of the PI function is normal on the right ear but shows mild rollover on the left ear. Speech thresholds agree with pure tone sensitivity results bilaterally. The PBT scores (Case 12-4B) are 14 dB HL on each ear.

Impedance audiometry (Case 12-4C) shows normal, type A, tympanograms and normal static compliance measures bilaterally. Crossed acoustic reflexes (Case 12-4A) on both ears are absent at equipment limits at all frequencies. In contrast, however, uncrossed reflexes on each ear are present at normal HLs. The reflex pattern (Case 12-4D) is characterized by a horizontal configuration of abnormality. Reflexes on both ears are consistently absent to crossed stimulation and consistently present to uncrossed stimulation.[23]

The SSI-ICM procedure (Case 12-4E) shows reduced performance on both ears. Average SSI-ICM scores (Case 12-4B) are 43% on the right ear and 53% on the left ear. In contrast to SSI-ICM performance, SSI-CCM performance (Case 12-4E) is normal on both ears. Average SSI-CCM scores (Case 12-4B) are 97% on the right ear and 100% on the left ear. The SSW test (Case

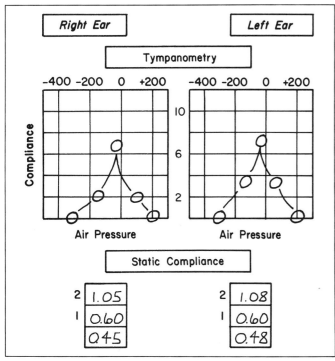

Case 12-4C

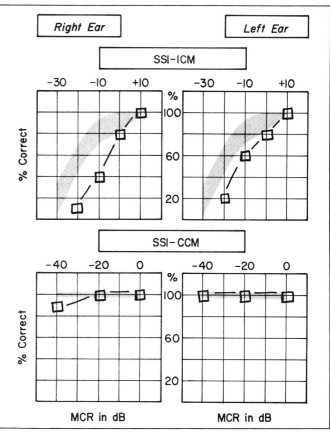

Case 12-4E

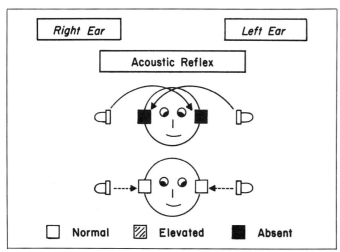

Case 12-4D

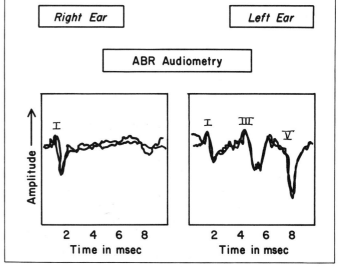

Case 12-4F

24. In this patient, notice that the SSI procedure is a more sensitive procedure than the SSW test in distinguishing the presence of a brain stem disorder (see also patient 2, Chapter 2, Cerebrovascular Disorders).

12-4B) shows normal performance on both ears. Average scores for the competing condition are 85% on the right ear and 88% on the left ear.[24]

Auditory brain stem evoked response (ABR) audiometry (Case 12-4F) shows abnormal results on both ears. On the left ear, wave I is at a normal latency (1.7 msec), but wave III is slightly delayed (4.2 msec) and wave V is considerably delayed (7.5 msec). On the right ear only wave I appears. No later waves can be observed.

Results from both ears were obtained at a click level of 80 dB HL.

Impression

Pure tone sensitivity within normal limits bilaterally. Tympanometry, static compliance measures, and uncrossed acoustic re-

25. Notice that performance deficits are more marked on the right ear, the ear opposite the most severely involved side of the brain stem.

flexes are consistent with normal middle ear function. Bone conduction measures are superimposed on air conduction thresholds bilaterally. Diagnostic test results are consistent with a central auditory disorder at the level of the brain stem. A brain stem site is supported by the presence of a horizontal reflex pattern, abnormal ABR results, and SSI-ICM deficits coupled with normal SSI-CCM performance. Performance deficits are observed on both ears. However, ABR and SSI-ICM results show slightly greater deficits on the right ear than on the left ear.[25]

CASE 5. A 9-YEAR-OLD FEMALE WITH AN EXTRA- AND INTRAAXIAL BRAIN STEM DISORDER, EXOPHYTIC TO THE RIGHT SIDE. AUTOPSY REVEALED A MASSIVE ASTROCYTOMA OF THE LOWER BRAIN STEM.

History

The patient is admitted to the hospital with a 2-month history of headaches accompanied by dizziness and vomiting. Her symptoms have increased in severity during the past 2 months. Presently, she also complains of unsteady balance.

Neurologic evaluation shows a bilaterally diminished corneal reflex, greater on the right; a bilateral absence of the gag reflex; and an ataxic gait. On Romberg testing, the patient falls to the left.

A left vertebral and right carotid angiogram and a CT scan reveal a brain stem mass involving the medulla, pons, mesencephalon, posterior thalamic structures, and peduncles of both cerebellar hemispheres. The mass is eccentrically larger on the right with exophytic projections to the right side.

The mother thinks that the patient's growth and development, including her speech and language, has been slow relative to her siblings. However, major milestones occurred within normal limits. The patient has no hearing complaints about either ear.

Results

The audiogram (Case 12-5A) shows normal pure tone sensitivity on both ears. The PTA scores (Case 12-5B) are 7 dB HL on the right ear and 12 dB HL on the left ear. Unmasked bone conduction thresholds (Case 12-5A) are superimposed on air conduction sensitivity bilaterally.

PI functions for PB-kindergarten (PB-K)

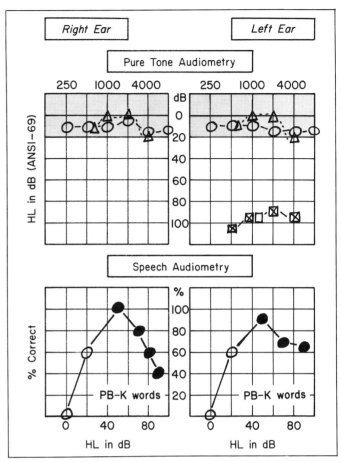

Case 12-5A

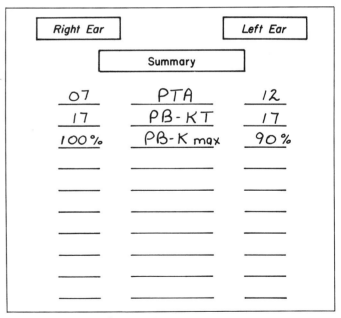

Case 12-5B

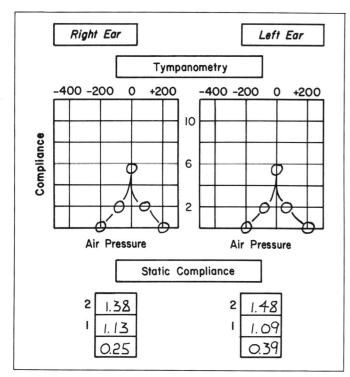

Case 12-5C

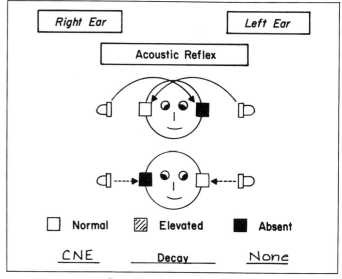

Case 12-5D

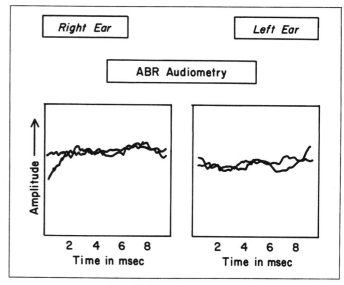

Case 12-5E

words show normal maximum intelligibility scores on both ears. The PB-K max scores (Case 12-5B) are 100% on the right ear and 90% on the left ear. Abnormal rollover is observed on both ears. The degree of rollover is 60% on the right ear and 26% on the left ear. Speech thresholds for PB-K words (PB-KT) (Case 12-5B) agree with pure tone sensitivity results bilaterally. The PB-KT scores are 17 dB HL on each ear.

Impedance audiometry (Case 12-5C) shows normal, type A, tympanograms on both ears. Static compliance measures are within normal limits on the left ear and slightly below the normal range on the right ear. With sound to the left ear, crossed and uncrossed acoustic reflexes (Case 12-5A) are present at normal HLs for all frequencies above 500 Hz. However, reflexes are elevated at 500 Hz and absent at equipment limits at 250 Hz. With sound to the right ear, both crossed and uncrossed acoustic reflexes are absent at equipment limits at all frequencies.

The reflex pattern at 1000 Hz (Case 12-5D) is characterized by a diagonal configuration of abnormality. Results are consistent with an abnormal sound effect on the right ear.[26] Reflex decay testing on the left ear at 500 Hz and 1000 Hz is within normal

26. Notice that the reflex pattern reflects only the relation between crossed and uncrossed reflexes. Results are confined to the frequency or frequencies (usually 1000 Hz, 2000 Hz, or both) yielding both crossed and uncrossed threshold measures. Consequently, as results in this patient illustrate, crossed reflex thresholds at other frequencies, such as 250 and 500 Hz, may be abnormal in an ear with a normal crossed vs uncrossed relation.

limits. At 500 Hz, results were obtained at 5 dB sensation level (SL), rather than the traditional 10 dB SL, due to the elevated threshold HL (105 dB). Reflex decay testing on the right ear could not be carried out.

Auditory brain stem evoked response testing (Case 12-5E) reveals no observable response to air- or bone-conducted clicks at equipment limits on either ear. No waves could be identified.

Impression

Normal pure tone sensitivity bilaterally. Diagnostic auditory test results are consistent with a brain stem disorder at the level of the eighth nerve or cochlear nucleus on the

27. A diagonal reflex pattern in this patient is considered a strong vote for eighth nerve abnormality. In a series of 17 patients with eighth nerve vs intraaxial brain stem sites, a diagonal pattern was always associated with eighth nerve involvement and a horizontal pattern was always associated with intraaxial brain stem site. There were no false positive findings in either group (Jerger and Jerger, 1977). Consequently, when one observes a diagonal configuration, the possibility of a pure intraaxial brain stem site is unlikely.

right side. Abnormal auditory symptoms are observed on both ears. A brain stem site is supported by the observation of abnormality on both ears for ABR audiometry, the roll-over index, and acoustic reflex thresholds at 250 and 500 Hz. Involvement of the eighth nerve on the right side is supported by the diagonal reflex pattern.[27]

SELECTED READINGS

Behrend, R. Epidemiology of Brain Tumors. In P. Vinken and G. Bruyn (eds.), *Handbook of Clinical Neurology*. Amsterdam: North-Holland, 1974. Pp. 56–87.

Green, J., Waggener, J., and Kriegsfeld, B. Classification and Incidence of Neoplasms of the Central Nervous System. In R. Thompson and J. Green (eds.), *Advances in Neurology*. New York: Raven Press, 1976. Pp. 51–55.

Jerger, J., and Jerger, S. Auditory findings in brain stem disorders. *Arch. Otolaryngol.* 99:342, 1974.

Jerger, S., and Jerger, J. Extra- and intra-axial brain stem auditory disorders. *Audiology* 14:93, 1975.

Jerger, S., and Jerger, J. Diagnostic value of crossed vs uncrossed acoustic reflexes. Eighth nerve and brain stem disorders. *Arch. Otolaryngol.* 103:445, 1977.

Klüver, H., and Bucy, P. Preliminary analysis of functions of the temporal lobes in monkeys. *Arch. Neurol. Psychiat.* 42:979, 1939.

Koos, W., and Miller, M. *Intracranial Tumors of Infants and Children.* St. Louis: Mosby, 1971. Pp. 9–27.

Kurland, L., Myrianthopoulos, N., and Lessell, S. Epidemiologic and Genetic Considerations of Intracranial Neoplasms. In W. Fields and P. Sharkey (eds.), *The Biology and Treatment of Intracranial Tumors.* Springfield, Ill.: Thomas, 1962. Pp. 5–43.

Lassman, L. Tumors of the Pons and Medulla Oblongata. In P. Vinken and G. Bruyn (eds.), *Handbook of Clinical Neurology.* Amsterdam: North-Holland, 1974. Pp. 693–706.

Neely, J., Alford, B., Templeton, T., and Neblett, C. Clinical correlates of neoplastic involvement of the eighth cranial nerve in man. *Surg. Forum* 28:508, 1977.

Northfield, D. *The Surgery of the Central Nervous System.* Oxford: Blackwell, 1973. Pp. 46–63.

Percy, A., Elveback, L., Okasaki, H., and Kurland, L. Neoplasms of the central nervous system: Epidemiologic considerations. *Neurology* 22:40, 1972.

Slager, T. *Basic Neuropathology.* Baltimore: Williams & Wilkins, 1970. Pp. 246–292.

Sparks, R., Goodglass, H., and Nickle, B. Ipsilateral versus contralateral extinction in dichotic listening resulting from hemispheric lesions. *Cortex* 6:249, 1970.

Stein, B. Clinical and Pathological Aspects of Posterior Fossa Tumors. In S. Wolpert (ed.), *Angiography of Posterior Fossa Tumors.* New York: Grune & Stratton, 1976. Pp. 20–30.

Strobos, R. Temporal Lobe Tumors. In P. Vinken and G. Bruyn (eds.), *Handbook of Clinical Neurology.* Amsterdam: North-Holland, 1974. Pp. 281–295.

Zulch, K. *Brain Tumors: Their Biology and Pathology.* London: Heinemann, 1965.

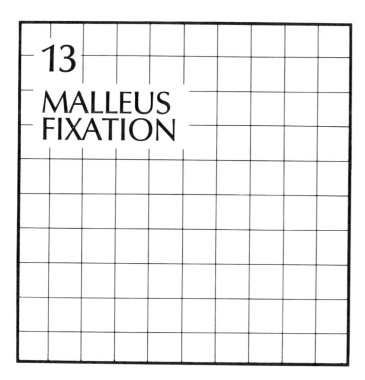

13
MALLEUS FIXATION

DESCRIPTION

Fixation of the malleus characteristically refers to an unusually firm attachment between the malleus and incus or between the malleus and roof or walls of the epitympanum. The malleus fixation may be congenital or acquired. Fixation may result from abnormal development, new bony growth, fibrous tissue, and/or soft tissue changes, such as calcification of the ligaments. Fixation of the malleus may occur as a consequence of chronic middle ear infection, trauma, surgical injury, or mechanical irritation between the malleus and epitympanic walls. On occasion, the fixation may appear to be of idiopathic origin. Malleus fixation may occur in conjunction with incus fixation, external ear abnormalities, discontinuity of the ossicular chain, and stapes fixation. In patients with malleus fixation and stapedial otosclerosis, the malleus fixation is generally not attributed to malleal otosclerosis, but to secondary formations resulting from mechanical irritations due to displacement of the ossicular chain, etc. (Goodhill, 1966).[1]

PATIENT CHARACTERISTICS

In patients with malleus fixation without concomitant stapes fixation due to otosclerosis, the onset of hearing loss usually occurs between 10 and 40 years of age

1. Fixation of the malleus and/or incus is reported in about 0.5% to 3.5% of patients undergoing middle ear surgery for the first time. Of these individuals, about 65% to 75% of patients have concomitant otosclerosis.

The incidence of malleus and/or incus fixation is increased in patients with a history of stapedectomy operations or congenital ear deformities. More specifically, epitympanic fixations occur in about 14% of patients that have previously undergone stapedectomies (Sleeckx et al., 1967).

In 16 patients with congenital middle ear deformities, the malleus was fixed in 38% of individuals (Scheer, 1967).

2. In a series of 18 patients with malleus or incus fixation without stapes fixation, the condition was unilateral in 94% of individuals (Sleeckx et al., 1967). A distinction between malleus fixation and stapes fixation due to otosclerosis is that the stapes condition is characteristically bilateral.

3. In conductive hearing loss, a rising audiometric contour may be referred to as a "stiffness tilt."

4. In human temporal bones, fixation of either the head of the malleus or the anterior crus of the stapes produces low frequency transmission loss. In contrast, fixation of the incudomalleal joint does not alter pure tone transmission at any frequency (Elpern et al., 1965). This latter observation may be due to the naturally rigid, interlocking position of the incudomalleal joint in man (Coats and Alford, 1977).

5. The possibility of a sensorineural component, particularly at high frequencies, is dramatized by a report (Goodhill, 1966) of two individuals with surgically confirmed fixed malleus syndrome who had sensorineural, rather than conductive or mixed, loss at all frequencies.

6. In patients with epitympanic fixation, the occurrence

(Guilford and Anson, 1967). Some affected persons report a family history of hearing loss. A sex ratio for malleus fixation is unreported. The condition is characteristically unilateral.[2]

CLINICAL COURSE

Slow, gradually progressive conductive or mixed hearing loss. However, in patients with traumatic malleus fixation, the onset of auditory symptoms is characteristically abrupt. The hearing loss may be accompanied by tinnitus. Treatment may involve reconstructive surgery of the middle ear.

SITE OF DISORDER

Middle ear.

GENERAL AUDIOLOGIC PATTERN

Pure tone sensitivity results characteristically show conductive or mixed hearing loss. The degree of loss is usually between 40 and 60 dB HL. The audiometric configuration is generally rising with greater loss in the low and mid frequency regions than in the high frequency region.[3] As a general rule, pure tone sensitivity results are similar to auditory findings in patients with fixation of the stapes due to otosclerosis.[4]

In some patients with malleus fixation, the rising audiometric contour may not stabilize above 1000 or 2000 Hz. Instead, pure tone sensitivity results may show greater loss for both the low and high frequency regions than for the mid frequency region. The audiogram in these patients shows a relatively rising contour to approximately 2000 Hz, then a downwardly sloping configuration. The sensitivity loss in the high frequency region may appear to be mixed or primarily sensorineural, rather than conductive, in nature.[5]

Maximum speech intelligibility scores are typically within normal limits, even in patients with some apparent high frequency sensorineural loss.

Impedance results characteristically show an abnormal tympanogram consistent with extreme restriction of mobility of the middle ear system. Static compliance measures are usually reduced.[6] Acoustic reflexes are typically abnormal with sound or probe to the affected ear. The reflex pattern may be char-

of tympanic membrane perforations and/or Eustachian tube patency may influence results of impedance audiometry. For a description of impedance results in the presence of these two abnormalities, see patient 1, Chapter 3, Cholesteatoma.

acterized by an inverted L-shaped configuration. Reflexes are normal only for uncrossed stimulation (sound and probe to the same ear) on the uninvolved ear.

Illustrative Patients

CASE 1. A 31-YEAR-OLD FEMALE WITH FIXATION OF THE MALLEUS AND INCUS ON THE LEFT EAR.

Surgical Findings

Upon surgical exploration of the middle ear, the malleus and the incus were immovable on palpation. The attic seemed foreshortened and filled with cortical bone. The middle ear was otherwise normal in appearance. There was no evidence of stapedial otosclerosis. The stapes appeared freely mobile.

History

The patient complains of a gradually progressive hearing loss in the left ear for approximately 10 months. For the past 2 months, she has noticed a feeling of fullness in the left ear. Approximately 6 years ago, she experienced a transient hearing loss in her left ear that resolved without medical attention. She does not have any hearing complaints about her right ear. She recalls frequent ear infections and temporary hearing loss during childhood.

On otorhinolaryngologic examination, the left tympanic membrane is noted to be unusually thin in the middle portion and unusually thick around the annulus. General tympanic membrane landmarks cannot be identified. The remainder of the examination is within normal limits.

Results

The audiogram (Case 13-1A) shows normal pure tone sensitivity on the right ear and a severe conductive loss on the left ear. The PTA scores (Case 13-1B) are 3 dB HL on the right ear and 65 dB HL on the left ear. Unmasked bone conduction thresholds (Case 13-1A) on the right ear are essentially superimposed on air conduction sensitivity. Masked bone conduction thresholds on the left ear show a conductive component of about 60 dB.[7]

The Weber test (Case 13-1B) at 500 Hz lateralizes to the left ear. The Bing test (not shown) at 500 Hz on the left ear shows no

7. In our Audiology Service, bone conduction measures are routinely obtained from the frontal bone. Bone vibrator placement seems critical in patients with malleus fixation. In these patients, bone conduction thresholds from the mastoid may be depressed relative to frontal bone conduction measures. A difference between mastoid and frontal bone conduction thresholds emphasizes the possible influence of mechanical middle ear

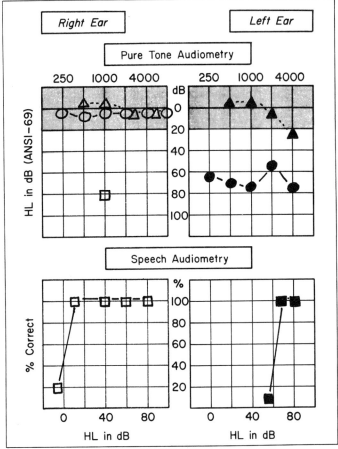

Case 13-1A

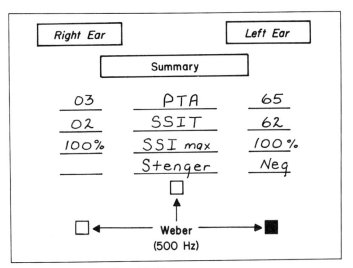

Case 13-1B

effects on bone conduction results. Postoperative air conduction sensitivity is best predicted by frontal bone conduction thresholds (Dirks and Malmquist, 1969).

benefit from occlusion. Bing results on the right ear could not be obtained because bone conducted signals at 500 Hz were heard in the non-test ear, even with maximum masking.

The PI-SSI functions (Case 13-1A) show normal maximum intelligibility scores of

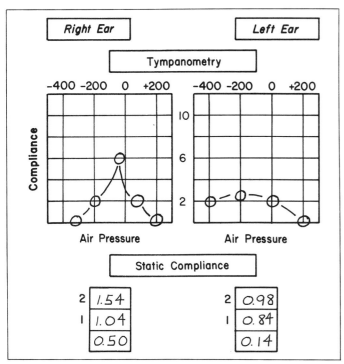

Case 13-1C

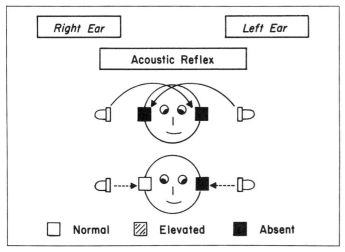

Case 13-1D

with sound to the left ear (Case 13-1A) are absent at all frequencies. With sound to the right ear, crossed reflexes are absent at 250 Hz through 4000 Hz. The uncrossed reflex at 1000 Hz, however, is within normal limits. The reflex pattern (Case 13-1D) is characterized by an inverted L-shaped configuration. Results suggest a combined probe effect (vertical pattern) and sound effect (diagonal pattern) on the left ear. Results are consistent with a moderate to severe conductive loss on the left ear. SPAR and reflex decay measures could not be evaluated on either ear.

Impression

RIGHT EAR: Normal pure tone sensitivity.

LEFT EAR: Severe conductive loss. Impedance audiometry is consistent with a middle ear disorder characterized by restricted mobility of the ossicular chain.

CASE 2. A 58-YEAR-OLD MALE WITH FIXATION OF THE MALLEUS AND INCUS ON THE RIGHT EAR.

Surgical Findings

The malleus and incus were completely fixed in the epitympanum. The rigidity of the incudomalleal complex appeared to produce fixation of the lateral ossicular chain. Good stapedial mobility was demonstrated by pericrural footplate palpation. There was no evidence of otosclerosis.

History

The patient complains of a gradually progressive hearing loss in both ears for the past 10 years. On occasion, he notices a high pitched ringing sound bilaterally. He reports numerous recurrences of otitis media.

Otorhinolaryngologic examination reveals a very prominent malleus and a retraction pocket on the anterior portion of the tympanic membrane on the right and left ears. Findings on the right ear are more pronounced than findings on the left ear. The remainder of the otorhinolaryngologic examination is within normal limits.

Results

The audiogram (Case 13-2A) shows a mild conductive loss on both ears.[9] PTA scores (Case 13-2B) are 40 dB HL on the right ear and 30 dB HL on the left ear. Bone conduction and SAL audiometry (Case 13-2A) show

9. One year after the present audiologic evaluation, surgery on the left ear revealed an attic cholesteatoma adherent to the malleus with partial erosion of the head. Remember, both malleus fixation and cholesteatoma may occur as a consequence of long-term middle ear infection.

Notice the masked air conduction thresholds in the presence of symmetric air conduction sensitivity. Remember, in determining "when to mask," the difference between ears is defined by the signal intensity to the test ear versus the bone conduction sensitivity of the non-test ear.

8. Some clinicians suggest that patients with unilateral hearing loss should be routinely screened for the possibility of functional disorder. In this circumstance, the speech Stenger test is a quick, efficient screening procedure for establishing the probable presence or absence of a functional component.

100% bilaterally. Rollover is not observed on either ear. SSIT scores (Case 13-1B) on both ears agree with pure tone sensitivity results. SSIT scores are 2 dB HL on the right ear and 62 dB HL on the left ear. The speech Stenger test (Case 13-1B) is negative for a functional component on the left ear.[8]

Tympanometry and static compliance measures (Case 13-1C) on the right ear are within normal limits. On the left ear, however, the tympanogram is a rounded, type B, shape. Static compliance is abnormally low. Crossed and uncrossed acoustic reflexes

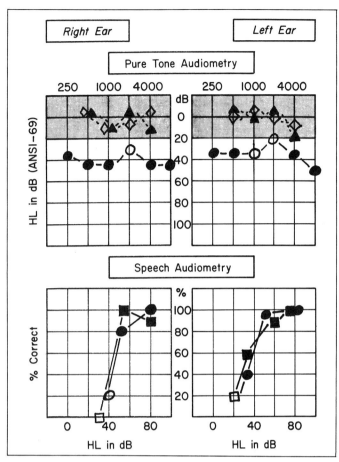

Case 13-2A

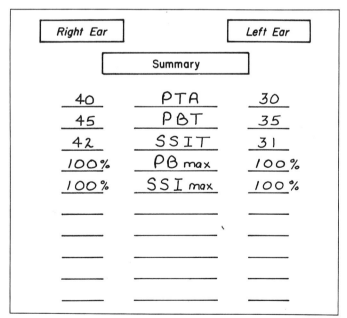

Case 13-2B

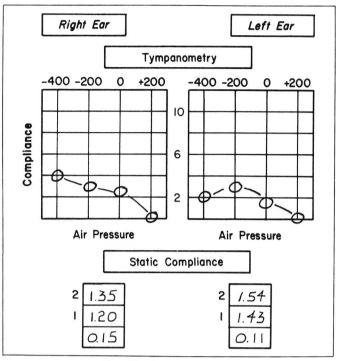

Case 13-2C

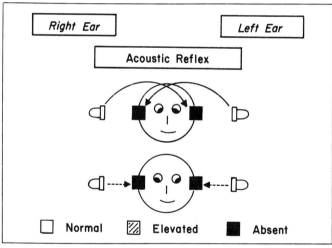

Case 13-2D

a conductive component of about 20 to 40 dB on both ears.

Speech audiometry (Case 13-2A) on both ears shows maximum intelligibility scores of 100% for both PB and SSI materials. Speech thresholds (Case 13-2B) agree with pure tone sensitivity results bilaterally. On the right ear, the PBT is 45 dB HL; the SSIT is 42 dB HL. On the left ear, the PBT is 35 dB HL; the SSIT is 31 dB HL.

Impedance audiometry (Case 13-2C) shows abnormal, type B, tympanograms on both ears. Static compliance measures are

10. Results in this patient illustrate the principle that audiometric test results may yield valuable information on the *site* of disorder (middle ear) but not on the *type* of disorder (malleus fixation on the right ear; cholesteatoma on the left ear). Notice also that impedance audiometry may yield important information on the *nature* of the conductive disorder (reduced mobility in both ears), but not on the *type* of disease process producing the altered middle ear function.

below normal limits bilaterally. Crossed and uncrossed acoustic reflexes (Case 13-2D) are absent at all frequencies on both ears.

Impression

Mild bilateral conductive hearing loss. Impedance audiometry on both ears is consistent with a middle ear disorder characterized by a type B tympanogram, reduced static compliance, and absent acoustic reflexes.[10]

SELECTED READINGS

Coats, A., and Alford, B. The Physiology of the Auditory and Vestibular Systems. In J. Ballenger (ed.), *Diseases of the Nose, Throat, and Ear.* Philadelphia: Lea & Febiger, 1977. Pp. 669–724.

Dirks, D., and Malmquist, C. Comparison of frontal and mastoid bone conduction thresholds in various conductive disorders. *J. Speech Hear. Res.* 12:729, 1969.

Elpern, B., Greisen, O., and Anderson, H. Experimental studies on sound transmission in the human ear. *Acta Otolaryngol.* 60:223, 1965.

Goodhill, V. External conductive hypacusis and the fixed malleus syndrome. *Acta Otolaryngol.* Suppl. 217:3, 1966.

Guilford, F., and Anson, B. Osseous fixation of the malleus. *Trans. Am. Acad. Ophthalmol. Otolaryngol.* 71:398, 1967.

Scheer, A. Correction of congenital middle ear deformities. *Arch. Otolaryngol.* 85:55, 1967.

Sleeckx, J., Shea, J., and Pitzer, F. Epitympanic ossicular fixation. *Arch. Otolaryngol.* 85:63, 1967.

Tos, M. Bony fixation of the malleus and incus. *Acta Otolaryngol.* 70:95, 1974.

viduals. The disease is rare in children.[2] The hearing loss is unilateral in approximately 80% of individuals. A hereditary predisposition for Meniere's disease may be indicated by occasional occurrences of episodic vertigo and hearing loss in families (Bernstein, 1965). A sex ratio for Meniere's disease is disputed.[3]

CLINICAL COURSE

The onset of Meniere's disease is typically characterized by a sudden episode of vertigo accompanied by nausea and vomiting. The onset of vertigo may be preceded by feelings of pressure or fullness in the ear. Briefly before or during the vertiginous episode, a loud roaring or ringing tinnitus may become apparent. Hearing sensitivity in the affected ear may decrease. However, information about hearing sensitivity during the vertiginous episode may be difficult to obtain because the symptoms of vertigo and loud, roaring tinnitus may be relatively more dramatic.

Following the acute episode, the vertigo may cease or subside into a sensation of unsteadiness. Feelings of unsteadiness may last for a period of days. The attack usually involves no neurologic symptoms other than those referable to the end organ. At the end of the attack, hearing sensitivity may improve. Tinnitus may lessen.

The initial attack of vertigo is characteristically followed by a period of remission. During this time, the patient may notice fluctuation in his hearing ability, in the tinnitus, and in the feelings of pressure or fullness within the ear. Subsequently, the above symptoms may be interrupted or exacerbated by another episode of spontaneous vertigo. The characteristic frequency of vertiginous attacks is variable among patients.

Gradually, a longer period of spontaneous or treatment-induced remission occurs. During remission, no symptoms may be noted other than a loss of hearing in the involved ear.[4] The clinical course is subsequently characterized by active periods of variable length interspersed with remission periods of variable length. Over time, the symptoms of vertigo, nausea, and vomiting tend to become less severe. In contrast, the hearing loss and tinnitus may become progressively worse (Haye and Quisthanssen, 1976).[5]

eas...
biochem...

sic symptoms of Meniere's disease are recurrent episodes of vertigo, fluctuating sensorineural hearing loss, and roaring tinnitus.

Histopathologic observations on temporal bones from individuals with Meniere's disease have consistently shown distention of the endolymphatic system. Dilatation of the membranous labyrinth may be accompanied by herniations, ruptures, fistulas, and/or total collapse. The organ of Corti appears normal in some specimens and abnormal in others (Kimura et al., 1976). In general, morphologic changes in the organ of Corti have been difficult to ascribe exclusively to Meniere's disease because similar changes may be found in non-Meniere's specimens, such as individuals with presbyacusis (Kimura et al., 1976).[1]

PATIENT CHARACTERISTICS

The initial onset of symptoms is between 40 and 60 years of age in about 50% of indi-

years of the disease and in individuals with fluctuating hearing threshold levels (Thomas and Harrison, 1971).

Although symptoms generally occur in a well-defined manner as described, variations in the clinical course occur in many individuals.

6. Although pure tone sensitivity tends to change in a well-defined manner as described, variations in the pattern of pure tone results may occur in many individuals.

In a series of 56 patients with Meniere's disease, 55% of individuals had a flat contour and 25% of persons had a rising configuration. The remaining patients had sloping or dome-shaped audiometric patterns (Dayal et al., 1970).

Treatment may involve drug therapy, diet modification, and/or surgery in patients with incapacitating and unsuccessfully treated vertiginous attacks.

SITE OF DISORDER

Cochlea.

GENERAL AUDIOLOGIC PATTERN

Pure tone sensitivity results characteristically show a unilateral, fluctuating sensorineural hearing loss. During the initial stages of Meniere's disease, the degree of loss may vary. However, over a period of years, the degree of loss usually progresses to a moderate to severe, permanent impairment. On rare occasions, a total loss of hearing may occur.

The audiometric configuration may vary with the time course of the disease. In the initial stages of Meniere's disease, the audiometric contour may be rising, with greater loss in the low frequency region than in the mid and high frequency regions. Subsequently, the audiometric configuration may change to a relatively flat contour with approximately the same degree of sensitivity loss at all frequencies. During a later stage of Meniere's disease, the audiogram may present a downwardly sloping configuration with greater loss in the high frequency region than in the low frequency region.[6]

Maximum speech intelligibility scores are usually reduced in a manner consistent with the degree and configuration of sensitivity loss.

Impedance results characteristically show normal, type A, tympanograms and normal static compliance measures. Acoustic reflexes are characteristically present at normal HLs and reduced sensation levels. No reflex decay is observed at 500 Hz or 1000 Hz.

In some patients with Meniere's disease, the loudness discomfort level or the intensity level where sounds are first reported as annoying, may occur at a reduced hearing level relative to the normal ear. Patients may report an intolerance to loud sounds. Consequently, auditory tests at loud intensity levels may not be obtainable. In addition, patients may complain of diplacusis or a difference of pitch sensation in the involved ear relative to the normal ear.

7. In Meniere's disease, exacerbation of symptoms may occur in some individuals under conditions of stress.

8. A glycerol test (Klockhoff, 1976) may be used in the diagnosis of Meniere's disease. Approximately 2½ hours after the ingestion of glycerol, patients with Meniere's disease may show temporarily improved pure tone sensitivity (at least 10 dB at 3 adjacent frequencies) and/or temporarily improved speech discrimination (at least 12%). Positive results (criteria in parentheses above) on a glycerol test indicate the presence of intralabyrinthine hydrops. Sensorineural losses of other origins do not improve after glycerol ingestion.

In some patients, electrocochleography may be a more sensitive indicator of cochlear changes secondary to glycerol dehydration than behavioral auditory tests (Moffat et al., 1978).

9. Notice how the two speech thresholds confirm a rising audiometric contour on the right ear. The speech threshold for PB words is consistent with high frequency

Illustrative Patients

CASE 1. A 26-YEAR-OLD MALE WITH MENIERE'S DISEASE ON THE RIGHT EAR.

History

The patient has a 5-year history of episodic vertigo accompanied by fluctuating tinnitus, hearing loss, and a feeling of fullness within the ear. Symptoms have been noticed on the right ear only. The patient's complaints have been satisfactorily relieved with medication therapy.

Recently, the patient changed jobs and moved to this city. His symptoms became more severe. He reports that his last episode of vertigo was accompanied by nausea and vomiting for the first time.[7]

This is the initial evaluation of this patient by the staff of the Neurosensory Center. Physical examination and neurologic evaluation are normal. X-rays of the internal auditory canal and skull are within normal limits. Computerized axial tomographic (CT) scanning shows no evidence of an intracranial mass lesion. The patient is presently referred for audiometric evaluation before and after the ingestion of glycerol.[8]

Results: Pre-glycerol Evaluation

The audiogram (Case 14-1A) on the right ear shows a mild sensorineural loss with a rising configuration. On the left ear, the audiogram shows normal pure tone sensitivity with the exception of a mild sensorineural loss at 8000 Hz. The PTA scores (Case 14-1B) are 39 dB HL on the right ear and −6 dB HL on the left ear. The Weber test (Case 14-1B) at 500 Hz lateralizes to the left ear.

Speech audiometry (Case 14-1A) on the right ear shows reduced maximum intelligibility scores for both PB words and SSI materials. The PB max score (Case 14-1B) is 80%; the SSI max score is 70%. The SSI function (Case 14-1A) shows mild rollover. On the left ear, PI-PB and PI-SSI functions are normal with 100% maximum intelligibility scores.

Speech thresholds (Case 14-1B) on both ears agree with average pure tone sensitivity results. On the left ear, the PBT is −3 dB HL; the SSIT is −6 dB HL. On the right ear, the PBT is 35 dB HL; the SSIT is 45 dB HL.[9]

Impedance audiometry (Case 14-1C) shows normal, type A, tympanograms and normal static compliance measures bilater-

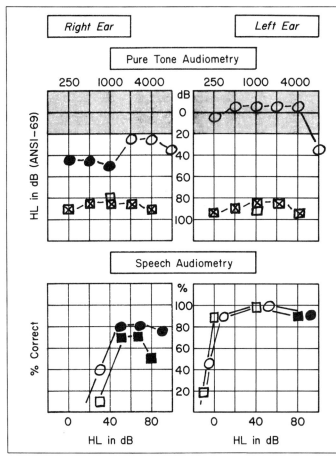

Case 14-1A. *Pre-glycerol evaluation.*

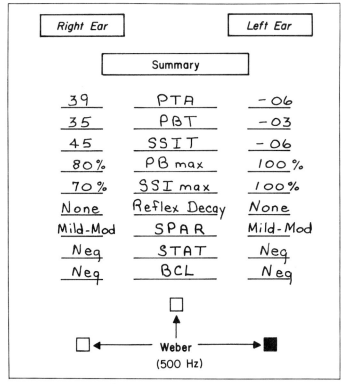

Case 14-1B

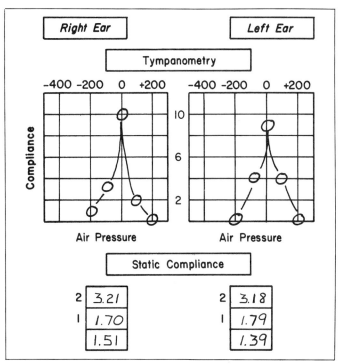

Case 14-1C

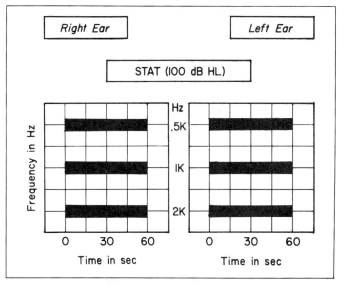

Case 14-1D

sensitivity levels. The speech threshold for SSI materials is consistent with low frequency sensitivity results.

10. On the right ear, notice the normal reflex HLs and reduced reflex sensation levels (SLs). For example, reflex HLs are 85 to 90 dB at all frequencies. How-

ally. Crossed and uncrossed acoustic reflexes (Case 14-1A) on both ears are present at normal HLs at all frequencies.[10] No reflex decay (Case 14-1B) is observed at 500 Hz or 1000 Hz on either ear. SPAR results predict a mild to moderate sensitivity loss at some audiometric frequency on both ears.

The STAT (Case 14-1D) is negative on both ears at all frequencies. BCL audiometry (Case 14-1E) yields a negative pattern on the right and left ears. Interrupted forward, con-

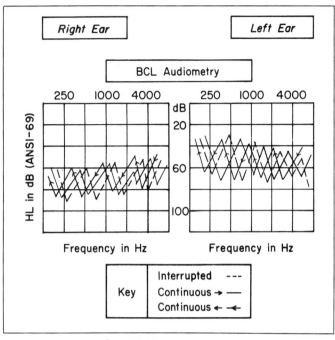

Case 14-1E

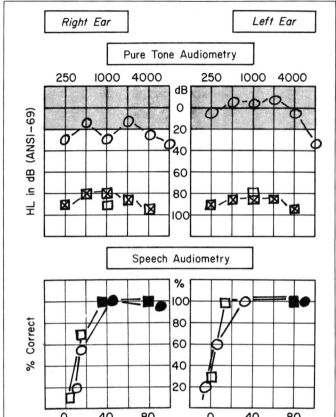

Case 14-1F. *Post-glycerol evaluation.*

Right Ear		Left Ear
	Summary	
18	PTA	−03
14	PBT	02
10	SSIT	03
100%	PB max	100%
100%	SSI max	100%

Case 14-1G

ever, reflex SLs are unusually small, ranging from only 35 dB at 1000 Hz to 65 dB at 4000 Hz. Normal reflex HLs and reduced reflex SLs are a hallmark of cochlear disorders.

tinuous forward, and continuous backward tracings are essentially superimposed across frequencies.

Impression

RIGHT EAR: Moderate sensorineural loss through 1000 Hz; mild sensorineural loss above 1000 Hz. Impedance audiometry indicates normal middle ear function. Diagnostic test results show no evidence of eighth nerve disorder. No abnormal adaptation is observed on STAT, BCL audiometry, or acoustic reflex testing.

LEFT EAR: Normal pure tone sensitivity with the exception of a mild sensorineural loss at 8000 Hz.

11. On the right ear, notice the substantial improvement in pure tone sensitivity at 250 Hz through 1000 Hz. For example, at 500 Hz, the pre-glycerol threshold is 45 dB; the post-glycerol threshold is 15 dB. Pure tone sensitivity results on the left ear are unchanged.

Post-glycerol Evaluation

Approximately 2 hours after the ingestion of glycerol, the audiogram (Case 14-1F) shows a mild sensorineural loss on the right ear. The audiogram on the left ear shows normal pure tone sensitivity except for a mild sensorineural loss at 8000 Hz.[11] The PTA scores (Case 14-1G) are 18 dB HL on the right ear and −3 dB HL on the left ear. Crossed and uncrossed acoustic reflexes (Case 14-1F) are present at normal HLs at all frequencies on both ears.[12]

Speech audiometry (Case 14-1F) on both ears shows normal maximum intelligibility scores (100%) for both PB words and SSI materials. Speech thresholds (Case 14-1G)

12. Notice that pure tone acoustic reflex thresholds on the right ear are essentially the same for

the pre- and post-glycerol evaluations. In contrast, the broadband noise reflex threshold on the right ear improved 10 dB relative to pre-glycerol results. An improvement in the noise reflex threshold but not pure tone reflex thresholds increased the absolute value of the SPAR measure. The predicted category of sensitivity loss did not change, however.

13. On the right ear, speech intelligibility performance improved 20% to 30% after the ingestion of glycerol. Speech thresholds improved about 20 dB to 35 dB relative to pre-glycerol results.

14. Improvement on pure tone and/or speech tests after glycerol ingestion may be observed in about 60% of individuals with Meniere's disease (Klockhoff, 1976).

agree with average pure tone sensitivity. On the right ear, the PBT is 14 dB HL; the SSIT is 10 dB HL. On the left ear, the PBT is 2 dB HL; the SSIT is 3 dB HL.[13]

Impression

RIGHT EAR: Mild sensorineural loss. Post-glycerol air conduction sensitivity is approximately 20 dB better than pre-glycerol sensitivity levels. Speech thresholds showed noticeable improvement. Maximum speech intelligibility scores increased to 100% for both PB words and SSI materials.[14]

LEFT EAR: Pure tone sensitivity and speech audiometry are essentially unchanged relative to pre-glycerol results.

CASE 2. A 37-YEAR-OLD FEMALE WITH MENIERE'S DISEASE ON THE RIGHT EAR.

History

Approximately 5 years ago, the patient had a sudden onset of vertigo, nausea, and vomiting. The vertigo subsided in about 8 hours. Approximately 2 weeks later, she experienced another vertiginous attack. During this episode, she noticed, for the first time, decreased hearing and a roaring tinnitus in her right ear. A physician in another city diagnosed her symptoms as Meniere's disease. She was treated with drug therapy. However, her symptoms continued. Approximately 3 years later, she underwent a surgical procedure for endolymphatic sac decompression on the right side. The surgery did not relieve her vertiginous attacks. Approximately 1 year later, drug therapy was resumed.

The present evaluation represents the patient's first visit to the Neurosensory Center, Houston. X-rays of the internal auditory canal and skull are normal. Brain scan and blood flow studies are within normal limits. EEG findings are normal. Otorhinolaryngologic and neurologic examinations are within normal limits, except for decreased hearing sensitivity on the right ear. At the initial evaluation, the patient complains of hearing loss and tinnitus in her right ear. She does not have any hearing complaints about her left ear.

Results

At the initial evaluation, the audiogram (Case 14-2A) shows a mild sensorineural loss with a rising configuration on the right

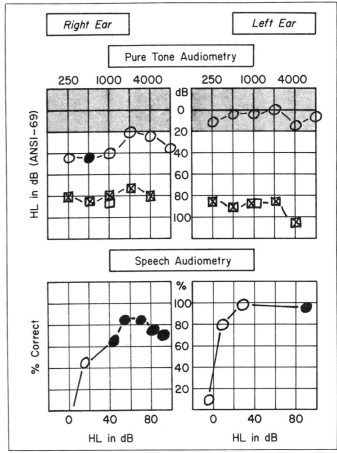

Case 14-2A

15. Remember, in patients with a rising audiometric contour, a difference between the PTA and PBT does not suggest the presence of a functional or nonorganic hearing disorder. Instead, the PTA vs PBT difference simply confirms the rising audiometric configuration. The PTA (36 dB HL) reflects the average loss at 500, 1000, and 2000 Hz. The PBT (24 dB HL) reflects the average loss at 2000 and 4000 Hz (Jerger and Jerger, 1976).

ear and normal pure tone sensitivity on the left ear. The PTA scores (Case 14-2B) are 36 dB HL on the right ear and 3 dB HL on the left ear.

The PI-PB function (Case 14-2A) on the right ear shows a reduced maximum intelligibility score and mild rollover. The PB max score (Case 14-2B) is 84%. The PBT score on the right ear, 24 dB HL, shows less sensitivity loss than the PTA score.[15] The PI-PB function (Case 14-2A) on the left ear is normal with a maximum intelligibility score of 100% correct. The PBT score, 2 dB HL, agrees with average pure tone sensitivity.

Impedance audiometry (Case 14-2C) shows normal, type A, tympanograms and normal static compliance measures bilaterally. Crossed and uncrossed acoustic reflexes (Case 14-2A) with sound to the right ear are present at normal HLs at all frequencies. With sound to the left ear, crossed and uncrossed acoustic reflexes are present at normal HLs at 250 Hz through 2000 Hz. However, the crossed reflex at 4000 Hz is elevated. No reflex decay (Case 14-2B) is

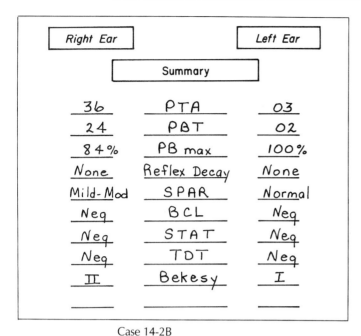

Case 14-2B

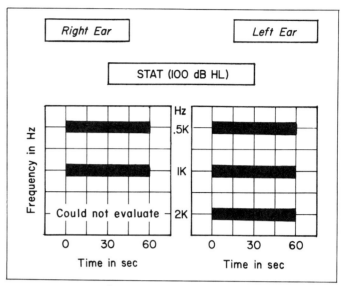

Case 14-2D

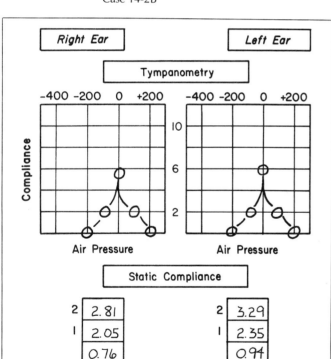

Case 14-2C

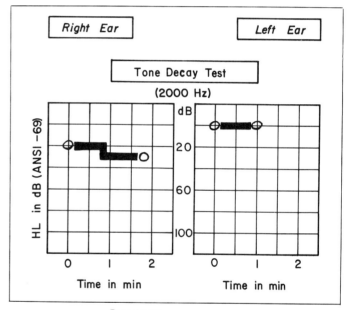

Case 14-2E

16. Recall that patients with Meniere's disease may have an intolerance for loud sounds. On STAT testing, sustained pure tone signals of 500 Hz and 1000 Hz at 100 dB HL did not seem to bother the patient. However, she refused to

observed at 500 Hz or 1000 Hz on either ear. The SPAR measure predicts a mild to moderate sensitivity loss on the right ear and normal sensitivity on the left ear.

The STAT at 500 Hz and 1000 Hz (Case 14-2D) and the threshold tone decay test at 500, 1000, and 2000 Hz (Case 14-2E) do not show abnormal adaptation on either ear.[16]

BCL audiometry (Case 14-2F) yields

tolerate a sustained 2000 Hz signal at 100 dB HL. When complete STAT results cannot be obtained, the threshold tone decay test becomes of increased benefit in determining the presence or absence of abnormal adaptation.

17. In a series of 172 patients with Meniere's disease who completed conventional threshold Bekesy audiometry, 94% had type II tracings and

negative results on both ears. Threshold Bekesy audiometry (Case 14-2G) shows a type II pattern on the right ear with no forward vs backward discrepancy. The Bekesy audiogram on the left ear is a type I pattern with interweaving forward and backward continuous tracings.[17]

Impression

RIGHT EAR: Moderate sensorineural loss through 1000 Hz; mild sensorineural loss above 1000 Hz. Diagnostic test results are most consistent with cochlear site. A cochlear disorder is supported by the presence of a type II Bekesy audiogram, acoustic reflex thresholds at normal HLs and

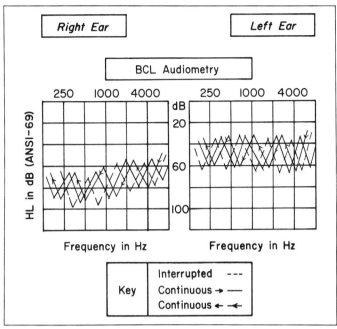

Case 14-2F

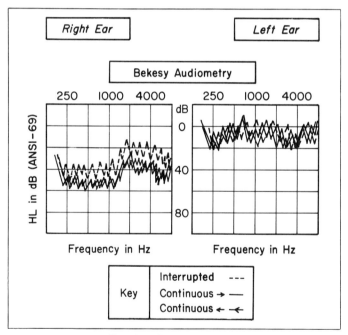

Case 14-2G

The attacks lasted 1 to 3 days at a time. They occurred at least monthly.

The patient underwent a vestibular nerve section on the right side. She was symptom-free for approximately 1 year. Now she is again noticing tinnitus in the right ear, feelings of imbalance and falling backward, and occasional mild episodes of rotational vertigo.

RESULTS. Case 14-2H presents two audiograms. Notice the results labeled "1." These findings were obtained at approximately the time the patient began to experience mild symptoms on the right ear after a relatively symptom-free year.

The audiogram ("1," Case 14-2H) shows a mild sensorineural loss on the right ear and normal pure tone sensitivity on the left ear. The PTA scores are 22 dB HL on the right ear and 3 dB HL on the left ear.[18]

PI-PB functions ("1," Case 14-2H) on both ears are normal. Maximum speech intelligibility scores are 96% on the right ear and 100% on the left ear.[19]

Impression

RIGHT EAR: Mild sensorineural loss with the exception of normal sensitivity at 2000 Hz and 4000 Hz. Pure tone results and speech intelligibility performance are slightly improved relative to previous findings.

LEFT EAR: Normal pure tone sensitivity. Results are unchanged from previous findings.

Audiologic Reevaluation

HISTORY. Approximately 2½ years later, the patient began to notice tinnitus and intermittent feelings of fullness in the left ear. This was the first time she had experienced any symptoms on the left ear. Approximately 1 month later, she noticed decreased hearing in the left ear. She thinks her hearing in the right ear is getting worse.

RESULTS. The audiogram (labeled "2," Case 14-2H) on the right ear shows a moderate sensorineural loss through 1000 Hz and a mild sensorineural loss above 1000 Hz. On the left ear, pure tone sensitivity is normal with the exception of a mild sensorineural drop at 250 Hz. The PTA scores are 42 dB HL on the right ear and 8 dB HL on the left ear.[20]

The PI-PB function ("2," Case 14-2H) is normal on the left ear, but shows a reduced

18. Notice that threshold sensitivity on the right ear is improved about 15 dB relative to results of the initial evaluation. Threshold sensitivity on the left ear is unchanged.

19. On the right ear, the PB max score is about 10% better than results of the initial evaluation.

20. Notice the decline in pure tone sensitivity on both ears. The right ear, after years of symptomatology, shows a decline of about 20 dB throughout the mid frequency range. The left ear, in the initial stages of symptomatology, shows a drop of 30 dB at 250 Hz only.

About 50% of patients eventually

6% had a type I pattern (Hedgecock, 1968).

reduced SLs, and a mild speech intelligibility loss. There is no evidence of abnormal adaptation on BCL audiometry, STAT, or threshold tone decay tests. No reflex decay is observed.

LEFT EAR: Normal pure tone sensitivity.

Audiologic Reevaluation

HISTORY. Approximately 7 months after the initial audiologic evaluation, the patient's vertiginous attacks became more severe.

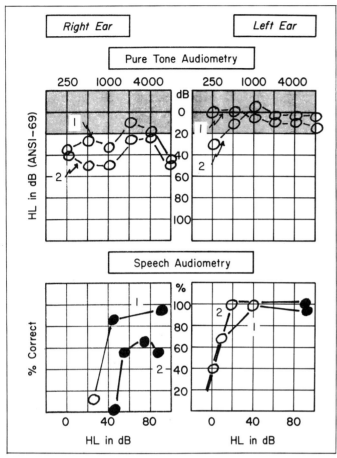

Case 14-2H. *Audiologic reevaluation 1½ years ("1") after the initial evaluation and approximately 4 years ("2") after the initial evaluation.*

vious results (Case 14-2A and "1," Case 14-2H). This finding highlights the possibility that speech discrimination may deteriorate to a greater degree than pure tone sensitivity in the later stages of Meniere's disease (Boles et al., 1975).

develop abnormal auditory symptoms on both ears. However, hearing sensitivity on the second ear may or may not be significantly impaired (Gibson, 1978).

In patients with bilateral Meniere's disease, about 50% of individuals have both ears affected simultaneously. In the remaining 50% of persons, the second ear may remain normal for many years (Friedmann, 1974).

21. Speech understanding ability on the right ear has declined more than 30% relative to pre-

maximum intelligibility score on the right ear. The PB max score is 100% on the left ear but only 64% on the right ear.[21]

Impression

RIGHT EAR: Moderate sensorineural loss through 1000 Hz; mild sensorineural loss above 1000 Hz. Pure tone sensitivity and speech intelligibility performance have declined relative to previous findings.

LEFT EAR: Normal pure tone sensitivity with the exception of a mild sensorineural loss at 250 Hz. A low frequency hearing loss is apparent for the first time. The maximum speech intelligibility score remains normal.

Comment

Diagnostic test results at this evaluation are unchanged from findings at the initial evaluation (see Case 14-2B).

SELECTED READINGS

Alford, B. Meniere's disease: Criteria for diagnosis and evaluation of therapy for reporting. *Trans. Am. Acad. Ophthalmol. Otolaryngol.* 86:683, 1977.

Alford, B., Cohn, A., and Igarashi, M. Current status of surgical decompression and drainage procedures upon the endolymphatic system. *Ann. Otol. Rhinol. Laryngol.* 86:683, 1977.

Bernstein, J. Occurrence of episodic vertigo and hearing loss in families. *Ann. Otol. Rhinol. Laryngol.* 74:1011, 1965.

Boles, R., Rice, D., Hybels, R., and Work, W. Conservative management of Meniere's disease. *Ann. Otol. Rhinol. Laryngol.* 84:513, 1975.

Dayal, V., Kane, N., and Mendelsohn, M. Patterns of pure tone hearing loss. A comparative study of presbyacusis, multiple sclerosis, Meniere's, and acoustic neuroma. *Acta Otolaryngol.* 69:329, 1970.

Friedmann, I. *Pathology of the Ear.* Oxford: Blackwell, 1974.

Gibson, W. The diagnosis and treatment of Meniere's disease. *Practitioner* 221:718, 1978.

Haye, R., and Quisthanssen, S. The natural course of Meniere's disease. *Acta Otolaryngol.* 82:289, 1976.

Hedgecock, L. Audiometric findings in Meniere's disease. *Otolaryngol. Clin. North Am* 1:489, 1968.

Jerger, J., and Jerger, S. Estimating speech threshold from the PI-PB function. *Arch. Otolaryngol.* 102:487, 1976.

Kimura, R., Ota, C., Schuknecht, H., and Takahashi, T. Electron microscopic cochlear observations in bilateral Meniere's disease. *Ann. Otol. Rhinol. Laryngol.* 85:791, 1976.

Klockhoff, I. Diagnosis of Meniere's disease. *Arch. Otorhinolaryngol.* 212:309, 1976.

Moffat, D., Gibson, R., Ramsden, R., Morrison, A., and Booth, J. Transtympanic electrocochleography during glycerol dehydration. *Acta Otolaryngol.* 85:158, 1978.

Shea, J. Definition of fluctuant hearing loss. *Otolaryngol. Clin. North Am.* 8:263, 1975.

Shea, J., and Bowers, R. Diagnosis and treatment of fluctuant hearing loss. *Otolaryngol. Clin. North Am.* 8:431, 1975.

Stahle, J., Stahle, C., and Arenberg, I. Incidence of Meniere's disease. *Arch. Otolaryngol.* 104:99, 1978.

Thomas, K., and Harrison, S. Long-term follow up of 610 cases of Meniere's disease. *Proc. R. Soc. Med.* 64:853, 1971.

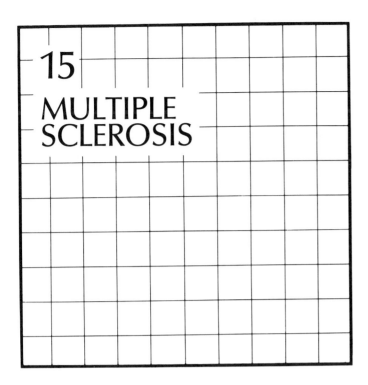

15
MULTIPLE SCLEROSIS

DESCRIPTION

1. The actual prevalence of MS is unknown. Estimates range from about 10 per 100,000 in the southern United States to about 50 to 75 per 100,000 in the northern United States.

Notice that the prevalence of MS varies geographically. MS is more common in cold and temperate climates than it is in the tropics and subtropics. An exception to this geographic pattern appears to exist in Japan, Africa, and Asia. In these countries, the occurrence of MS is uniformly low.

A survey of United States army veterans indicates that MS is less frequent in blacks than in whites (Kurtzke et al., 1975).

MS may be termed *disseminated* sclerosis or *insular* sclerosis.

Multiple sclerosis (MS) is a chronic, basically progressive disease of the central nervous system. Pathologically, a primary feature of MS is destruction of the myelin sheath (demyelinization) of nerve fibers. Sclerotic plaque formations may occur throughout the brain and spinal cord. The plaques are most numerous in the white matter of the cerebrum, brain stem, cerebellum, and spinal cord. Clinically, MS is characterized by episodes of localized central nervous system disorders. A cause(s) of MS is unknown.[1]

In individuals with MS, abnormalities of the auditory system may include disorders of the eighth nerve, brain stem, and temporal lobe. However, involvement of the cerebrum rarely occurs until a late stage of the disease (Merritt, 1963). Involvement of the eighth nerve is thought to be limited to the central nervous system portion of the nerve. In histologic studies of a 48-year-old woman with MS (Ward et al., 1965), the peripheral (neurilemmal) portion of the eighth nerve appeared normal. Demyelinating lesions appeared to be confined to the central (neuroglial) portion of the nerve.

PATIENT CHARACTERISTICS

The initial onset of symptoms occurs between 20 and 40 years of age in approxi-

mately 65% of patients. Onset of symptoms below the age of 10 and above the age of 60 is uncommon.

2. In three areas where MS is relatively rare (Hawaii, South Africa, and Western Australia), the female-to-male ratio is substantially changed, more than 2 : 1 (Acheson, 1977).

MS is more prevalent in females than in males. The disease tends to become apparent at a slightly earlier age in females than in males. The female-to-male ratio is approximately 1.4 : 1.[2]

Approximately 10% of patients with MS have another closely related member of the family affected with the disease. A hearing loss, if present, is bilateral in about 55% of individuals (Noffsinger et al., 1972).

CLINICAL COURSE

3. During the early stages of MS, patients may be thought to have acute labyrinthitis due to the transient episodes of vertigo and unsteadiness of gait (Merritt, 1963).

The initial onset of MS is characteristically acute. Initial symptoms vary depending on the foci of the central nervous system abnormality. Initial neurologic deficits may include paresthesia, a feeling of heaviness or deadness in the legs or one arm, diplopia, impaired vision, ataxia, or vertigo.[3]

The clinical course in about 60% of patients is subsequently characterized by periods of remission and exacerbation of symptoms (Merritt, 1963). In some individuals, remission of symptoms may last for as long as 2 years. In contrast to patients with a waxing and waning of symptoms, approximately 10% of patients develop a progressively downhill course from the onset (McDonald and Halliday, 1977). A progressive course is more frequent when the onset of symptoms is after 40 years of age (Merritt, 1963). The remaining about 30% of patients have a basically downhill course with intermittent periods of exacerbation and partial remission of symptoms.

As a rule, over the years, each exacerbation of symptoms in patients with MS leaves some evidence of a permanent neurologic deficit. Succeeding acute manifestations are superimposed on the previous permanent deficits.

4. In a series of 46 patients with a diagnosis of MS confirmed at autopsy, 52% had a history of euphoria, depression, or lability of mood (Merritt, 1963). Mental and/or emotional symptoms may complicate the audiologic evaluation of some patients.

5. In patients with MS, a commonly cited estimate of the

Classic symptomatology of MS may include visual problems, nystagmus, dysarthria, ataxia, bladder dysfunction, paraplegia, a weakness or spasticity of extremities, and alterations in emotional response.[4] Subjective auditory complaints are rare, occurring in less than 10% of individuals (Noffsinger et al., 1972).[5] The preferred treatment of MS varies.

prevalence of hearing loss (for at least one frequency) is about 50% of individuals. Estimates range from about 1% to 85% of persons (Noffsinger et al., 1972).

6. In studies of patients with hearing loss due to MS . . . PTA scores at 500, 1000, and 2000 Hz were within normal limits (≤25 dB HL) in 88% of ears (Noffsinger et al., 1972) . . . the audiometric contour was downwardly sloping with greater loss in the high frequency region in about 65% of patients (Dayal et al., 1970) . . . the degree of loss at impaired frequencies was mild in about 60% of ears, moderate in about 20% of ears, and severe in about 20% of ears (Noffsinger et al., 1972).

7. In a series of patients with MS, about 20% of individuals showed unusual performance deficits for degraded monotic PB word materials relative to unaltered PB word performance. The performance deficits were unilateral in about 85% of persons (Noffsinger et al., 1972).

SITE OF DISORDER

Eighth nerve and/or auditory pathways at the level of the brain stem. In patients with a relatively late stage of MS, a temporal lobe disorder may be apparent. An exception involves patients with normal auditory function and no apparent retrocochlear involvement.

GENERAL AUDIOLOGIC PATTERN

Pure tone sensitivity results may vary widely in patients with MS. As a broad rule of thumb, pure tone sensitivity results characteristically show a bilateral, sensorineural hearing loss for at least one frequency. The degree of loss is generally mild. The audiometric contour frequently shows a sloping configuration with greater high frequency loss than low and mid frequency loss. A notable exception, however, is the patient with normal pure tone sensitivity or with low frequency sensitivity loss.[6]

Maximum speech intelligibility scores for monosyllabic (PB) words are generally within normal limits. However, some patients may show abnormal PI-PB functions with an unusually slow rise to maximum performance and rollover at loud intensity levels.

In contrast to the characteristically normal performance on routine speech intelligibility tests, performance for degraded speech intelligibility tests may be strikingly abnormal. Speech signals may be degraded by filtering, temporal alteration, and competing noise or speech messages. In general, patients with a disorder at the level of the eighth nerve or brain stem show greater performance deficits for degraded monotic speech tasks than for difficult dichotic speech messages. Unusual performance deficits on degraded monotic speech tasks may be observed on one ear only or on both ears.[7]

Impedance audiometry characteristically shows normal tympanograms, normal static compliance measures, and abnormal acoustic reflexes. Reflex abnormalities may include reduced amplitudes, abnormal temporal patterns, or elevated or absent threshold measures.

Reflex threshold abnormalities may be characterized by a diagonal or horizontal pattern. In the diagonal configuration, crossed and uncrossed acoustic reflexes are

8. In 3 of 4 patients with reflex recovery, threshold HLs returned to normal limits at 500 Hz and 1000 Hz, but remained abnormally elevated at 2000 Hz and 4000 Hz (Bosatra et al., 1975).

9. Of 88 patients with MS, abnormal amplitude and/or latency measures for wave V on ABR audiometry were observed in 79% of persons with neurologic evidence of a brain stem lesion and in 51% of individuals without other neurologic evidence of a brain stem lesion (Robinson and Rudge, 1977).

abnormal with sound to the affected ear. In the horizontal pattern, reflexes on both ears are abnormal in the crossed condition and normal in the uncrossed condition. The diagonal pattern is consistent with eighth nerve site; the horizontal pattern is consistent with an intraaxial brain stem disorder.

During periods of remission, pure tone sensitivity and speech intelligibility performance for degraded speech tasks may return to within the normal range. Acoustic reflex measures may show systematic recovery. However, improvement of reflex measures may be delayed relative to improvement of pure tone sensitivity. In some patients, reflex thresholds may not recover to within normal limits at all frequencies.[8]

Other abnormalities associated with MS may include deficits on masking level difference (MLD) tasks; adaptation tests such as Bekesy audiometry, STAT and TDT; and auditory brain stem evoked response (ABR) audiometry.[9] In general, abnormality on auditory tests is more likely to be observed in patients with apparently widespread central nervous system involvement.

DIAGNOSIS OF MS

Currently, there is no specific diagnostic test for MS. Instead, the diagnosis of MS is generally a clinical judgment. For a clinical diagnosis of MS, some physicians require that periods of exacerbation and remission be documented or that lesions at two or more distinct sites within the central nervous system be demonstrated (Poskanzer and Adams, 1974). As a consequence, a diagnosis of MS is rarely made at the time of the first patient evaluation (Merritt, 1963).

The following three patients represent three different stages in the clinical course of MS. In the first two patients, a clinical diagnosis of MS was not made at the time of the audiologic evaluation. The first patient, a 26-year-old male, represents an initial early stage of MS. He has approximately a 3-week history of neurologic signs and symptoms. The second patient, a 32-year-old female, represents an intermediate early stage of MS. She has approximately a 2-year history of neurologic symptomatology.

In the third patient, a 29-year-old male, a clinically definite diagnosis of MS was made before the time of the audiologic evaluation.

He had about a 4-year history of central nervous system symptomatology. His clinical course was characterized by periods of exacerbation and partial remission.

Illustrative Patients

CASE 1. A 26-YEAR-OLD MALE WITH MS.

History

The patient reports an intermittent ringing tinnitus in the right ear for several years. About 3 weeks ago, the loudness of the tinnitus increased, accompanied by episodes of lightheadedness and disequilibrium. At this time, the patient noticed particular difficulty understanding conversations on the telephone with his right ear. During the next few days, he experienced numbness on the right side of his lower face and on the tip of his tongue.

Neurologic examination is consistent with involvement of cranial nerves five, seven, and eight on the right side. Facial nerve studies reveal mild facial nerve dysfunction on the right side. No weakness of the facial musculature is apparent, however. The Romberg test is positive with a tendency to fall to the right. X-rays of the internal auditory canals, computerized axial tomographic (CT) scanning, vertebral angiograms, and EEG findings are within normal limits. The patient does not have any hearing complaints about his left ear.

Results

The audiogram (Case 15-1A) shows an apparent low frequency sensorineural loss on the right ear and normal pure tone sensitivity on the left ear. The PTA scores (Case 15-1B) are 17 dB HL on the right ear and −2 dB HL on the left ear.[10] Bone conduction thresholds (Case 15-1A) are superimposed on air conduction thresholds bilaterally.

The PI-PB and PI-SSI functions (Case 15-1A) are normal on the left ear, but show substantial rollover on the right ear. PB max and SSI max scores (Case 15-1B) on the left ear are normal (100%). On the right ear, the PB max score is normal (92%), but SSI max performance is unusually reduced (60%).[11]

Speech thresholds agree with average pure tone sensitivity measures bilaterally. On the right ear, the PBT is 17 dB HL; the SSIT is 20 dB HL. On the left ear, the PBT is −2 dB HL; the SSIT is 3 dB HL.

10. On the right ear, notice the profound sensitivity loss at 250 Hz. An unusual low frequency loss has been a predominant finding in patients with MS for at least 45 years (Mygind, 1933).

11. On the right ear, a PB max vs SSI max difference of 32% coupled with rollover of the PI functions suggests further tests for the evaluation of retrocochlear site.

Notice that PB word testing at a single intensity level of 40 dB above the speech threshold may have shown normal performance

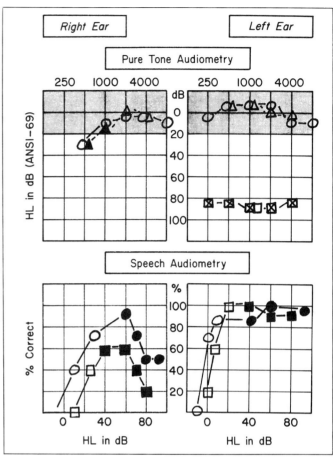

Case 15-1A

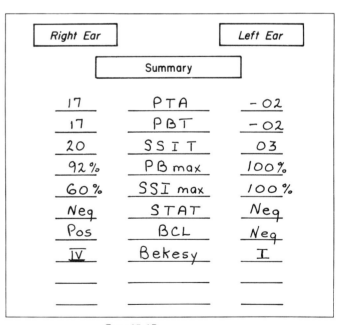

Case 15-1B

112

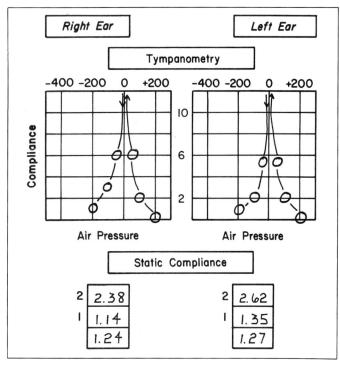

Case 15-1C

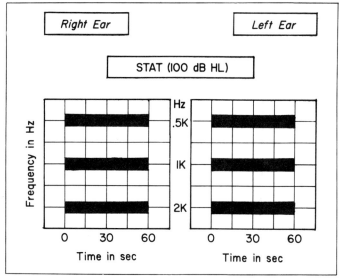

Case 15-1E

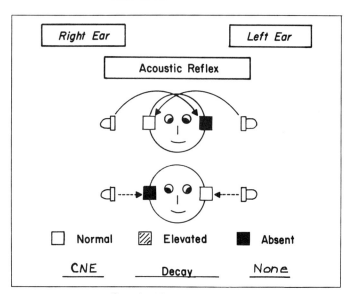

Case 15-1D

and no suggestion of retrocochlear disorder on the right ear.

12. Remember, the presence of type A_D tympanograms and no air-bone gap (Case 15-1A) suggests the possibility of unusually flaccid tympanic membranes, rather than discontinuity of the ossicular chain.

Tympanometry (Case 15-1C) shows unusually deep, type A, tympanograms on both ears.[12] Static compliance measures are within normal limits bilaterally. Crossed and uncrossed acoustic reflexes (Case 15-1A) with sound to the right ear are absent at equipment limits at all frequencies. With sound to the left ear, crossed and uncrossed reflexes are present at normal HLs at all frequencies. The reflex pattern (Case 15-1D) is characterized by a diagonal configuration.

13. On the right ear, notice that threshold Bekesy and BCL tracings start at 500 Hz, rather than 250 Hz. Remember, with masking to the left ear, this patient did not respond to 250 Hz signals at equipment limits.

Reflex decay testing on the left ear at 500 Hz and 1000 Hz is within normal limits. The reflex decay test could not be administered on the right ear.

The STAT (Case 15-1E) does not show abnormal adaptation at any frequency on either ear. BCL audiometry (Case 15-1F) yields a positive pattern on the right ear and negative results on the left ear. Conventional threshold Bekesy audiometry (Case 15-1G) is a type IV tracing on the right ear with a forward vs backward discrepancy. The Bekesy audiogram on the left ear is a type I pattern with interweaving continuous forward vs backward tracings.[13]

Impression

RIGHT EAR: Sensorineural loss at 250 Hz and 500 Hz; normal pure tone sensitivity above 500 Hz. Diagnostic test results are consistent with eighth nerve site. An eighth nerve disorder is indicated by abnormal adaptation on BCL audiometry and conventional threshold Bekesy audiometry, absent acoustic reflexes with sound to the right ear, unusually poor maximum intelligibility score on PI-SSI testing, and abnormal rollover of the PI-PB and PI-SSI functions.

LEFT EAR: Normal pure tone sensitivity.

CASE 2. A 32-YEAR-OLD FEMALE WITH MS.

History

Approximately 2 years ago, the patient noticed a weakness of the left arm, visual

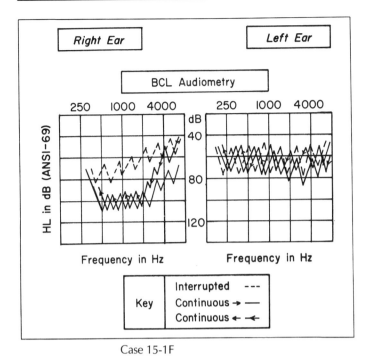

Case 15-1F

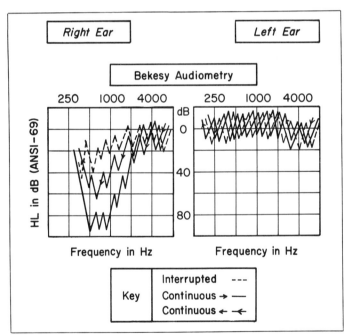

Case 15-1G

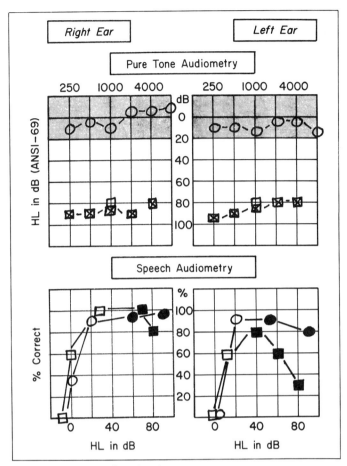

Case 15-2A

difficulties, and dizziness. The symptoms have gradually worsened. At this time, she complains of a progressive weakness of the left arm and leg, a tingling-type sensation (paresthesia) on the left side of the body, an impaired sensation of touch (dysesthesia) on the left side, episodes of jerking-type movements of the thumb and fingers on the left hand, diplopia, and dizziness. She has no nausea, vomiting, or headaches.

14. Some patients with central auditory disorder may notice a hearing problem for the first time when using a telephone on the affected ear (see Comment, Chapter 2, Cerebrovascular Disorders).

Neurologic examination notes left hemiparesis, hyperreflexia, left extensor plantar reflex, spastic gait, and bilateral weakness on upward gaze. Right carotid and left vertebral angiograms, skull x-rays, and EEG findings are within normal limits.

The patient does not notice any hearing problem on either ear. However, on structured questioning, the patient admits difficulty hearing on the telephone with her left ear.[14]

Results

The audiogram (Case 15-2A) shows normal pure tone sensitivity on both ears. The PTA scores (Case 15-2B) are 3 dB HL on the right ear and 9 dB HL on the left ear.

Speech audiometry (Case 15-2A) on the right ear shows essentially normal PI functions for both PB word and SSI materials. The PB max score (Case 15-2B) is 96%; the SSI max score is 100%. PI functions (Case 15-2A) on the left ear show a slight difference between PB max and SSI max perfor-

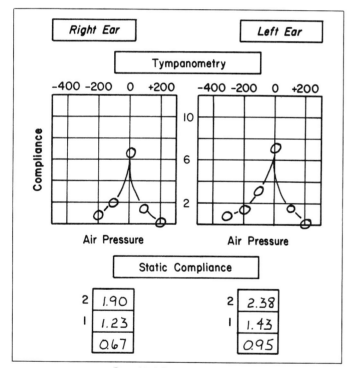

Right Ear		Left Ear
	Summary	
03	PTA	09
06	PBT	12
−02	SSIT	10
96%	PB max	92%
100%	SSI max	80%
None	Reflex Decay	None
63%	SSI - ICM	37%
100%	SSI - CCM	100%

Case 15-2B

Right Ear   **Left Ear**

Tympanometry

Static Compliance

2	1.90		2	2.38
1	1.23		1	1.43
	0.67			0.95

Case 15-2C

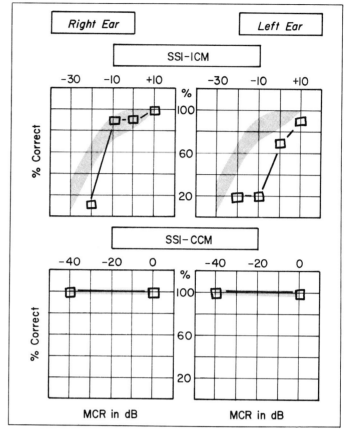

Right Ear   **Left Ear**

SSI-ICM

% Correct

SSI-CCM

% Correct

MCR in dB   MCR in dB

Case 15-2D

shows normal, type A, tympanograms and normal static compliance measures bilaterally. Crossed and uncrossed acoustic reflexes (Case 15-2A) are present at normal HLs at all frequencies. Reflex decay testing (Case 15-2B) at 500 Hz and 1000 Hz is normal on both ears. Results do not show any decline in reflex amplitude during a 10-sec test period.

SSI-ICM scores (Case 15-2D) are essentially normal on the right ear but show unusually poor performance on the left ear at all message-to-competition ratios (MCRs). Average SSI-ICM performance (Case 15-2B) is 63% on the right ear and 37% on the left ear. In contrast to SSI-ICM performance, SSI-CCM performance (Case 15-2D) is normal on both ears. SSI-CCM scores (Case 15-2B) are 100% at all test conditions.

Impression

Pure tone sensitivity within normal limits bilaterally. Impedance audiometry is consistent with normal middle ear function on both ears. Diagnostic test results indicate a

over. Without PI-SSI functions, the patient's performance is remarkably unsuspicious.

In a series of 61 patients with MS, PB max scores were at least 90% in about 90% of individuals (Noffsinger et al., 1972).

mance and severe rollover of the SSI function. The PB max score (Case 15-2B) is 92%; the SSI max score is 80%.

Speech thresholds on both ears agree with average pure tone sensitivity. On the right ear, the PBT is 6 dB HL; the SSIT is −2 dB HL. On the left ear, the PBT is 12 dB HL; the SSIT is 10 dB HL.[15]

Impedance audiometry (Case 15-2C)

15. Notice that the possibility of a central auditory disorder is suggested by a slight difference in PB max vs SSI max scores and SSI roll-

16. Remember, in patients with abnormal speech findings on one ear only, the site of the brain stem disorder is usually opposite the ear yielding the abnormal results (Jerger, 1973).

central auditory disorder involving the brain stem auditory pathways on the right side.

A brain stem site is supported by a substantial SSI-ICM performance deficit in the presence of normal SSI-CCM performance. Performance deficits on the left ear indicate a disorder on the opposite, right, side of the brain stem.[16] The possibility of eighth nerve involvement is rendered unlikely by the normal, relatively symmetric pure tone sensitivity, relatively normal acoustic reflex thresholds, and no reflex decay.

CASE 3. A 29-YEAR-OLD MALE WITH MS.

History

17. In a late stage of MS, nystagmus, intention tremor, and scanning speech may appear. This triad of signs may be referred to as *Charcot's triad* (Merritt, 1963).

This patient has a 4-year history of MS. The patient's first symptoms were diplopia, blurred vision, and right facial numbness. During subsequent exacerbations, he has complained of weakness of all four extremities, incoordination, intention tremor, difficulty with balance, numbness and tingling of the body, urinary problems, blurred vision, diplopia, dysarthria, and scanning speech.[17]

Presently, the patient's chief complaints are increased fatigue, slowed speech, dizziness, and clonus for the past 6 weeks. Neurologic examination reveals slight dysarthria, ataxic gait, and mild dysmetria of the upper extremities, greater on the right side. Plantar responses are extensor bilaterally. Clonic responses are noted in the ankles and knees. Reflexes in the upper extremities are hyperactive. Visual evoked responses show no recordable response to pattern stimuli with either binocular or monocular stimulation. Results are compatible with bilateral optic nerve dysfunction. The patient denies having any hearing problems on either ear.

Results

The audiogram (Case 15-3A) shows normal pure tone sensitivity on both ears. The PTA scores (Case 15-3B) are 8 dB HL on the right ear and 10 dB HL on the left ear. Unmasked bone conduction thresholds (Case 15-3A) do not show an air-bone gap on either ear.

18. Once again, on the right ear, notice the value of comparing PB max and SSI max scores as a screening procedure for possible retrocochlear disorder.

PI-SSI functions (Case 15-3A) show slightly reduced maximum intelligibility scores on both ears. The SSI max (Case 15-3B) is 80% on the right ear and 90% on the left ear. In contrast to SSI performance, maximum intelligibility scores for PB word materials are 100% on both ears.[18] No roll-

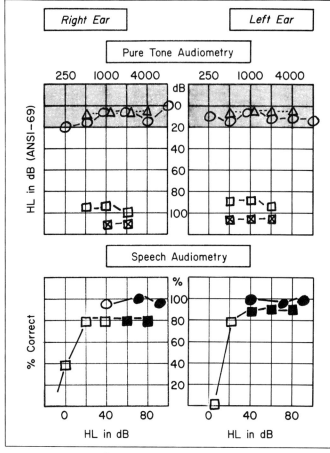

Case 15-3A

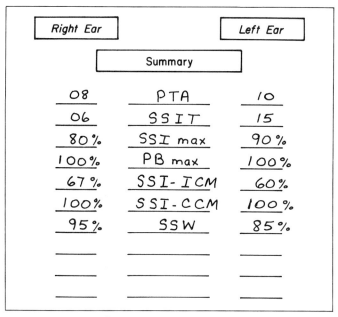

Right Ear		Left Ear
	Summary	
08	PTA	10
06	SSI IT	15
80%	SSI max	90%
100%	PB max	100%
67%	SSI-ICM	60%
100%	SSI-CCM	100%
95%	SSW	85%

Case 15-3B

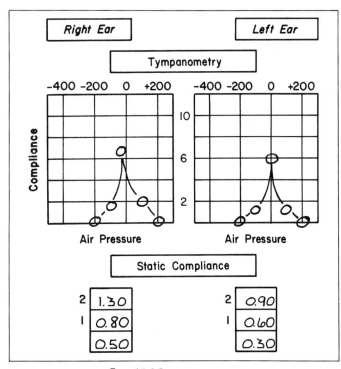

Case 15-3C

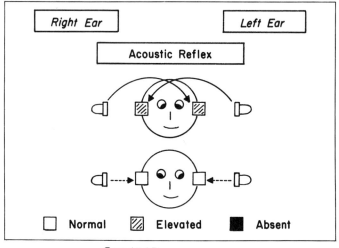

Case 15-3D

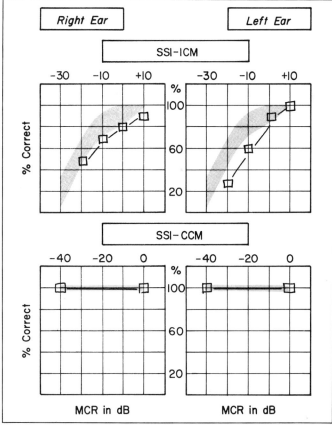

Case 15-3E

over is observed for either SSI or PB word tasks. The SSIT scores, 6 dB HL for the right ear and 15 dB HL for the left ear, agree with average pure tone sensitivity bilaterally.

Impedance audiometry (Case 15-3C) shows type A tympanograms and normal static compliance measures on both ears. Acoustic reflexes (Case 15-3A) on both ears are abnormally elevated in the crossed condition and present at normal HLs in the uncrossed condition. With sound to the right ear, crossed reflexes are absent at 250 Hz, 500 Hz, and 4000 Hz, and elevated at 1000 Hz and 2000 Hz. With sound to the left ear, crossed reflexes are absent at 250 Hz and 4000 Hz and elevated at 500 Hz, 1000 Hz, and 2000 Hz. In contrast, uncrossed reflexes on both ears are present at HLs within the normal range at 500 Hz, 1000 Hz, and 2000 Hz. Uncrossed reflex thresholds were not measured at 250 Hz and 4000 Hz. The reflex pattern (Case 15-3D) is characterized by a horizontal configuration. On both ears, reflex thresholds are elevated on crossed stimulation and within normal limits on uncrossed stimulation.[19]

SSI-ICM functions (Case 15-3E) show slightly reduced performance on both ears. Average SSI-ICM scores (Case 15-3B) are 67% on the right ear and 60% on the left

19. Acoustic reflex thresholds may be abnormal in about 30% to 70% of patients with MS (Bosatra et al., 1975; Coletti, 1975).

ear. SSI-CCM performance (Case 15-3E) is unimpaired on either ear. SSI-CCM scores (Case 15-3B) are 100% at all test conditions.

SSW results (Case 15-3B) are within normal limits for all test conditions on both ears. Average performance scores for the competing condition are 95% for the right ear and 85% for the left ear.

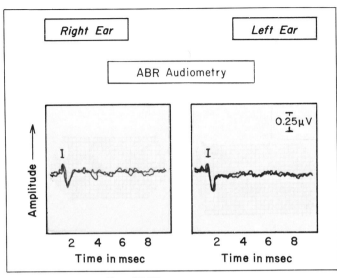

Case 15-3F

Auditory brain stem evoked response (ABR) audiometry yields no observable wave V response on either ear. As seen in Case 15-3F, ABR results showed a repeatable wave I on both ears at normal latencies. However, waves II through V were absent bilaterally. ABR results are consistent with bilateral brain stem auditory pathway involvement.

Impression

Pure tone sensitivity within normal limits bilaterally. Diagnostic test results are consistent with a central auditory disorder at the level of the brain stem. A brain stem disorder is supported by abnormal results on ABR audiometry and abnormal crossed acoustic reflexes in the presence of normal uncrossed reflexes (a horizontal configuration). Abnormal auditory findings are observed on both ears.[20]

sults may be normal (see patient 3, Chapter 12, Intracranial Tumors Affecting the Central Auditory System). This observation stresses the importance of a battery of test procedures for precise site prediction.

20. Notice that the SSI-ICM vs SSI-CCM procedure is not as helpful in this patient as ABR audiometry and acoustic reflex results. In other patients with brain stem site, however, the reverse may be true. Speech audiometric results may identify the presence of brain stem disorder and ABR results and acoustic reflex re-

SELECTED READINGS

Acheson, E. Epidemiology of multiple sclerosis. *Br. Med. Bull.* 33:9, 1977.

Bosatra, A., Russolo, M., and Poli, P. Modifications of the stapedius muscle reflex under spontaneous and experimental brain-stem impairment. *Acta Otolaryngol.* 80:61, 1975.

Coletti, V. Stapedius reflex abnormalities in multiple sclerosis. *Audiology* 14:63, 1975.

Dayal, V., Kane, N., and Mendelsohn, M. Patterns of pure tone hearing loss. *Acta Otolaryngol.* 69:329, 1970.

Jerger, J. Diagnostic Audiometry. In J. Jerger (ed.), *Modern Developments in Audiology.* New York: Academic Press, 1973. Pp. 75–115.

Kurtzke, J., Beebee, G., and Norman, J. Epidemiology of Multiple Sclerosis in the United States: Preliminary Data. Scientific Program of American Academy of Neurology, 27th Annual Meeting. May 1–3, 1975.

McDonald, W., and Halliday, A. Diagnosis and classification of multiple sclerosis. *Br. Med. Bull.* 33:4, 1977.

Merritt, H. *A Textbook of Neurology.* Philadelphia: Lea & Febiger, 1963. Pp. 670–692.

Mygind, S. Investigation of the aural function in certain brain diseases. *Acta Psychiatr. Neurol. Scand.* 8:173, 1933.

Noffsinger, D., Olsen, W., Carhart, R., Hart, C., and Sahgal, V. Auditory and vestibular aberration in multiple sclerosis. *Acta Otolaryngol.* Suppl. 303:1, 1972.

Percy, A., Nobrega, F., Okazaki, O., Glattre, E., and Kurland, L. Multiple sclerosis in Rochester, Minn. *Arch. Neurol.* 25:105, 1971.

Poskanzer, D., and Adams, R. Multiple Sclerosis and Other Demyelinating Diseases. In M. Wintrobe, G. Thorn, R. Adams, E. Braunwald, K. Isselbacher, and R. Petersdorf (eds.), *Harrison's Principles of Internal Medicine* (7th ed.). New York: McGraw-Hill, 1974. Pp. 1815–1821.

Robinson, K., and Rudge, P. Abnormalities of the auditory evoked potentials in patients with multiple sclerosis. *Brain* 100:19, 1977.

Von Leden, H., and Horton, B. Auditory nerve in multiple sclerosis. *Arch. Otolaryngol.* 48:51, 1948.

Ward, P., Cannon, D., and Lindsay, J. The vestibular system in multiple sclerosis. A clinical-histopathological study. *Laryngoscope* 75:1031, 1965.

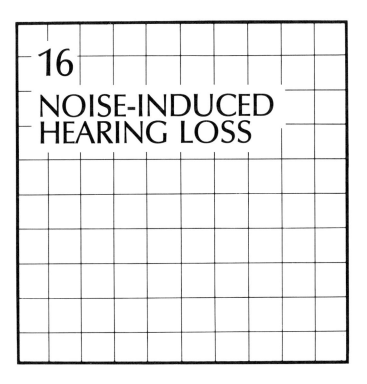

16

NOISE-INDUCED HEARING LOSS

DESCRIPTION

Exposure to noises of sufficiently high intensity may result in a temporary or permanent loss of hearing. The hearing loss may occur in two different ways: either from long-term exposure to a hazardous noise environment (noise-induced hearing loss) or from short-term exposure to a single blast of intense noise (acoustic trauma). The probability that a noise may damage hearing is related to the overall sound pressure level, the frequency spectrum, and the temporal pattern of a noise vs the duration of exposure. Tables of damage risk criteria (Kryter, 1970) describe the relation between noise environments and the probability of incurring hearing impairment.

Specific causes of noise-induced hearing loss and acoustic trauma are unknown. Hearing loss from acoustic trauma may be caused by exceeding the physiologic limits of the auditory system. The tympanic membrane may rupture. The ossicular chain may be dislocated. The organ of Corti may be partially or completely destroyed.[1] In contrast to acoustic trauma, hearing loss from habitual exposure to hazardous noise may be caused by microtrauma or metabolic, vascular, ischemic, and ionic disorders.[2]

Temporal bone findings in animals and humans with acoustic trauma or noise-induced hearing loss may range from mild swelling and condensation (pyknosis) of

1. Rupture of middle ear structures may be a safety valve mechanism that decreases the amount of energy transmitted to the cochlea.

2. In Denmark, noise-induced hearing loss occurs in about 28 per 100,000 individuals (Ewertsen, 1973). About 6% of military draftees in Norway have high frequency sensorineural dips (Bentzen, 1972).
   A United States

Public Health survey estimates that 10 million American industrial employees may have hearing loss due to hazardous noise exposure (Snow, 1976).

Fox (1977) estimates that about 40% of American industries have hazardous noise environments.

The Occupational Safety and Health Act and the Noise Control Act require the development of hearing conservation programs in industries with noise levels of greater than or equal to 90 dB (A) (see glossary).

After aging, noise is thought to be the second most common cause of sensorineural hearing loss (Gilad and Glorig, 1979).

3. In surveys of persons with noise-induced hearing loss, about 80% to 90% of individuals are males (Ewertsen, 1973; Surjan et al., 1973).

4. Recently, some clinicians have modified the idea that conductive hearing loss may be a built-in protection against the occurrence of noise-induced hearing loss. For example, in a series of patients with active middle ear infections, the conductive disorder seemed to precipitate, rather than delay, the appearance of a sensorineural loss (Tonndorf, 1976).

In persons with sensorineural hearing loss, powerful hearing aids may be a source of hazardous noise exposure (Macrae, 1968).

outer hair cells to a complete absence of the organ of Corti. Secondary degeneration of ganglion cells and nerve fibers may be observed. The abnormalities are typically more pronounced in the basal coil of the cochlea than in the apical region.

PATIENT CHARACTERISTICS

Acoustic trauma may occur at any age. In contrast, noise-induced hearing loss occurs primarily in adults. The incidence of noise-induced hearing loss is higher in males than in females.[3] The degree of loss tends to be more severe in males than in females (Gallo and Glorig, 1964). A difference between the sexes may reflect different susceptibility between males and females or may be related to differences in noise-exposure patterns.

In both sexes, large individual variations in susceptibility to noise-induced hearing loss occur. Reasons for individual variations are not clearcut. A person's susceptibility to hearing damage from noise may be influenced by illness, age, hereditary factors, and concomitant exposure to other agents such as drugs. Preexisting hearing loss may change an individual's susceptibility to noise- induced hearing loss. For example, in a hazardous noise environment, persons with preexisting conductive loss may be less susceptible to sensorineural damage than normal hearing persons. In contrast, individuals with preexisting sensorineural loss may be more susceptible to further sensorineural impairment than normal hearing persons.[4]

Hearing loss from acoustic trauma may be unilateral or bilateral. Noise-induced hearing loss is characteristically bilateral.

CLINICAL COURSE

The onset of hearing loss in acoustic trauma is characteristically instantaneous. In contrast, the onset of noise-induced hearing loss is characteristically insidious. In the latter circumstance, the clinical course is initially characterized by a temporary loss of hearing. A temporary hearing loss may be accompanied by a high pitched, ringing tinnitus, a feeling of fullness within the ear, and a sensation of "muffled" hearing.

During the initial stages of noise-induced hearing loss, the temporary hearing loss characteristically recovers within a few hours or a few days. Subsequently, however, if exposure to hazardous noise continues, the threshold shift may no longer show recovery. A permanent sensorineural hearing loss may occur. Subjective complaints of hearing loss are generally not reported by patients until a hearing loss of more than 25 dB HL (ANSI-69) occurs at a frequency below 3000 Hz.

Conventional methods for the conservation of hearing sensitivity may include ear plugs, semi-inserts, and ear muffs.[5] In addition to personal protection, noise-induced hearing loss may be controlled or prevented by modifying the noise environment.

SITE OF DISORDER

Cochlea. In some patients with acoustic trauma, the middle ear may be involved along with the cochlea.

GENERAL AUDIOLOGIC PATTERN

Pure tone sensitivity results characteristically show a bilateral, symmetric sensorineural hearing loss. The audiometric contour is generally a downwardly sloping configuration with greater loss in the high frequency region than in the low and mid frequency regions.

The degree of loss is usually progressive. For example, initial pure tone sensitivity results characteristically show a mild loss at a frequency(ies) between 3000 Hz and 6000 Hz. Usually, the maximum threshold sensitivity loss occurs at 4000 Hz.[6] With further noise exposure, the 4000 Hz notch may become deeper and wider. Finally, the high frequency hearing loss tends to stabilize at approximately 60 to 70 dB HL. Subsequently, the hearing sensitivity at lower frequencies may become impaired. A greater degree of hearing loss at high frequencies may occur.

Speech intelligibility results vary depending on the frequencies affected by the noise-induced hearing loss. When a hearing loss is confined to frequencies above 3000 Hz, maximum speech intelligibility scores are usually within normal limits. As the frequencies below 3000 Hz become involved, maximum speech intelligibility scores usually diminish in accordance with the degree of pure tone impairment.

Impedance audiometry characteristically shows normal, type A, tympanograms and normal static compliance measures. Acoustic reflexes are generally present at normal HLs for all frequencies. An exception may involve patients with steeply sloping audiometric contours. In these individuals, reflexes may be absent in the high frequency region even though the degree of high frequency sensitivity loss does not exceed 80 dB HL (ANSI-69).

COMPUTATION OF HEARING IMPAIRMENT

The American Academy of Ophthalmology and Otolaryngology has established standard methods for computing the degree of hearing impairment in individuals with unilateral and bilateral hearing loss (Snow, 1976). For computation of hearing impairment, hearing threshold measures should be obtained only after the patient has been removed from the noise environment for a sufficient period of time to minimize the occurrence of temporary threshold shifts. The Bureau of Employees Compensation recommends a 6-week period free of noise exposure before hearing tests are carried out.[7]

Illustrative Patient

CASE 1. A 34-YEAR-OLD MALE WITH NOISE-INDUCED HEARING LOSS ON BOTH EARS.

History

The patient's chief complaint is a constant ringing tinnitus in both ears for the past 2 weeks. He denies any difficulty hearing on either ear. He does not remember any previous serious illnesses, accidents, unusual or atypical drug use, or problems with his ears. He denies dizziness and nausea. For the past 5 years, the patient has been employed as an aircraft mechanic. He states that he wears hearing protective devices during his work. The patient is not exposed to other hazardous noises, such as gunfire. Information about the patient was obtained through a Spanish interpreter. The patient does not understand English.

Results

Case 16-1A presents results for two audiologic evaluations. Notice the results labeled "1." The audiogram ("1," Case 16-1A) shows normal pure tone sensitivity

5. Ear defenders are capable of attenuating most noises up to about 40 dB. However, in a survey of 126 textile mill workers, only about 45% of individuals routinely used the provided ear protectors (Flodgren and Kylin, 1960).

6. Human temporal bone studies report maximum damage approximately 5 to 15 mm from the oval window. This area corresponds to the 4000 Hz to 6000 Hz receptor region. Causes of the unusual vulnerability of this region to noise damage are unknown. Reasons may be related to the blood supply of the cochlea, mechanical and anatomic characteristics of the cochlea, or the resonance characteristics of the external ear–middle ear system.

7. In the determination of the degree of occupational noise-induced hearing loss in older individuals, some clinicians propose age correction factors. The purpose of age correction factors is to counteract hearing loss due to the normal physiologic processes of aging (Corso, 1976).

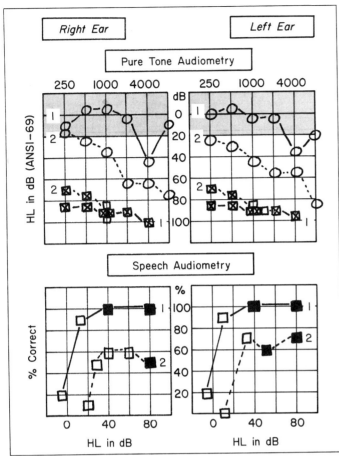

Case 16-1A. *Pure tone audiogram and speech audiometry. "1" initial evaluation, history of 5 years of noise exposure; "2" audiologic reevaluation, history of 8 years of noise exposure.*

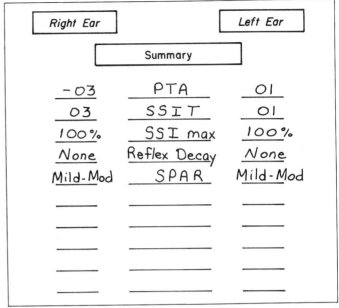

Case 16-1B. *Summary of test results for initial evaluation ("1").*

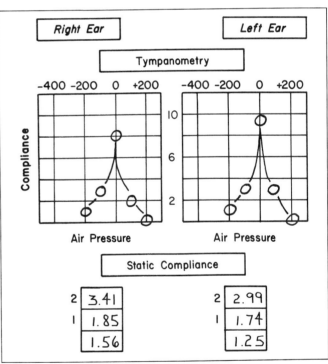

Case 16-1C. *Impedance audiometry; tympanometry and static compliance measures (in cc) for evaluations "1" and "2."*

8. A 4000 Hz notch may be referred to as a *boilermaker's notch.*

9. Notice the value of Spanish speech materials in a patient that does not speak English. Remember, with the SSI procedure, the tester is not required to interpret a verbal response from the patient. Instead, the patient responds by pushing a button corresponding to the sentence he thinks he heard.

on both ears with the exception of a mild high frequency sensorineural notch at 4000 Hz.[8] The PTA scores (Case 16-1B) are −3 dB HL on the right ear and 1 dB HL on the left ear.

PI-SSI functions ("1," Case 16-1A) for Spanish materials are normal on both ears. The SSI max scores (Case 16-1B) are 100% bilaterally. SSIT scores, 3 dB HL on the right ear and 1 dB HL on the left ear, agree with average pure tone sensitivity.[9]

Tympanometry and static compliance measures (Case 16-1C) are within normal limits on both ears. Crossed and uncrossed acoustic reflexes ("1," Case 16-1A) on both ears are present at normal HLs at all frequencies. No reflex decay (Case 16-1B) at 500 Hz or 1000 Hz is observed on either ear. The SPAR measure predicts a mild to moderate sensitivity loss on both ears.

Impression

On both ears, sensitivity is within normal limits except for a mild, sensorineural notch at 4000 Hz. Impedance audiometry indicates normal middle ear function. The au-

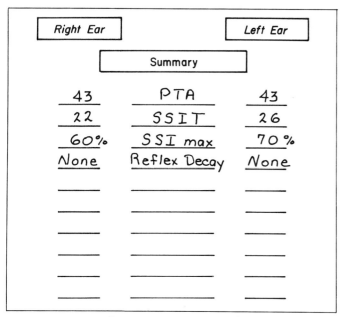

Right Ear		Left Ear
	Summary	
43	PTA	43
22	SSIT	26
60%	SSI max	70%
None	Reflex Decay	None

Case 16-1D. *Summary of test results for audiologic reevaluation ("2").*

10. Notice that until this evaluation, this patient seemed unconcerned about his hearing. At the initial evaluation, he had no hearing complaints. He did not return for yearly monitoring of hearing sensitivity. Remember, subjective complaints of hearing loss may not be reported until a loss of more than about 25 dB HL (ANSI-69) occurs at a frequency(ies) below 3000 Hz.

11. Comparison of the first audiogram (5 years of noise exposure) and the second audiogram (8 years of noise exposure) illustrates two characteristics of noise-induced hearing loss: (1) hearing loss progresses more slowly at low frequencies than at high frequencies; (2) most of the noise-induced hearing loss at 4000 Hz is produced in the first 5 years of exposure (Ward, 1973).

diometric contour is consistent with the patient's history of noise exposure.

Recommendation

Monitoring of hearing sensitivity at yearly intervals or before if patient notices any change in his auditory symptoms.

Audiologic Reevaluation

HISTORY. Approximately 3 years after the initial audiologic evaluation, the patient returned for a retest of his hearing. At this time, he complains of a hearing loss in both ears. He seems concerned about his hearing problems.[10]

RESULTS. The audiogram ("2," Case 16-1A) on both ears shows a mild sensorineural loss through 1000 Hz and a moderate sensorineural loss above 1000 Hz. The PTA scores (Case 16-1D) are 43 dB HL bilaterally.[11]

PI-SSI functions ("2," Case 16-1A) for Spanish materials show reduced maximum intelligibility scores on both ears. The SSI max scores (Case 16-1D) are 60% on the right ear and 70% on the left ear. No rollover is observed on either ear.[12] SSIT scores (Case 16-1D) are 22 dB HL on the right ear and 26 dB HL on the left ear.[13]

Tympanometry and static compliance measures are the same as results previously obtained (Case 16-1C). Crossed and un-

12. Speech intelligibility performance has declined 30% to 40% on both ears relative to results of the first evaluation.

13. On both ears, speech thresholds show less sensitivity loss than average pure tone results. Remember, however, the most important frequencies for understanding SSI materials are in the region of about 750 Hz. SSIT scores in this patient agree with low frequency sensitivity.

When the performance plateau is at or near the 50% intelligibility level, remember that speech thresholds are more accurately obtained on a steeper part of the function, such as the 25% intelligibility level.

crossed acoustic reflexes ("2," Case 16-1A) on both ears are present at normal HLs from 250 Hz through 1000 Hz. However, acoustic reflexes are absent at 2000 Hz and 4000 Hz bilaterally. No reflex decay (Case 16-1D) is observed at 500 or 1000 Hz on either ear.

IMPRESSION. On both ears, a mild sensorineural loss through 1000 Hz; a moderate sensorineural loss above 1000 Hz. Pure tone sensitivity has decreased approximately 40 dB since the first evaluation. Speech intelligibility scores for Spanish synthetic sentence identification (SSI) materials have decreased 30% to 40% bilaterally. Impedance audiometry is consistent with normal middle ear function on both ears.

Comment

An Industrial Accident Board awarded the patient financial compensation for noise-induced hearing loss.

SELECTED READINGS

Bentzen, O. The audiological examination, treatment and education in the five Scandinavian countries. *Scand. Audiol.* 1:89, 1972.

Corso, J. Presbyacusis as a Competing Factor in Evaluating Noise Induced Hearing Loss. In D. Henderson, R. Hamernik, D. Dosanjh, and J. Mills (eds.), *Effects of Noise on Hearing.* New York: Raven Press, 1976. Pp. 497–524.

Ewertsen, H. Epidemiology of professional noise-induced hearing loss. *Audiology* 12:453, 1973.

Flodgren, E., and Kylin, B. Sex differences in hearing in relation to noise exposure. *Acta Otolaryngol.* 52:358, 1960.

Fox, M. Industrial Noise Exposure and Hearing Loss. In J. Ballenger (ed.), *Diseases of the Nose, Throat, and Ear.* Philadelphia: Lea & Febiger, 1977. Pp. 963–987.

Gallo, R., and Glorig, A. Permanent threshold shift changes produced by noise exposure and aging. *Am. Ind. Hyg. Assoc. J.* 25:237, 1964.

Gilad, O., and Glorig, A. Presbyacusis: The aging ear. *J. Am. Audiol. Soc.* 4:207, 1979.

Igarashi, M., Schuknecht, H., and Myers, E. Cochlear pathology in humans with stimulation deafness. *J. Laryngol.* 78:115, 1964.

Johnson, L., and Hawkins, J. Degeneration patterns in human ears exposed to noise. *Ann. Otol. Rhinol. Laryngol.* 85:725, 1976.

Kryter, K. *The Effects of Noise on Man.* New York: Academic Press, 1970. Pp. 139–205.

Lipscomb, D. What is the audiogram really telling us? Part I: Audiometrics vs cochlear damage. Maico Audiological Library Series, vol. 13:1, 1975.

Macrae, J. Determination of the residual hearing of children with sensorineural deafness. *Acta Otolaryngol.* 66:33, 1968.

Moller, A. Noise as a health hazard. *AMBIO* 4:6, 1975.

Snow, J. Otological Considerations in Noise-Induced Hearing Loss. In D. Henderson, R. Hamernik, D. Dosanjh, and J. Mills (eds.), *Effects of Noise on Hearing*. New York: Raven Press, 1976. Pp. 467–478.

Surjan, L., Devald, J., and Palfalvi, L. Epidemiology of hearing loss. *Audiology* 12: 396, 1973.

Tonndorf, J. Relationship Between the Transmission Characteristics of the Conductive System and Noise-Induced Hearing Loss. In D. Henderson, R. Hamernik, D. Dosanjh, and J. Mills (eds.), *Effects of Noise on Hearing*. New York: Raven Press, 1976. Pp. 159–177.

Ward, W. Noise-Induced Hearing Damage. In M. Paparella and D. Shumrick (eds.), *Otolaryngology* (vol. 2). Philadelphia: Saunders, 1973. Pp. 377–390.

Zakrisson, J. The role of the stapedius reflex in poststimulatory auditory fatigue. *Acta Otolaryngol.* 79:1, 1975.

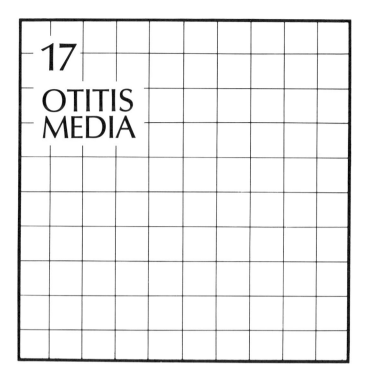

17
OTITIS MEDIA

DESCRIPTION

Otitis media refers to an accumulation of fluid in the middle ear space. The disease characteristically results from inflammation of the mucoperiosteal lining of the middle ear cleft.

In some individuals, otitis media may be related to inadequate aeration of the tympanic cavity due to dysfunction or obstruction of the Eustachian tube. When middle ear ventilation is impaired, the static air in the middle air space may be absorbed by blood vessels in the mucosal lining. A negative pressure is created in the tympanic cavity. The tympanic membrane may become retracted. Reduced middle ear pressure may result in edema of the mucosa and secretion of fluid from the mucoperiosteum (Friedmann, 1974). The fluid may be watery (serous otitis media) or mucoid (secretory otitis media).[1]

Some causes of Eustachian tube malfunction include allergy, enlarged adenoids, barotrauma, cleft palate, and developmental factors.[2]

In addition to Eustachian tube dysfunction, another factor in the development of otitis media may be a spread of infection into the middle ear. An acute infectious otitis media may occur. A common mechanism for acute infectious otitis media is a spread of upper respiratory infections through the Eustachian tube. The middle ear

mucoperiosteum may react to the invasion with hyperemia, edema, and cellular infiltration (Friedmann, 1974). A pus-like fluid (suppurative otitis media) may collect in the middle ear space.[3]

In contrast to an acute course, suppurative otitis media may be chronic in some individuals. Chronic suppurative otitis media may result in pathologic changes or destruction of the middle ear mucosa, ossicles, and mastoid bone. Perforation of the tympanic membrane and a discharge of pus from the ear may occur.

In some individuals, the different types of otitis media may not occur as distinct entities. For example, a prolonged accumulation of serous fluid within the middle ear space may result in increased vulnerability of the ear to bacteria and viruses. If allowed to progress uninterrupted, serous otitis media may progress to chronic infectious otitis media.[4]

Complications of otitis media may include tympanosclerosis, tympanic membrane perforation, and cholesteatoma. If the inflammation spreads to adjacent structures in the temporal bone or inside the cranial cavity, complications may include labyrinthitis, mastoiditis, facial paralysis, brain abscess, and meningitis. A permanent sensorineural hearing loss may develop in some individuals.

PATIENT CHARACTERISTICS

Otitis media may occur at any age. However, the disease appears to be more common in children between 6 and 24 months and between 4 and 6 years of age. Approximately 80% of patients are children less than 5 years old. Chronic suppurative otitis media most often has its onset between 5 and 10 years of age. The disease is characteristically bilateral. A sex ratio for otitis media is unsettled.[5]

CLINICAL COURSE

Fluctuating, conductive hearing loss. The onset of otitis media may be acute or insidious. Otitis media of acute onset may be accompanied by earache, hearing loss, and rupture of the tympanic membrane. If spontaneous rupture of the eardrum occurs, the pain characteristically subsides.

Otitis media of insidious onset is charac-

---

1. Serous or secretory otitis media may be referred to as *middle ear effusion* or *middle ear catarrh*. A severe form of secretory otitis may be referred to as *glue ear*.

In a survey of 704 4-year-olds, serous otitis media was present in about 20% of children (Gerwin and Read, 1974).

2. In children, the ventilatory, protective, and drainage functions of the Eustachian tube may be inefficient due to developmental immaturity. Relative to the adult Eustachian tube, the cartilaginous portion of a child's Eustachian tube is shorter, less stiff, and in a more horizontal position (Bluestone, 1975).

3. In a series of 704 4-year-olds, suppurative otitis media was present in 2% of children (Gerwin and Read, 1974).

4. Estimates of an annual incidence rate for otitis media range from about 10% to 20% of children (McEldowney and Kessner, 1972).

In a series of 2500 children less than 2 years old, 42% had occasional (less than three episodes) otitis media and 33% had recurring (more than three episodes) otitis media. Only 25% of children had no evidence of middle ear disease during the 2-year period (Klein, 1979).

The incidence of severe otitis media may vary as a function of racial or socioeconomic factors. Estimates, based on evidence of a perforated eardrum and conductive hearing loss, range from about 5% of American Indian children to approximately 30% of Alaskan Eskimo children (Hinchcliffe, 1972).

5. Some studies (Anderson and Wedenberg, 1970) report no difference between the sexes in the prevalence of otitis media; other studies (McEldowney and Kessner, 1972) report a higher prevalence of acute middle ear infections in males than in females; still other studies (Bjuggren and Tunevall,

1952) report that the male-to-female ratio varies with age.

teristically not accompanied by substantial ear pain. Symptomatology may include hearing loss, a feeling of fullness in the ear, a low pitched, pulsating or continuous tinnitus, crackling or popping sounds within the ear, chills, and fever. A patient's voice may sound unusually loud and/or hollow to him (autophony). Subjective symptomatology accompanying otitis media of insidious onset may be difficult to elicit from children.

In some persons, otitis media may recur over a period of years. Severe, recurrent otitis media in the first 3 years of life may be associated with delayed language development in some children (Lewis, 1976; Zinkus et al., 1978).[6]

6. In newborn experimental animals, sound deprivation due to conductive hearing loss appears to be associated with morphologic abnormalities in the central auditory system (Webster and Webster, 1977).

Treatment may include drug therapy, inflation techniques, allergy management, and surgery. Ventilation (PE) tubes may be placed in the tympanic membrane(s).

SITE OF DISORDER

Middle ear. On rare occasions, the cochlea may also be involved.

GENERAL AUDIOLOGIC PATTERN

7. Estimates of the prevalence of hearing loss in otitis media range from about 25% to 95% of children. A wide range probably reflects the variations in degree of loss that may occur with the stages and types of otitis media.

Pure tone sensitivity results characteristically show bilateral conductive hearing loss. The degree of loss is typically between 20 dB to 40 dB HL. However, variations in the degree of loss may occur with the different stages of the disease. Initial stages of otitis media may be associated with normal hearing; more advanced stages of otitis media may be associated with a hearing loss of greater than 40 dB HL.[7]

The audiometric contour may vary with the progression of the disease. Initially, as middle ear pressure is reduced, the tympanic membrane and ossicular chain may become increasingly stiff. During this stage, the audiometric contour may be rising with greater loss in the low frequency region than in the high frequency region. Subsequently, as fluid accumulates, high frequency sensitivity may become impaired due to mass loading of the ossicular chain. In this stage, the audiometric contour is characteristically flat.

Bone conduction audiometry is typically within normal limits. However, bone conduction thresholds may become abnormal depending on the duration and severity of

8. In a survey of 171 children with otitis media, about 4% of persons had sensorineural loss on one ear and about 1% of individuals had sensorineural loss on both ears (Friedmann, 1974).

the disease.[8] In patients with a sensorineural component, the audiometric contour may be flat or downwardly sloping.

Speech intelligibility scores are generally within normal limits.

Impedance audiometry characteristically shows abnormal tympanograms, reduced static compliance measures, and absent acoustic reflexes. The shape of the tympanogram may change in a predictable manner as the disease progresses and subsides. In the initial stages of otitis media, the peak of the tympanogram may show slight positive pressure. Subsequently, as the air in the middle ear space is exhausted, the peak of the tympanogram may occur at an increasing degree of negative pressure. The tympanogram in this stage is a type C configuration. Gradually, the amplitude of the negative peak may decrease. The peak may become rounded or blunted. Subsequently the tympanogram is a flattened shape. The characteristic pattern at this stage is a type B configuration. As the otitis media resolves, the tympanogram tends to recover systematically through reversal of the same sequence of events.[9]

9. Tympanometry may be of unique value in evaluating patients with otitis media. Substantial negative middle ear pressure and fluid may exist within the middle ear space without significant air conduction sensitivity loss.

In patients with otitis media, Eustachian tube function may be evaluated with an impedance audiometer. Procedures for patients with intact tympanic membranes characteristically determine changes in the peak of tympanometric pressure with swallowing. Procedures for patients with perforated tympanic membranes evaluate the ability to sustain or evacuate induced positive or negative pressure in the middle ear cavity, with or without swallowing (Bluestone, 1975).

Illustrative Patients

CASE 1. A 10-YEAR-OLD FEMALE WITH BILATERAL RECURRENT OTITIS MEDIA.

History and Surgical Findings

The patient was initially evaluated 7 years ago for bilateral otitis media. Subsequent to that evaluation she had a tonsillectomy, adenoidectomy, and bilateral myringotomies with insertion of ventilation (PE) tubes in both ears.

During the past 7 years, the child has had recurrent episodes of bilateral otitis media, usually more severe on the right ear. Oto-

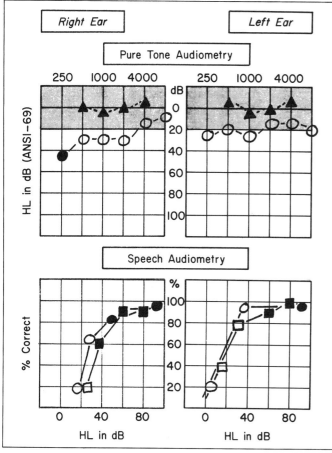

Case 17-1A

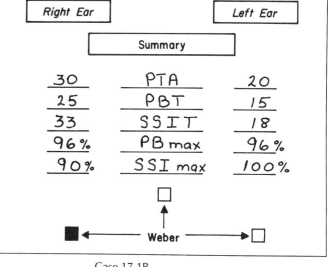

Case 17-1B

rhinolaryngologic examinations have revealed tympanosclerosis on the right ear and a large central perforation of the tympanic membrane on the left ear. Tympanoplasties have been performed on both ears.

Presently, otorhinolaryngologic examination reveals bilateral adhesive otitis media. There is no evidence of cholesteatoma or tympanic membrane perforation on either ear.

The patient is presently in the fifth grade. She receives satisfactory grades. She complains of a mild hearing loss and a high pitched ringing tinnitus in both ears.

Results

The audiogram (Case 17-1A) shows a mild conductive loss on both ears. The PTA scores (Case 17-1B) are 30 dB HL on the right ear and 20 dB HL on the left ear. Bone conduction audiometry (Case 17-1A) shows a conductive component of approximately 30 dB on the right ear and 20 dB on the left

10. On the left ear, notice the sharp peak at −400 mm H_2O air pressure. This sharp peak distinguishes the tympanogram as a type C, rather than a type B, pattern. Theoretically, if the air pressure is extended beyond −400 mm H_2O, the characteristic type C shape would emerge. As a rule, however, we do not test beyond −400 mm H_2O air pressure.

ear. On the Weber test (Case 17-1B) the 500 Hz tone is heard in the right ear.

Speech audiometry (Case 17-1A) shows normal maximum intelligibility scores on both ears. On the right ear, the PB max (Case 17-1B) is 96%; the SSI max is 90%. On the left ear, the PB max is 96%; the SSI max is 100%. No rollover is observed on either ear. Speech thresholds on both ears agree with average pure tone sensitivity. On the right ear, the PBT is 25 dB HL; the SSIT is 33 dB HL. On the left ear, the PBT is 15 dB HL; the SSIT is 18 dB HL.

Impedance audiometry (Case 17-1C) shows abnormal tympanograms on both ears. The pattern is a type B shape on the right ear and a type C configuration on the left ear.[10] Static compliance measures are slightly below normal limits on the right ear and within normal limits on the left ear. Crossed and uncrossed acoustic reflexes (Case 17-1D) are absent on both ears.

Impression

Mild conductive loss on both ears. On the right ear, impedance audiometry is consistent with extreme restriction of mobility of the middle ear system. On the left ear, impedance audiometry shows severe negative pressure within the middle ear space.

CASE 2. A 19-YEAR-OLD FEMALE WITH BILATERAL, RECURRENT OTITIS MEDIA.

History

The patient has noticed a fluctuating hearing loss on both ears for almost her entire life.

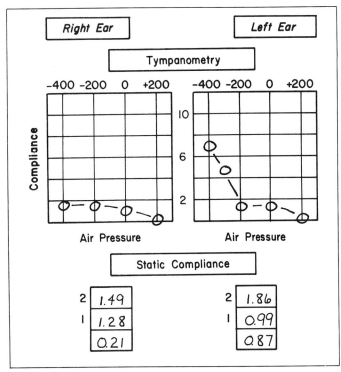

Case 17-1C

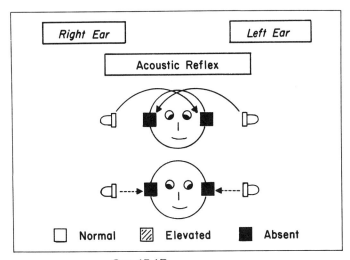

Case 17-1D

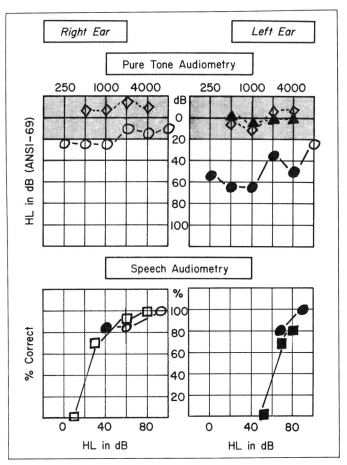

Case 17-2A

11. Otitis media may occur in as many as 50% of persons with cleft palate (Yules, 1970). Serious sequelae of otitis media may be present in about 33% of persons with cleft palate (Moller, 1975).

She reports a previous tonsillectomy, two previous adenoidectomies, and multiple placements of ventilation (PE) tubes into both ears. She has a congenital submucous cleft of the palate.[11]

At the present time, otorhinolaryngologic examination is consistent with serous otitis media on the right ear and secretory (glue ear) otitis media on the left ear.

Results

The audiogram (Case 17-2A) shows a mild conductive loss on the right ear and a mod-

12. Notice, on the right ear, the unique contribution of SAL audiometry in quantifying the degree of conductive component.

erate conductive loss on the left ear. The PTA scores (Case 17-2B) are 18 dB HL on the right ear and 55 dB HL on the left ear. SAL audiometry (Case 17-2A) shows a conductive component of approximately 20 dB on the right ear and 40 dB to 60 dB on the left ear. Bone conduction responses on the left ear interweave with SAL results. Bone conduction audiometry on the right ear could not be obtained. All bone conducted signals to the right ear were consistently heard in the left ear, even with maximum masking.[12] The Weber test (Case 17-2B) shows that, at 500 Hz, the bone conducted signal lateralizes to the left ear. The Bing test (not shown) at 500 Hz on the left ear shows no benefit from occlusion. Bing test results on the right ear could not be obtained.

PI-SSI functions (Case 17-2A) and PB testing at high intensity levels show maximum intelligibility scores within normal limits on both ears. No rollover is observed on either ear. On the right ear, SSI max (Case 17-2B) and PB max scores are 100%.

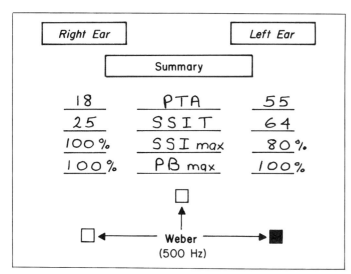

Case 17-2B

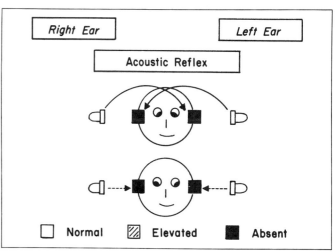

Case 17-2D

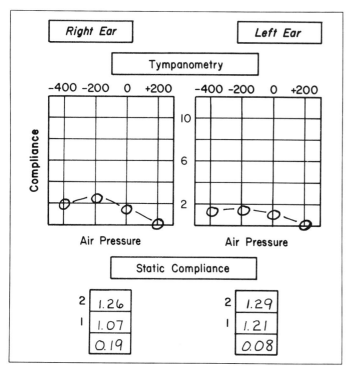

Case 17-2C

PB and SSI scores is not interpreted as a suggestion of central auditory disorder.

Notice that speech results at high intensity levels on the right ear are not recorded with masked symbols. In this patient, masking out the crossed speech signal on the left ear is a problem due to the large conductive component on the left ear (for further discussion of this masking dilemma, see patient 1, Chapter 18, Otosclerosis).

Impression

Mild conductive loss on the right ear; moderate conductive loss on the left ear. On both ears, impedance audiometry shows abnormal, type B, tympanograms, reduced static compliance measures, and absent crossed and uncrossed acoustic reflexes. Impedance results are consistent with extreme restriction of mobility of the middle ear system.

SELECTED READINGS

Alford, B. Complications of Suppurative Otitis Media. In M. Paparella and D. Shumrick (eds.), *Otolaryngology* (vol. 2). Philadelphia: Saunders, 1973. Pp. 156–157.

Anderson, H., and Wedenberg, E. Genetic aspects of hearing impairments in children. *Acta Otolaryngol.* 69:77, 1970.

Bjuggren, G., and Tunevall, G. Otitis in childhood. *Acta Otolaryngol.* 42:311, 1952.

Bluestone, C. Assessment of Eustachian Tube Function. In J. Jerger (ed.), *Handbook of Clinical Impedance Audiometry.* Dobbs Ferry, N.Y.: Morgan Press, 1975. Pp. 127–148.

Brydoy, B., and Ellekjaer, E. Otogenic meningitis: A five year study. *J. Laryngol. Otol.* 86:871, 1972.

Eagles, E. L., Wishik, S., and Doerfler, L. Hearing sensitivity and ear disease in children: A prospective study. *Laryngoscope* 77:1, 1967. (Monograph).

Friedmann, I. *Pathology of the Ear.* Oxford: Blackwell, 1974. Pp. 25–83.

Gerwin, K., and Read, C. Causes of Ear Disease in the Callier Study. In K. Gerwin and A. Glorig (eds.), *Detection of Hearing Loss and Ear Disease in Children.* Springfield, Ill.: Thomas, 1974. Pp. 173–187.

13. On the left ear, the PI-SSI function is still rising at equipment limits. In this circumstance, the maximum SSI score may not represent maximum performance. Notice that when a performance plateau is not established, a difference between

On the left ear, the SSI max at 80 dB HL is 80%; the PB max is 100%.[13] SSIT scores agree with average pure tone sensitivity bilaterally. The SSIT is 25 dB HL on the right ear and 64 dB HL on the left ear.

Impedance audiometry (Case 17-2C) yields abnormal, type B, tympanograms, reduced static compliance measures, and absent crossed and uncrossed acoustic reflexes (Case 17-2D) on both ears.

Hinchcliffe, R. Epidemiological Aspects of Otitis Media. In A. Glorig and K. Gerwin (eds.), *Otitis Media.* Proceedings of the National Conference, Callier Hearing and Speech Center. Springfield, Ill.: Thomas, 1972.

Klein, J. The Changing Challenge of Otitis Media. *Hearing Aid J.* 32:11, 1979.

Lewis, N. Otitis media and linguistic incompetence. *Arch. Otolaryngol.* 102:387, 1976.

Lim, D. Infectious and Inflammatory Auditory Disorder. In D. Tower (ed.), *The Nervous System.* Vol. 3: *Human Communication and Its Disorders.* New York: Raven Press, 1975. Pp. 263–271.

McEldowney, D., and Kessner, D. Review of the Literature: Epidemiology of Otitis Media. In A. Glorig and K. Gerwin (eds.), *Otitis Media.* Proceedings of the National Conference, Callier Hearing and Speech Center. Springfield, Ill.: Thomas, 1972. Pp. 11–25.

Moller, P. Long-term otologic features of cleft palate patients. *Arch. Otolaryngol.* 101:605, 1975.

Webster, D., and Webster, M. Neonatal sound deprivation affects brain stem auditory nuclei. *Arch. Otolaryngol.* 103:392, 1977.

Yules, R. Hearing in cleft palate patients. *Arch. Otolaryngol.* 91:319, 1970.

Zinkus, P., Gottlieb, M., and Shapiro, M. Developmental and psycho-educational sequelae of chronic otitis media. *Am. J. Dis. Child.* 132:1100, 1978.

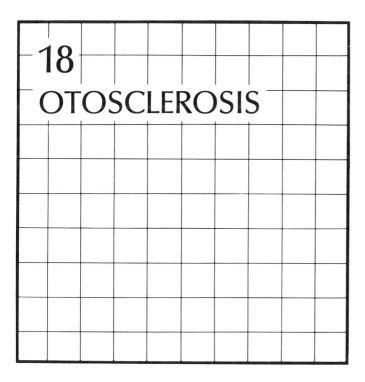

18
OTOSCLEROSIS

DESCRIPTION

Otosclerosis is a focal disease of the otic capsule. The disease is characterized by excessive resorption of bone. Abnormal new bone tissue is formed. The new bone formation is soft, hypervascular tissue that may gradually change into a dense sclerotic mass.

Otosclerosis may occur anywhere within the petrous bone. In about 70% to 90% of ears, otosclerotic foci occur in the angle formed by the anterior part of the stapes footplate, the cochleariform process, and the bulge of the promontory. In about 30% to 50% of ears, otosclerotic bone is found in the region of the round window.[1]

In some patients, the cochlea may be damaged by an extension of otosclerotic foci into the bony capsule and/or by the presence of associated endolymphatic hydrops. On rare occasions, otosclerotic foci may extend into the internal auditory canal.[2]

The etiology of otosclerosis is obscure. Proposed theories involve genetic, metabolic, vascular, and infectious disturbances.

PATIENT CHARACTERISTICS

In 90% of individuals, the onset of hearing loss is between 15 and 45 years of age (Booth, 1978). The occurrence of hearing loss due to otosclerosis is rare in children less than 15 years old. About 40% to 50%

1. Some clinicians consider the term *otosclerosis* a misnomer. They prefer the term *otospongiosis* as a more accurate description of the disease process.

The prevalence of otosclerosis varies with race. Histologic evidence of otosclerosis is present in about 10% of whites and about 1% of blacks. The disease is rare in Orientals.

2. Of 90 patients with surgically confirmed stapedial otosclerosis, tomographic evidence of otosclerotic foci within the cochlea was present in about 37% of individuals (Naunton and Valvassori, 1969). In a series of 490 patients with otosclerosis, about

4% had associated endolymphatic hydrops (McCabe, 1966).

3. An initial awareness of hearing loss or an accelerated progression of existing hearing loss may be noted during or immediately following pregnancy in about 50% of women.

4. Otosclerosis may be asymptomatic in many individuals. In a series of 81 ears with histologic evidence of otosclerosis, the disease did not seem to cause hearing loss unless stapes fixation occurred. Stapes fixation was observed in only 12% of ears (Guild, 1944).

5. Some clinicians suggest that otosclerosis may be treated with sodium fluoride therapy. In a series of 1536 individuals, stapes fixation was 4 times more frequent in areas with a low fluoride content in the drinking water than in areas with a high fluoride water content (Daniel, 1969).

of patients report a family history of otosclerosis. The disease affects twice as many females as males. The condition is bilateral in about 80% of men and 90% of women (Booth, 1978).[3]

CLINICAL COURSE

The onset of otosclerosis is characteristically insidious. Waves of bone destruction and new bone formation may continue indefinitely or may be interrupted by quiescent, sclerotic periods.

A gradually progressive conductive hearing loss may occur if the otosclerotic foci encroach upon the oval window and fix the stapes footplate. The rate of progression of the hearing loss varies substantially among patients. In some patients, the hearing loss may become relatively stable after a period of time.[4]

Tinnitus may be reported in about 50% to 65% of patients. The patient may notice that he can hear better in noisy environments than in quiet (paracusis willisiana).

There is no standard medical treatment for otosclerosis.[5] Restorative surgery may improve hearing sensitivity in most patients. However, a hearing loss may recur after surgery in some individuals due to regrowth of otosclerotic foci. On rare occasions, a complication of surgery may be the development of a fistula in the membrane covering the oval window. In this circumstance, a sensorineural hearing loss may occur.

SITE OF DISORDER

Middle ear. In some individuals, the cochlea may be involved.

GENERAL AUDIOLOGIC PATTERN

The audiologic signature of otosclerosis primarily involves results of impedance audiometry. As a rule, type A, probably shallow, tympanograms, normal or low static compliance measures, absent acoustic reflexes, and conductive hearing loss are considered pathognomonic of ossicular fixation.

An exception to the above pattern involves acoustic reflex results in the initial stages of otosclerosis. In patients with early stapes fixation, acoustic reflex thresholds are characteristically present at relatively normal or slightly elevated HLs. In contrast to

6. Negative deflections at the onset of reflex eliciting signals are present in many normal ears and are considered nondiagnostic.

7. A sensorineural hearing loss may develop in about 20% of patients with stapedial otosclerosis (Lindsay, 1973).

8. In our experience, patients with an apparently sensorineural loss or normal sensitivity during the initial stages of otosclerosis may show an abnormal reflex time course with an unusual negative deflection at the offset of the reflex eliciting signal.
   Patients with consistent sensorineural hearing loss may be diagnosed as having cochlear otosclerosis (Shambaugh, 1978).

9. In patients with a fistula due to post-surgical complications, speech intelligibility scores characteristically show unusual fluctuation and reduced maximum performance.

normal reflex thresholds, however, the reflex time course is generally characterized by an unusual negative deflection at the offset of the reflex eliciting signal. Negative deflections accompanying the termination of reflex eliciting signals seem unique to ossicular chain fixation.[6]

Pure tone sensitivity results characteristically show a bilateral conductive hearing loss. The degree of loss is generally a mild to moderate impairment. The maximum air-bone gap rarely exceeds 50 dB. In the initial stages of otosclerosis, the audiometric contour is generally rising with greater loss in the low frequency region than in the high frequency region. As the stapes footplate becomes more severely fixed, the audiometric contour gradually flattens. In some patients, a conductive hearing loss may progress over time to a mixed or primarily sensorineural loss.[7]

On rare occasions, pure tone sensitivity results in patients with otosclerosis may not show a conductive disorder. Instead, a sensorineural hearing loss may be apparent. In some patients, a sensorineural hearing loss is observed during the initial stages of otosclerosis. However, as the disease progresses, a conductive component (mixed hearing loss) becomes apparent. In other patients, a sensorineural hearing loss is observed at all stages of the disease.[8]

Speech intelligibility scores are generally within the normal range, even in the presence of mixed or sensorineural hearing impairment.[9]

Illustrative Patients

CASE 1. A 23-YEAR-OLD FEMALE WITH OTOSCLEROSIS.

History

The patient reports a 5-year history of tinnitus in both ears, greater on the right ear. During the past year, she has noticed a feeling of pressure and a gradually increasing hearing loss in her right ear. She has no hearing complaints about her left ear.

Otorhinolaryngologic examination reveals normal tympanic membranes bilaterally. A pinkish glow from the promontory (Schwartz sign) is noted on both ears. The oral cavity, nasopharynx, larynx, hypopharynx, and neck are clear. The patient's fa-

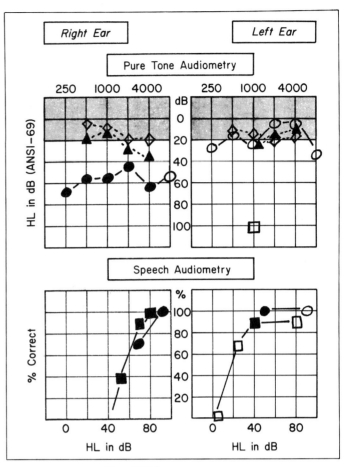

Case 18-1A

ther has a hearing loss due to otosclerosis.

Results

The audiogram (Case 18-1A) shows a moderate, primarily conductive, loss on the right ear and a very mild sensorineural loss on the left ear. The PTA scores (Case 18-1B) are 55 dB HL on the right ear and 16 dB HL on the left ear. Bone conduction and SAL audiometry (Case 18-1A) on the right ear show a conductive component of approximately 50 dB in the low frequencies and 25 dB in the high frequencies. On the left ear, bone conduction and SAL results are superimposed on air conduction.

The Weber test (Case 18-1B), at 500 Hz shows that the bone conducted signal lateralizes to the right ear. The Bing test (not shown) at 500 Hz on the right ear shows no difference between occluded and unoccluded thresholds. The Bing test could not be obtained on the left ear. At 500 Hz, all

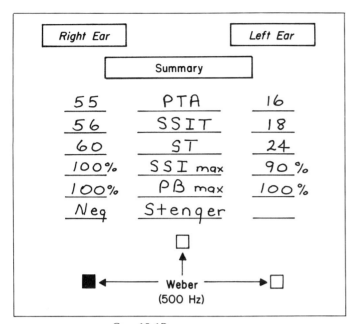

Case 18-1B

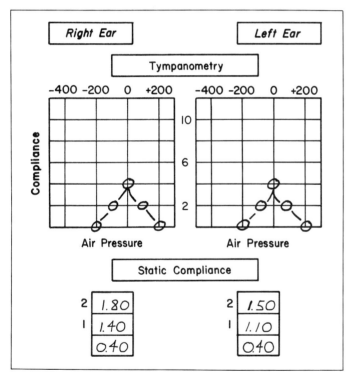

Case 18-1C

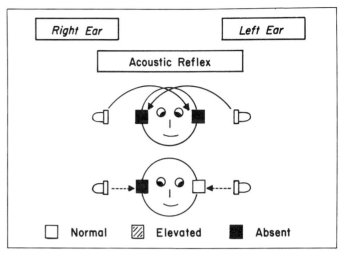

Case 18-1D

bone conducted signals were referred to the right ear, even with maximum masking.

PI-SSI functions and PB testing at high intensity levels (Case 18-1A) show normal maximum intelligibility scores on both ears. On the right ear, the SSI max and PB max scores (Case 18-1B) are 100%. On the left ear, the SSI max is 90%; the PB max is

10. Notice that speech results on the left ear at 80 and 90 dB HL are not recorded with masked symbols. A speech signal to the left ear of 80 dB HL may be heard in the right ear at about 40 dB HL due to crossover. In this patient, masking out the crossed speech signal on the right ear is a problem. The masking noise presented to the right ear by air conduction is attenuated by the large conductive component. Theoretically, the remaining masking noise may be insufficient to mask out a crossed speech signal of 40 dB HL.

11. In our experience, reflex amplitude between the double negative deflections may vary substantially among patients. For example, in some individuals, reflex amplitude may remain completely below the baseline during the signal presentation interval.

100%.[10] SSIT scores agree with pure tone sensitivity results bilaterally. SSIT scores are 56 dB HL on the right ear and 18 dB HL on the left ear.

Impedance audiometry (Case 18-1C) shows slightly shallow, type A, tympanograms and normal static compliance measures on both ears. Crossed and uncrossed acoustic reflexes (Case 18-1A) with sound to the right ear are absent at all frequencies at equipment limits. With sound to the left ear, crossed acoustic reflexes are absent at 500 Hz through 4000 Hz. However, the uncrossed reflex at 1000 Hz is present at an HL within the normal range.

The reflex pattern (Case 18-1D) is characterized by an inverted L-shaped configuration. Results indicate a combined probe effect (vertical pattern) and sound effect (diagonal pattern) on the right ear.

With sound and probe to the left ear (uncrossed test condition), the reflex time course (Case 18-1E) is characterized by large negative deflections at both the onset and offset of the reflex eliciting signal. With probe to the right ear, no reflexes could be obtained.[11]

Speech thresholds for spondee words (STs) (Case 18-1B) agree with average pure tone sensitivity bilaterally. The ST scores are 60 dB HL on the right ear and 24 dB HL on the left ear. A speech Stenger test is negative for a functional component on the right ear.

Impression

RIGHT EAR: Moderate, primarily conductive loss. Impedance audiometry is consistent

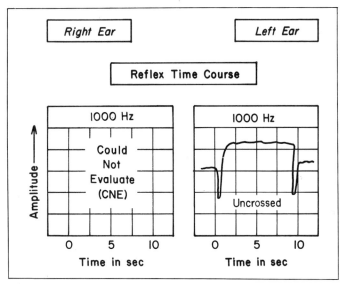

Case 18-1E

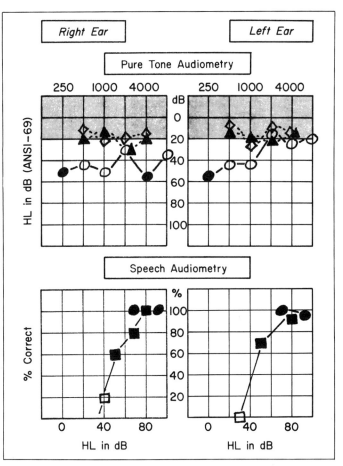

Case 18-2A

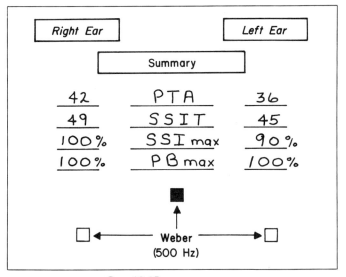

Case 18-2B

12. Remember, results of impedance audiometry describe the alteration or modification of middle ear function, not the particular disease process producing the abnormality. Consequently, impedance results are interpreted as consistent with ossicular chain fixation, rather than otosclerosis. Other disorders producing ossicular fixation may produce the same pattern of results.

with fixation of the ossicular chain. Slightly shallow, type A, tympanograms, normal static compliance measures, and absent acoustic reflexes were observed.[12]

LEFT EAR: Mild sensitivity loss with no apparent air-bone or air-SAL gap. Impedance audiometry is consistent with early fixation of the ossicular chain. With probe to the left ear, the acoustic reflex time course shows unusual negative deflections at the offset of reflex eliciting signals.

CASE 2. A 48-YEAR-OLD FEMALE WITH OTOSCLEROSIS.

History

The patient has noticed a gradually increasing hearing loss in both ears for approximately 1 year. Occasionally, she notices a roaring tinnitus bilaterally. She denies dizziness and headaches. She reports no known previous otologic disease. However, her mother and brother have hearing loss due to otosclerosis. The patient has three children.

Findings of general physical examination, otorhinolaryngologic evaluation, and routine laboratory studies are consistently within normal limits, except for decreased hearing sensitivity on both ears.

A right stapedectomy was performed.

Results

The audiogram (Case 18-2A) on the right ear shows a moderate conductive loss. On the

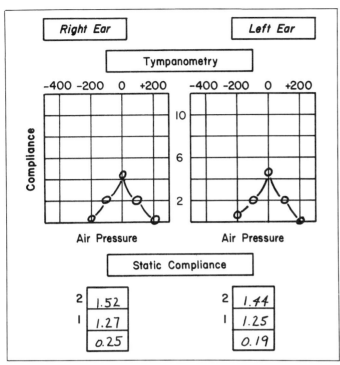

Case 18-2C

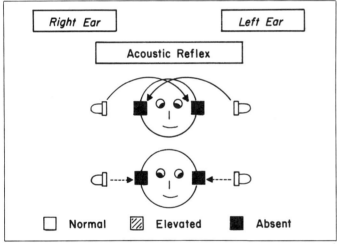

Case 18-2D

chanical depression of bone conduction sensitivity, maximal at 2000 Hz (Carhart's notch).

14. Remember, in ears with no threshold improvement from occlusion, SAL results at 500 Hz and 1000 Hz are corrected by the amount of the occlusion effect observed in normal ears. A correction is necessary in order for SAL results to agree with conventional unoccluded bone conduction thresholds.

The Bing test (not shown) at 500 Hz shows no occlusion effect (no enhancement of occluded bone conduction sensitivity relative to unoccluded sensitivity) on either ear. Results suggest a middle ear disorder on both ears.[14]

PI-SSI functions (Case 18-2A) are normal on both ears. SSI max scores (Case 18-2B) are 100% on the right ear and 90% on the left ear. SSIT scores, 49 dB HL on the right ear and 45 dB HL on the left ear, agree with low frequency sensitivity on both ears. PB testing at high intensity levels (Case 18-2A) shows normal intelligibility scores and no rollover. PB max scores are 100% on each ear.

Impedance audiometry (Case 18-2C) shows slightly shallow, type A, tympanograms and low static compliance on both ears. Acoustic reflexes (Case 18-2D) are not observed on either ear at equipment limits.

Impression

RIGHT EAR: Moderate conductive loss.

LEFT EAR: Moderate conductive loss through 1000 Hz; very slight conductive loss above 1000 Hz.

On both ears, impedance audiometry is consistent with fixation of the ossicular chain.

SELECTED READINGS

Booth, J. Otosclerosis. *Practitioner* 221:710, 1978.
Carhart, R. Atypical configurations associated with otosclerosis. *Ann. Otol. Rhinol. Laryngol.* 71:744, 1962.
Daniel, H. Stapedial otosclerosis and fluoride in the drinking water. *Arch. Otolaryngol.* 90:585, 1969.
Djupesland, G. Use of impedance indicator in diagnosis of middle ear pathology. *Int. Aud.* 8:570, 1969.
Guild, S. Histologic otosclerosis. *Ann. Otol. Rhinol. Laryngol.* 53:246, 1944.
Lindsay, J. Otosclerosis. In M. Paparella and D. Shumrick (eds.), *Otolaryngology* (vol. 2). Philadelphia: Saunders, 1973. Pp. 205–230.
McCabe, B. Otosclerosis and vertigo. *Trans. Pac. Coast Otoophthalmol. Soc. Annu. Meet.* 47:37, 1966.
Nager, G. Histopathology of otosclerosis. *Arch. Otolaryngol.* 89:341, 1969.
Naunton, R., and Valvassori, G. Sensorineural hearing loss in otosclerosis. *Arch. Otolaryngol.* 89:372, 1969.

13. In patients with conductive hearing loss, a rising audiometric contour may be referred to as a *stiffness tilt*, because the increase in acoustic impedance of the middle ear mechanism affects sensitivity as a function of frequency in this characteristic fashion.
Note the me-

left ear, the audiogram shows a moderate conductive loss through 1000 Hz and a very slight conductive loss above 1000 Hz. PTA scores (Case 18-2B) are 42 dB HL on the right ear and 36 dB HL on the left ear. The left ear has a rising audiometric contour with greater loss in the low frequency region than in the high frequency region.[13]

The Weber test (Case 18-2B) at 500 Hz is reported as midline. Results suggest a bilateral symmetric conductive component at 500 Hz.

Ruedi, L. Otosclerotic lesion and cochlear degeneration. *Arch. Otolaryngol.* 89:364, 1969.

Schuknecht, H. *Pathology of the Ear.* Cambridge: Harvard University Press, 1974. Pp. 351–369.

Shambaugh, G. *Surgery of the Ear.* Philadelphia: Saunders, 1959. Pp. 437–459.

Shambaugh, G. Sensorineural deafness due to cochlear otospongiosis: Pathogenesis, clinical diagnosis, and therapy. *Otolaryngol. Clin. North Am.* 11:135, 1978.

Terkildsen, K., Osterhammel, P., and Bretlau, P. Acoustic middle ear muscle reflexes in patients with otosclerosis. *Arch. Otolaryngol.* 98:152, 1973.

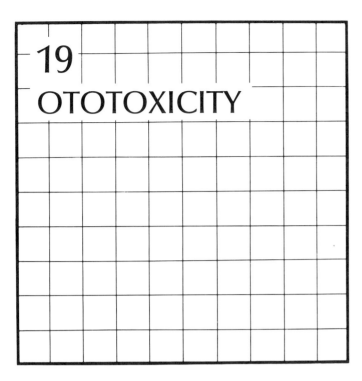

19
OTOTOXICITY

DESCRIPTION

1. About 1 million Americans are hospitalized annually for drug-induced disorders. Of individuals with adverse drug reactions, about 20% have neurologic complaints (Cluff and Caldwell, 1974).

Estimates of the prevalence of ototoxicity due to gentamicin, streptomycin, kanamycin, or neomycin range from about 2% of individuals receiving gentamicin to about 8% of persons receiving neomycin (Archieri et al., 1970).

Gorbach (1979) estimates that about 5% to 10% of persons have at least a 15 dB loss following a course of aminoglycoside therapy.

2. Ototoxic drugs, noise trauma, and presbyacusis produce similar histologic changes in the cochlea.

Ototoxicity refers to the occurrence of an undesired toxic reaction in the auditory or vestibular systems. Ototoxic reactions may be caused by a great variety of substances; e.g., aminoglycoside antibiotics, diuretics, arsenic, alcohol, tobacco, lead, carbon monoxide, mercury, aspirin, quinine, and nitrogen mustard. Factors that may influence the development of a hearing loss from ototoxic agents include the potential toxicity of the agent, the absolute dosage, the duration and method of exposure, the normalcy of kidney function, simultaneous or previous use of other ototoxic drugs, and individual susceptibility.[1]

The main findings from histopathologic studies in animals and humans with hearing loss from ototoxic substances are sensory cell damage in the cochlea and subsequent neural degeneration. Damage is characteristically more marked in outer hair cells than in inner hair cells. The abnormalities are characteristically more pronounced in the basal coil of the cochlea than in the apical region.[2]

A cause(s) of hearing loss from ototoxic agents is not clearcut. Toxic substances reach the inner ear through the bloodstream and accumulate in inner ear fluids. Some proposed theories of cochlear dysfunction suggest that toxic substances may inhibit oxidative and metabolic enzymes of af-

3. Of 84 children who received streptomycin in infancy, about 50% developed high frequency sensorineural loss (Székely and Draskovich, 1965).

Of 1131 ears with sensorineural hearing loss due to toxicity, the peak prevalence occurred in patients between 55 and 65 years of age (Surjan et al., 1973).

In experimental animals with spontaneous unilateral otitis media, the concentration of ototoxic antibiotics found in the inner ear was substantially increased in the ear with middle ear disorder relative to the opposite normal ear (Voldrich, 1965).

4. Temporary hearing loss from an ototoxic reaction to aspirin tablets may be more prevalent in females than in males (Miller, 1978).

5. Recovery of hearing is more commonly associated with toxic reactions to aspirin or diuretics than to antibiotics.

Of 38 patients receiving large doses of aspirin, 89% of persons developed hearing loss or tinnitus. When the medication was discontinued, however, all individuals demonstrated recovery from auditory symptoms (Jager and Always, 1946).

6. Threshold testing at ultra-high fre-

fected cells, may alter membrane permeability, or may interfere with protein synthesis.

PATIENT CHARACTERISTICS

A hearing loss from ototoxic agents may be congenital or acquired. Congenital hearing loss may occur from the mother's ingestion of ototoxic drugs during pregnancy, especially during the first trimester. Acquired hearing loss from ototoxic substances may occur at any age.

Individual susceptibility to ototoxic agents varies substantially for all ages. As a general rule, an increased sensitivity to ototoxic substances may be observed in infants, elderly individuals and persons with preexisting sensorineural loss or active middle ear disease (Bergstrom and Thompson, 1976; Lafton and Charachon, 1959).[3]

The incidence of hearing loss due to ototoxic drugs is equal for males and females (Surjan et al., 1973).[4] The hearing loss is characteristically bilateral.

CLINICAL COURSE

The onset of acquired hearing loss may be rapid or insidious. The hearing loss may occur during exposure to an ototoxic agent or may not appear until months after the ototoxic exposure is discontinued. The loss may be preceded or accompanied by a high pitched, ringing tinnitus. If the vestibular system is damaged, the patient may report dizziness and an unsteady gait.

The initial degree of loss may be unstable. For example, after exposure to an ototoxic agent has ceased, the hearing loss in some individuals may recover to within normal limits. In other individuals, however, the loss may progress to a more severe impairment.[5]

Serial audiograms may be an integral part of an ototoxic drug administration program. Pure tone sensitivity is characteristically monitored during treatment and for several months after administration of the ototoxic agent has stopped. During treatment, if tinnitus or a hearing loss develops, the therapy may be discontinued or changed.[6]

As a rule, the administration of ototoxic drugs is avoided whenever possible. If ototoxic drug therapy is necessary for medical reasons, the drug is characteristically discontinued from use as soon as possible.

quencies (above 8000 Hz) may indicate the occurrence of hearing loss due to ototoxicity as much as 75 days before testing at standard audiometric frequencies (Jacobson et al., 1969).

There is no preferred treatment for hearing loss due to ototoxicity.

SITE OF DISORDER

Cochlea. An exception involves patients with congenital hearing loss from ototoxic agents. Congenital abnormalities may include external and middle ear malformations, aplasia of the cochlea, and degeneration of the eighth nerve.

GENERAL AUDIOLOGIC PATTERN

Pure tone sensitivity results characteristically show an unstable, bilateral sensorineural hearing loss. On occasion, a unilateral sensorineural loss may occur. The initial degree of loss may vary from mild to profound impairment. In many patients, the degree of loss may be asymmetric.

7. In some patients with hearing loss due to ototoxicity from diuretics, the audiogram may show greater loss in the low and mid frequency regions than in the high frequency region.

The audiometric configuration varies substantially. As a general rule, the initial stage of hearing loss due to ototoxicity shows a high frequency sensorineural loss. A sloping audiometric contour is present. Subsequently, the audiometric configuration may change to a relatively flatter contour with sensitivity loss at all frequencies. In patients with severe sensitivity loss, the audiogram usually shows a greater loss in the high frequency region than in the low frequency region.[7]

Maximum speech intelligibility performance varies. In some patients, maximum speech intelligibility scores are consistent with the degree of sensitivity loss. In other patients, however, speech intelligibility scores are disproportionately reduced relative to pure tone sensitivity results. In contrast to variable maximum intelligibility performance, the shape of the PI function is characteristically normal (no rollover phenomenon).

Impedance results usually show normal, type A, tympanograms and normal static compliance measures. Acoustic reflexes are characteristically present at normal HLs and reduced sensation levels. No reflex decay is observed at 500 Hz or 1000 Hz. In individuals with severe hearing loss due to ototoxicity, reflex thresholds cannot be measured because signals cannot be presented at sufficiently high intensity levels.

8. Monitoring of pure tone sensitivity during ototoxic drug administration was not requested in this patient. Remember, however, in patients that are too ill for behavioral audiometric testing, acoustic reflex predictive methods like the SPAR procedure may be helpful in monitoring auditory sensitivity.

In monkeys with hearing loss due to ototoxic drugs, acoustic reflex measures consistently reflected the approximate degree of cochlear damage found in subsequent histologic studies (Jerger et al., 1978).

Illustrative Patient

CASE 1. A 19-YEAR-OLD MALE WITH HEARING LOSS ON BOTH EARS DUE TO OTOTOXICITY.

History

The patient complains of a hearing loss and tinnitus on both ears. He denies feelings of dizziness or disequilibrium. Approximately 3 months ago, the patient was crushed between pipes in an accident on an oil pipeline. Following the accident, he was unconscious for 1 month. He received ototoxic drug therapy for lifesaving purposes. The antibiotic regimen consisted of chloramphenicol for 7 days, gentamicin sulfate for 5 days, and chloramphenicol for 6 days. Other medications during hospitalization included Demerol, Tylenol, and Phenergan.[8]

The patient reports that he had no hearing complaints before the accident. He has approximately a 2-year history of noise exposure from industrial machinery. The patient says that a hearing test performed 2 days before the accident showed a very slight loss for high pitched sounds on both ears.

Results

Case 19-1A presents results of two audiologic evaluations. Notice the results labeled "1." These findings were obtained at the initial evaluation, approximately 3 months after the patient's ototoxic drug therapy began.

The audiogram ("1," Case 19-1A) on the right ear shows a mild sensorineural loss through 1000 Hz and a moderate sensorineural loss above 1000 Hz. On the left ear, the audiogram shows a moderate sensorineural loss at all frequencies. The PTA scores (Case 19-1B) are 37 dB HL on the right ear and 57 dB HL on the left ear.

The Weber test (Case 19-1B) at 500 Hz lateralizes to the right ear, the ear with the better pure tone sensitivity.

The shape of the PI-PB functions ("1," Case 19-1A) is normal on both ears. The PB max scores (Case 19-1B) are 88% on the right ear and 48% on the left ear. Speech thresholds on both ears agree with average pure tone sensitivity. The PBT scores are 34 dB HL on the right ear and 50 dB HL on the left ear.

Impedance audiometry (Case 19-1C)

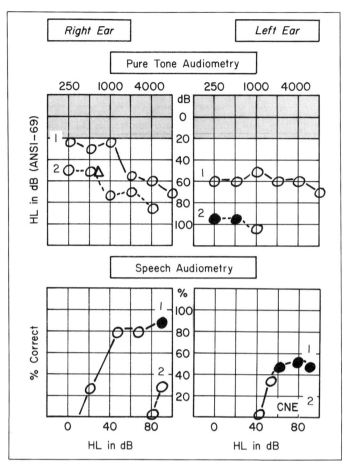

Case 19-1A. *Pure tone audiogram and speech audiometry. "1" initial evaluation, approximately 3 months after first ototoxic drug therapy; "2" audiologic reevaluation, approximately 2 years after initial evaluation, 19 months after repeated ototoxic drug administration. Acoustic reflex thresholds are not shown.*

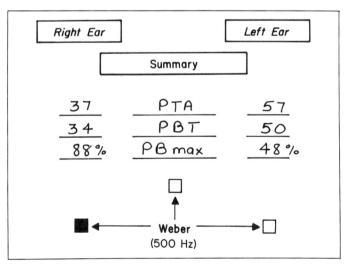

Case 19-1B. *Summary of test results and Weber test for initial evaluation ("1").*

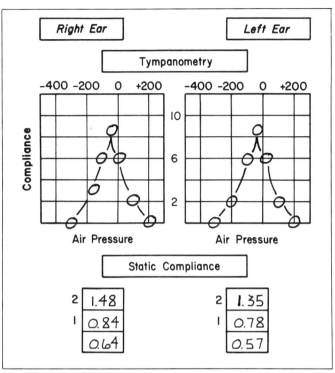

Case 19-1C. *Impedance audiometry: tympanometry and static compliance measures (in cc) for evaluations "1" and "2."*

9. More specifically, for all frequencies between 250 Hz and 4000 Hz, reflex thresholds were present at normal HLs and reduced sensation levels bilaterally.

shows normal, type A, tympanograms and normal static compliance measures bilaterally. The reflex pattern (Case 19-1D) shows normal reflex thresholds for both crossed and uncrossed stimulation on both ears.[9] No reflex decay is observed at 500 Hz or 1000 Hz on either ear. The SPAR measure predicts a mild to moderate sensitivity loss on both ears.

Impression

RIGHT EAR: Mild sensorineural loss through 1000 Hz; moderate sensorineural loss above 1000 Hz.

LEFT EAR: Moderate sensorineural hearing loss.

On both ears, impedance audiometry indicates normal middle ear function.

Recommendations

Monitoring of pure tone sensitivity at regular intervals.

Audiologic Reevaluation

HISTORY. The patient's hearing sensitivity was monitored at regular intervals for a 2-

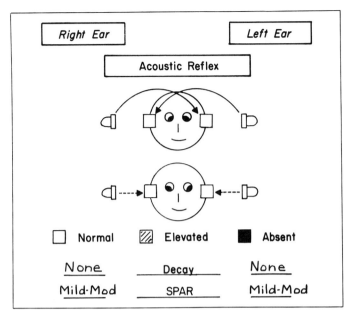

Case 19-1D. *Impedance audiometry: acoustic reflex pattern, sensitivity prediction from the acoustic reflex, and reflex decay results for initial evaluation ("1").*

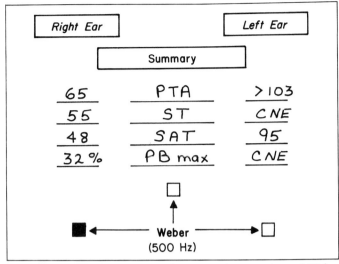

Case 19-1E. *Summary of test results and Weber test for audiologic reevaluation ("2").*

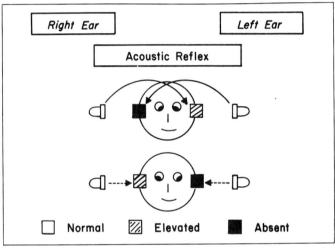

Case 19-1F. *Impedance audiometry: acoustic reflex pattern (crossed vs uncrossed conditions) for audiologic reevaluation ("2").*

year period. The patient's medical history during this period was noncontributory with one exception. Approximately 5 months after the initial audiologic evaluation, the patient had serious medical complications that required additional ototoxic drug therapy. He received tobramycin for approximately 8 days.

Case 19-1A ("2") presents results of an audiologic evaluation obtained approximately 2 years after the initial test.

Results

10. During a 2-year observation period, pure tone sensitivity declined about 30 dB on the right ear and more than 50 dB on the left ear.

The audiogram ("2," Case 19-1A) on the right ear shows a moderate sensorineural loss through 500 Hz and a severe sensorineural loss above 500 Hz. The audiogram on the left ear shows a profound sensorineural loss. The PTA scores (Case 19-1E) are 65 dB HL on the right ear and greater than 103 dB HL on the left ear.[10]

The Weber test (Case 19-1E) at 500 Hz lateralizes to the right ear. The unmasked bone conduction threshold ("2," Case 19-1A) at 500 Hz is superimposed on the air conduction threshold of the right ear. With masking to the right ear, bone conduction sensitivity at 500 Hz on the left ear is beyond equipment limits. At frequencies above 500 Hz, there is no observable re-

11. During the observation period, maximum speech intelligibility performance on the right ear declined about 55%.

12. Notice that when PB testing cannot be carried out or when PB max is reduced to the extent that a PBT score may not be obtained, an ST or SAT score provides

sponse to unmasked bone conducted signals at equipment limits.

Speech audiometry ("2," Case 19-1A) on the right ear shows a PB max score of 32%.[11] A speech threshold for spondee words (ST) and a speech awareness threshold (SAT) on the right ear agree with average pure tone sensitivity or low frequency sensitivity. The ST score (Case 19-1E) is 55 dB HL; the SAT score is 48 dB HL. Speech intelligibility testing ("2," Case 19-1A) on the left ear could not be evaluated (CNE) due to the severity of the pure tone sensitivity loss. The SAT score (Case 19-1E) on the left ear is 95 dB HL.[12]

a useful crosscheck on pure tone sensitivity results.

13. More specifically, with sound to the right ear, acoustic reflexes are present at normal HLs at 250 Hz and 500 Hz. Above 500 Hz, reflex thresholds are elevated or absent at all frequencies. With sound to the left ear, acoustic reflex thresholds are absent at all frequencies.

Tympanometry and static compliance measures are the same as results of the initial evaluation (Case 19-1C). The reflex pattern (Case 19-1F) shows elevated or absent reflex thresholds for both crossed and uncrossed stimulation on both ears.[13] Results are consistent with a severe sensorineural loss on both ears.

Impression

RIGHT EAR: Moderate sensorineural loss through 500 Hz; severe sensorineural loss above 500 Hz.

LEFT EAR: Profound sensorineural loss.

On both ears, pure tone sensitivity and maximum speech intelligibility performance have declined relative to results of the initial evaluation.

SELECTED READINGS

Archieri, G., Falco, F., Smith, H., and Hobson, L. Clinical research experience with gentamicin: Incidence of adverse reactions. *Med. J. Aust.* Suppl. 1:30, 1970.

Ballantyne, J. Ototoxicity: A clinical review. *Audiology* 12:325, 1973.

Bergstrom, L., and Thompson, P. Ototoxicity. In J. Northern (ed.), *Hearing Disorders*. Boston: Little, Brown, 1976. Pp. 136–152.

Cluff, L., and Caldwell, J. Reactions to Drugs. In M. Wintrobe, G. Thorn, R. Adams, E. Braunwald, K. Isselbacher, and R. Petersdorf (eds.), *Harrison's Principles of Internal Medicine* (7th ed.). New York: McGraw-Hill, 1974. Pp. 375–381.

Glorig, A. The effect of dihydrostreptomycin hydrochloride and sulfate on the auditory mechanism. *Ann. Otol. Rhinol. Laryngol.* 60:327, 1951.

Gorbach, S. Discussion on the Frequency of Ototoxicity—a Review of the Literature. In R. Richardson (ed.), *Round-Table Discussion on Gentamicin and Tobramycin*. London: Royal Society of Medicine, 1979. P. 53.

Jacobson, E., Downs, M., and Fletcher, J. Clinical findings in high-frequency thresholds during known ototoxic drug usage. *J. Aud. Res.* 9:379, 1969.

Jager, B., and Always, R. The treatment of acute rheumatic fever with large doses of sodium salicylate. *Am. J. Med. Sci.* 211:273, 1946.

Jerger, J., Mauldin, L., and Igarashi, M. Impedance audiometry in the squirrel monkey: Sensori-neural losses. *Arch. Otolaryngol.* 104:559, 1978.

Lafton, H., and Charachon, R. Le rôle de la barrière hémolabyrinthique dans la pathogénie des accidents cochléaires du à la streptomycine. *J. Franc. Otorhinolaryngol.* 8:965, 1959.

Miller, R. Deafness due to plain and long-acting aspirin tablets. *J. Clin. Pharmacol.* 18:468, 1978.

Schuknecht, H. *Pathology of the Ear.* Cambridge: Harvard University Press, 1974. Pp. 273–288.

Stupp, H., Rauch, S., Brun, J., and Lagler, F. Kanamycin dosage and levels in ear and other organs. *Arch. Otolaryngol.* 86:515, 1967

Surjan, L., Devald, J., and Palfalvi, L. Epidemiology of hearing loss. *Audiology* 12:396, 1973.

Székely, T., and Draskovich, E. Die Wirkung des Streptomycins auf das Gehörorgan von Kleinkindern. *Z. Laryngol. Rhinol.* 44:15, 1965. Cited in J. Ballantyne, Ototoxicity: A clinical review. *Audiology* 12:325, 1973.

Voldrich, L. The kinetics of streptomycin, kanamycin, and neomycin in the inner ear. *Acta Otolaryngol.* 60:243, 1965.

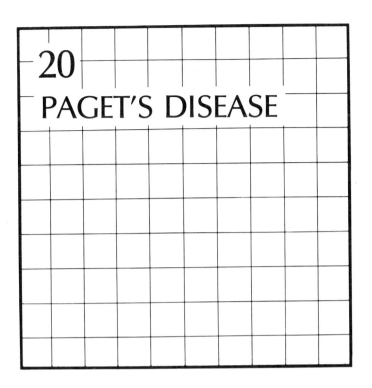

20

PAGET'S DISEASE

DESCRIPTION

1. Paget's disease may be referred to as *osteitis deformans*.

An estimate of the prevalence of Paget's disease in persons over 40 years of age is about 3%. Prevalence appears to increase with age. In persons over 89 years of age, the disease is present in about 5% to 10% of individuals.

The prevalence of Paget's disease seems higher in persons of Anglo-Saxon descent. The disease is most common in the United Kingdom, Australia, and New Zealand. Paget's disease is rare in the Middle East, Africa, Asia, South America, and India.

Some clinicians suggest that otosclerosis may be a localized form of Paget's disease. In a series of 463 patients with Paget's disease, 4% had concurrent otosclerosis (Harner et al., 1978).

Paget's disease is a chronic bone disease. The condition may affect only one bone or many bones. Paget's disease is asymptomatic and undetected in many individuals. Pathologically, Paget's disease is characterized by excessive resorption of bone. The bone marrow is replaced by vascular, fibrous connective tissue. New bone tissue is formed. The newly formed pagetoid bone is generally structurally abnormal. The new bone mass may be larger than normal. Characteristic sites of involvement in patients with Paget's disease include the spine, pelvis, femur, tibia, and skull.

The etiology of Paget's disease is unknown. Proposed theories include vascular, endocrine, and metabolic disturbances; viral or genetic factors; and neoplastic or inflammatory processes.[1]

In patients with Paget's disease involving the temporal bone, histologic studies may show abnormality of the external auditory canal, middle ear cavity, and cochlea. Findings may include stenosis of the external auditory canal, bony spurs in the epitympanic region of the middle ear space, pagetoid changes in the ossicles, ossification of the stapedial tendon, fibrotic or bony changes in the annular ligament, and destruction and/or fracture of the bony labyrinth. Morphologic changes within the

Beethoven's deafness was probably due to Paget's disease (Naiken, 1972).

2. In patients with clinically evident Paget's disease, the skull and temporal bones may be involved in about 50% to 70% of individuals.

cochlea may include atrophy of receptor cells, nerve fibers, ganglion cells, and stria vascularis. On rare occasions, in patients with widespread involvement of the petrous pyramid, narrowing and distortion of the internal auditory canal may be observed.[2]

Complications of Paget's disease may include fractures, arthritis, neoplasms, and cardiovascular disease.

PATIENT CHARACTERISTICS

In about 85% to 95% of individuals, a diagnosis of Paget's disease is made after 49 years of age. The disease is rare in persons less than 40 years old. The diagnosis is made as an incidental finding in about 38% of patients (Galbraith et al., 1977).

In individuals with an advanced stage of Paget's disease, physical findings may include a markedly enlarged skull, a sunken chest, a curved back, and a waddling gait. A family history of Paget's disease may be reported by about 7% of patients with clinically evident disease.

Paget's disease is more prevalent in males than in females at all ages. The male-to-female ratio is approximately 4:3. A hearing loss, when present, is characteristically bilateral.

CLINICAL COURSE

3. Of patients with Paget's disease, more than 5% but less than 25% have hearing loss that may be attributed to the disease (Harner et al., 1978).

In a series of 111 patients with Paget's disease, hearing loss was the second most frequent symptom. A hearing loss was present in 14% of individuals (Rosenkrantz et al., 1952).

The onset of Paget's disease is characteristically insidious. Waves of bone destruction and new bone formation may continue indefinitely or may be interrupted by quiescent, sclerotic periods. Clinical symptoms in patients with Paget's disease involving the skull may include headache, facial pain, numbness, tingling, visual impairment, and hearing loss. The hearing loss is slowly progressive in most people. The loss is accompanied by tinnitus and dizziness in 20% to 35% of patients.[3] The treatment of Paget's disease may involve drug therapy and surgery. The treatment of choice varies depending on the site, extent, and activity of the lesion.

SITE OF DISORDER

Middle ear and cochlea. The external auditory canal may be involved in some patients.

GENERAL AUDIOLOGIC PATTERN

4. In a series of 319 patients with Paget's disease, 70% of ears had sensorineural hearing loss. However, relative to findings in a normal control group of the same age, the hearing loss could be explained by presbyacusis in most patients. Further, in about 75% of individuals, the disease did not appear to involve the skull (Harner et al., 1978).

The auditory characteristics of Paget's disease are difficult to define. The problem is that in a disease primarily affecting older individuals, it is difficult to determine whether a hearing loss is age related or disease related. A sensorineural hearing loss is frequently observed in patients with Paget's disease. However, many persons with sensorineural loss have no evidence of temporal bone involvement due to Paget's disease. Instead, the loss seems proportional to the patient's age and/or history of noise exposure. In this circumstance, the hearing loss is generally not attributed to Paget's disease.[4]

In our experience, patients with Paget's disease of the skull and hearing loss that cannot be explained solely by presbyacusis have the following auditory characteristics.

Pure tone sensitivity results usually show a bilateral mixed hearing loss. The degree of loss may vary from mild to severe impairment. In most patients, the degree of loss progresses over time.

The audiometric contour is usually a downwardly sloping configuration with greater loss in the high frequency region than in the low frequency region. The air-bone gap is usually greater at low frequencies than at high frequencies. The degree of conductive component in the low frequency region may be about 20 to 30 dB. In some individuals, the conductive component may diminish over time. The mixed hearing loss may progress to a pure sensorineural loss at all frequencies.

Speech intelligibility scores for monosyllabic (PB) words are generally within the normal range or consistent with the degree of peripheral sensorineural impairment.

Impedance audiometry usually shows abnormal tympanograms, abnormal static compliance measures, and absent acoustic reflexes.

Illustrative Patient

CASE 1. A 63-YEAR-OLD MALE WITH PAGET'S DISEASE INVOLVING THE TEMPORAL BONE.

History

Approximately 1 month ago the patient's dentist noted abnormal mouth x-rays on routine examination. He referred the patient

5. In some patients, hearing sensitivity may improve during calcitonin therapy (Hsu, 1977).

6. Masked frontal bone conduction thresholds and SAL results could not be determined in this patient at 2000 Hz and 4000 Hz due to the severity of the sensorineural loss. In this circumstance, unmasked mastoid bone conduction measures were obtained. Remember, although frontal bone conduction thresholds usually offer clinical advantages over mastoid bone conduction measures, the greater vibrational output required to reach threshold at the frontal bone relative to the mastoid may be a practical limitation in some patients with substantial sensorineural loss.

7. Notice that a difference between PB max and SSI max scores on the right

to a physician. The patient claims to be in good health. He denies any difficulties except for hearing loss.

The patient has noticed a gradually progressive loss of hearing in both ears for the past 10 years. The progression of the loss seems greater during the past year. He reports an occasional buzzing tinnitus in each ear. The patient notices difficulty understanding people who talk rapidly or who "slur their speech." He has more difficulty understanding in noisy places.

Physical examination reveals a normocephalic male with no gross asymmetry or deformity. Neurologic and otorhinolaryngologic examinations are within normal limits, except for the hearing loss. The tympanic membranes are intact and clear bilaterally. There is no suggestion of mass or fluid on otoscopic examination.

Results of x-ray and bone scan studies are consistent with Paget's disease involving the skull, mandible, spine, and possibly the left distal femur. Laboratory studies reveal elevated serum alkaline phosphatase levels. The patient is receiving calcitonin therapy.[5]

Results

The audiogram (Case 20-1A) on both ears shows a moderate mixed loss through 1000 Hz and a severe mixed loss above 1000 Hz. The PTA scores (Case 20-1B) are 60 dB HL on the right ear and 53 dB HL on the left ear. Bone conduction and SAL audiometry (Case 20-1A) on both ears show a conductive component of about 40 dB at 500 Hz and 20 dB at 1000 Hz. Unmasked bone conduction thresholds at 2000 Hz and 4000 Hz suggest a conductive component on at least one ear of 10 dB to 20 dB.[6]

The Weber test (Case 20-1B) at 500 Hz does not lateralize to either ear. The signal is heard in the midline. The Bing test (not shown) at 500 Hz shows no difference between occluded and unoccluded thresholds on either ear.

Speech audiometry (Case 20-1A) on both ears shows reduced maximum intelligibility scores for both PB words and SSI materials. On the right ear, the PB max score (Case 20-1B) is 60%; the SSI max score is 40%. On the left ear, the PB max and SSI max scores are 60%. No rollover is observed on either ear.[7]

Speech thresholds (Case 20-1B) on both

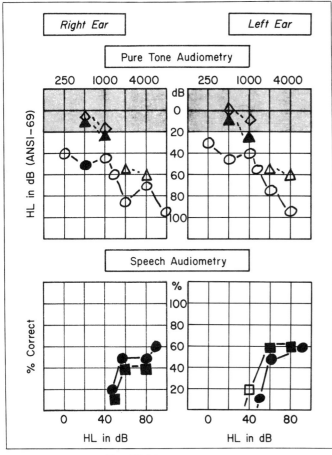

Case 20-1A

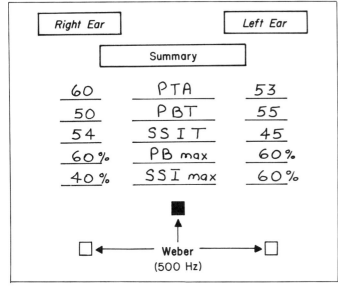

Case 20-1B

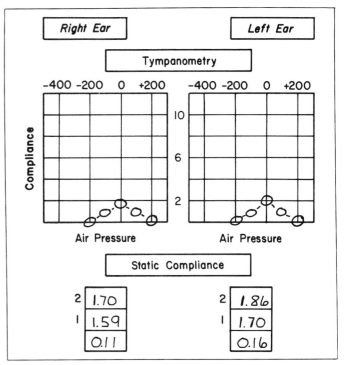

Case 20-1C

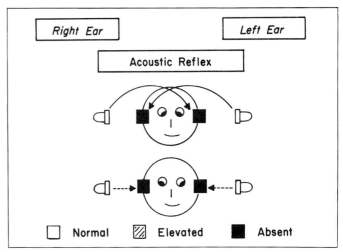

Case 20-1D

ear is related to a difference in the maximum intensity level used for each test. For PI-PB functions, the maximum test intensity is 90 dB HL. For PI-SSI functions with a competing speech message at a message-to-competition ratio of 0 dB, the maximum intensity is 80 dB HL. In this circum- ears agree (± 10 dB) with average pure tone sensitivity. On the right ear, the PBT score is 50 dB HL; the SSIT score is 54 dB HL. On the left ear, the PBT score is 55 dB HL; the SSIT score is 45 dB HL.

Impedance audiometry (Case 20-1C) shows unusually shallow, type A, tympanograms and abnormally reduced static compliance measures bilaterally. Crossed and uncrossed acoustic reflexes (Case 20-1D) on both ears are absent at equipment limits at all frequencies.

stance, a difference between PB max and SSI max performance is not interpreted as a suggestion of central auditory disorder.

8. In patients with Paget's disease of the skull, serial hearing tests may be used to monitor the progression of the disease.

Impression

On both ears, a moderate mixed loss through 1000 Hz; a severe mixed loss above 1000 Hz. Middle ear involvement is supported by the presence of an air-bone and air-SAL gap, abnormally shallow tympanograms, abnormally reduced static compliance measures, absent acoustic reflexes, and no difference between occluded and unoccluded bone conduction thresholds. The pattern of impedance results on both ears is consistent with fixation of the ossicular chain.[8]

SELECTED READINGS

Barker, D., Clough, P., Guyer, P., and Gardner, M. Paget's disease of bone in 14 British towns. *Br. Med. J.* 7:1181, 1977.

Clarke, C., and Harrison, M. Neurological manifestations of Paget's disease. *J. Neurol. Sci.* 38:171, 1978.

Collins, D. Paget's disease of bone: Incidence and subclinical forms. *Lancet* 2:6933, 1956.

Davies, G. Paget's disease of the temporal bone. *Acta Otolaryngol.* Suppl. 242:1, 1968.

Galbraith, H., Evans, E., and Lacey, J. Paget's disease of bone—a clinical and genetic study. *Postgrad. Med. J.* 53:33, 1977.

Hamdy, R. The signs and treatment of Paget's disease. *Geriatrics* 32:89, 1977.

Harner, S., Rose, D., and Facer, G. Paget's disease and hearing loss. *Trans. Am. Acad. Ophthalmol. Otolaryngol.* 86:869, 1978.

Hsu, T. Current diagnosis and management of Paget's disease. *Md. State Med. J.* 27:48, 1977.

Lindsay, J., and Suga, F. Paget's disease and sensori-neural deafness: Temporal bone histopathology of Paget's disease. *Laryngoscope* 86:1029, 1976.

Nager, G. Paget's disease of the temporal bone. *Ann. Otol. Rhinol. Laryngol.* 84, Suppl. 22:1, 1975.

Naiken, V. Paget's disease and Beethoven's deafness. *Clin. Orthop.* 89:103, 1972.

Rosenkrantz, J., Wolf, J., and Kaicher, J. Paget's disease (osteitis deformans). *Arch. Intern. Med.* 90:610, 1952.

Schuknecht, H. *Pathology of the Ear.* Cambridge: Harvard University Press, 1974. Pp. 374–378.

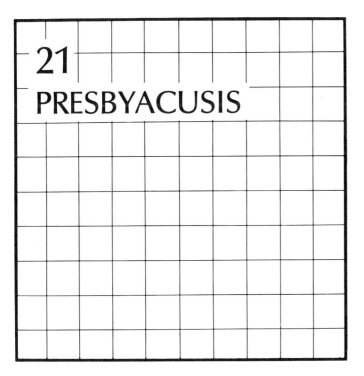

21
PRESBYACUSIS

DESCRIPTION

1. Estimates of the prevalence of presbyacusis in persons at least 65 years of age range from about 5% to 20%.
In individuals over 65 years of age with deteriorated health, hearing problems may be observed in about 60% of persons (Kronholm, 1968).

Presbyacusis refers to hearing disorders due to senescent changes in the auditory system. Current theories of presbyacusis include both environmental and genetic factors. Theories oriented around environmental factors stress that aging within the auditory system is primarily due to "wear and tear." A gradual loss of function may occur from the cumulative effects of environmental influences, e.g., infections, toxins, and traumas. Theories oriented around genetic factors stress that aging is primarily due to hereditary processes. Gradual retrogressive changes in cell function, cell structure, and in the number of cells may occur due to the effects of natural genetic factors within each individual.[1]

2. The senescent changes of the external and middle ear systems are generally not associated with measurable hearing loss. However, senescent changes of the external ear may be associated with an erroneous conductive hearing loss due to collapse of the ear canal under earphones. Remember, about one-third of patients with col-

Physical findings and histopathologic studies in elderly individuals reveal senescent changes in all parts of the auditory system. In the external and middle ear systems, alterations may include decreased elasticity and increased size of the pinna, atrophy or increased flaccidity of the external auditory canal wall, excessive accumulation of cerumen, thickening of the tympanic membrane, and arthritic changes of the ossicular joints.[2]

In the inner ear, senescent changes may be noted in any of the morphologic structures of the cochlea. Degeneration of the

lapsing ear canal are 65 years of age or older (see Chapter 4, Collapsing Ear Canal).

The prevalence of otitis media is increased in elderly persons relative to young adults (see Chapter 17, Otitis Media).

3. In elderly individuals, auditory dysfunction may be related to specific cerebrovascular disorders (see Chapter 2, Cerebrovascular Disorders).

4. Some studies (Lowell and Paparella, 1977) report no difference between the sexes. Other studies (Surjan et al., 1973) report a higher prevalence of presbyacusis in males (53%) than in females (47%), even though the general population over 65 years of age has approximately 20% more females than males. In contrast to these observations, Hayes and Jerger (1979) noted that the prevalence of central auditory disorders due to aging seems greater in females than in males.

eighth nerve may occur. Schuknecht (1974) classifies senescent alterations of the inner ear into four basic types: sensory, neural, metabolic, and mechanical. Sensory presbyacusis reflects the atrophy and degeneration of the hair cells and supporting cells of the organ of Corti. Neural presbyacusis refers to a loss of auditory neurons. In both sensory and neural types of presbyacusis, abnormalities are typically more pronounced in the basal coil of the cochlea than in the apical region.

Metabolic presbyacusis is based on vascular and atrophic changes in the stria vascularis. Finally, mechanical presbyacusis reflects the atrophic changes in the physical properties of the cochlear duct, especially the basilar membrane and the spiral ligament. In elderly persons, the four general types of alterations may occur singly or in any combination.

In the central auditory system, senescent changes have been observed in the cochlear nucleus, superior olivary nucleus, lateral lemniscus, inferior colliculus, medial geniculate body, and auditory cortex (Kirikae et al., 1964; Corso, 1977). These changes may include a reduction in the number and size of ganglion cells, a decrease in the number of myelinated axons, and irregularity in the shape of nerve cells.[3]

PATIENT CHARACTERISTICS

The age of onset of presbyacusis varies among individuals. As a general rule, some degree of presbyacusis may be observed in males after the age of 32 years and in females after the age of 37 years (Corso, 1977). However, large individual variations in susceptibility to presbyacusis occur. A sex distribution for presbyacusis is unsettled.[4] The hearing loss is characteristically bilateral.

CLINICAL COURSE

The onset of presbyacusis is characteristically insidious. Affected individuals generally report a gradually progressive, bilateral hearing loss. A high pitched, ringing tinnitus may accompany the loss in many persons. The rate of progression of the hearing loss may vary widely among patients. As a general rule, however, as age increases from 20 to 90 years, average pure tone sensitivity may decline about 30 dB (Lebo and Reddell, 1972) and average speech intelligibility (PB max) performance may decline approximately 35% (Jerger, 1973). Subjective complaints of hearing loss are generally not reported by patients until a hearing loss of more than 25 dB HL (ANSI-69) occurs at a frequency below 3000 Hz.

Frequently, subjective awareness of the loss occurs at a time when the individual is experiencing increasing personal stress due to retirement, socioeconomic change, etc. In some individuals, consequences of presbyacusis may include depression and withdrawal.

In addition to hearing loss, elderly persons may have personality changes due to senescent alterations in the central nervous system. Individuals may exhibit increased irritability, reduced attention span, reduced alertness, lowered emotional and intellectual strengths, and loss of memory.

The treatment of presbyacusis centers primarily around aural rehabilitation, psychological counseling, and amplification.[5]

SITE OF DISORDER

Cochlea, eighth nerve, and/or central auditory system.[6]

GENERAL AUDIOLOGIC PATTERN

Pure tone sensitivity results characteristically show a gradually progressive, bilateral sensorineural loss. The sensitivity loss is generally symmetric. The average degree of loss for 500 Hz, 1000 Hz, and 2000 Hz is usually between 15 dB HL to 60 dB HL.

The audiometric contour is characteristically sloping. However, the frequency region affected by presbyacusis usually increases over time. In the initial stages, the hearing loss is typically confined to frequencies above 2000 Hz. However, with increasing age, the hearing loss eventually involves progressively lower frequencies.

On occasion, pure tone sensitivity results may not conform to the above general pattern. Notable exceptions include patients with normal pure tone sensitivity or with approximately the same degree of sensitivity loss at all frequencies (a flat audiometric configuration).[7]

5. The effective use of hearing aids in elderly persons with peripheral hearing loss is frequently limited by the presence of a central auditory disorder superimposed on the peripheral auditory deficit. In this circumstance, realistic counseling concerning the possible benefits and limitations of amplification is of critical importance.

6. The relative importance of peripheral vs central auditory dysfunction in presbyacusis seems unresolved. Some clinicians (Schuknecht, 1974) have emphasized the peripheral changes. Others (Hinchcliffe, 1962; Kirikae et al., 1964) have stressed the central auditory alterations.

7. In a series of 55 elderly individuals with hearing loss due to presbyacusis, the audiometric contour was sloping in 65% and flat in 31% of persons (Dayal et al., 1970).

8. Our observation of an unusual degree of low frequency sensitivity loss in elderly females is supported by data of the United States Health and Nutrition Examination survey (Leske, 1979), and by studies in the Mabaan tribe of Africa (Rosen et al., 1962). The Mabaan tribe seems unique in that they do not incur significant hearing loss with increasing age. However, in both of the above reports, audiometric studies show poorer low frequency sensitivity in elderly women than in elderly men.

In our experience, the pattern of hearing loss due to presbyacusis frequently differs between the sexes. For example, in the high frequency region of the audiogram, the degree of loss is characteristically greater in males than in females. In contrast, in the low frequency region of the audiogram, the degree of loss is generally greater in females than in males.[8]

Maximum speech intelligibility varies depending on the site and severity of the auditory disorder. In patients with cochlear site, maximum speech intelligibility scores are usually consistent with the degree of sensitivity loss. In patients with retrocochlear site, however, maximum speech intelligibility performance may be unusually poor relative to the degree of sensitivity loss. Abnormal speech intelligibility performance may be observed in some persons with normal pure tone sensitivity. Abnormalities may include unusually reduced maximum intelligibility scores, rollover of the PI function, and a disproportionate speech threshold loss relative to average pure tone sensitivity results.

In contrast to the variable performance on routine speech intelligibility tests, performance on degraded speech tests is characteristically abnormal on both ears. Performance deficits may be observed for speech signals that are temporally interrupted, accelerated, filtered, or presented in the presence of a competing speech message.

Impedance audiometry usually shows normal, type A, tympanograms and normal static compliance measures. Acoustic reflex results vary, however, depending on the site of disorder and degree of sensitivity loss. As a general rule, in patients with cochlear site, reflexes are present at normal HLs and reduced sensation levels. An exception involves patients with steeply sloping audiometric configurations. In these individuals, acoustic reflexes may be absent at high frequencies even though the degree of sensitivity loss is not severe. In contrast to patients with cochlear site, patients with retrocochlear involvement characteristically show elevated threshold HLs and/or an abnormal time course during reflex decay testing.

Other abnormalities associated with presbyacusis may include aberrant results on adaptation tests, such as STAT, and on au-

9. On ABR audiometry, elderly individuals may show an increased wave V latency (about 0.2 msec) and a decreased wave V amplitude (about 15%) relative to results in young adults (Jerger and Hall, 1980).

10. Remember, the testing of elderly individuals may be complicated by some of the symptoms of brain damage, such as shortened attention span (see Clinical Course). In particular, elderly individuals may be disadvantaged on tests that have short respond intervals. For example, Feldman and Reger (1967) observed that the reaction time to a 500 Hz pure tone signal increased about 0.3 sec as age increased from 20 to 80 years.

ditory brain stem evoked response (ABR) audiometry.[9]

In order to ensure accurate results on behavioral auditory tests, some elderly patients may need modification of test instructions and test techniques.[10]

Illustrative Patients

CASE 1. A 66-YEAR-OLD FEMALE WITH PRESBYACUSIS.

History

The patient is concerned about several fainting episodes that she has experienced during the past 2 years. The episodes are characterized by nausea, shortness of breath, and unconsciousness.

On admission to the hospital, general physical examination is within normal limits. Neurologic examination reveals no abnormality except for slightly diminished hearing bilaterally. Results of routine laboratory studies, skull x-rays, CT scan, brain scan, blood flow studies, and EEG studies are within normal limits. The final medical diagnosis is syncope, probably a hyperventilation syndrome.

During hospitalization, the patient asked to have her hearing evaluated. She reports that her hearing in both ears has decreased gradually during the past 5 years. She notices particular difficulty understanding speech in noisy situations. The patient denies tinnitus and ear tenderness on both ears. She does not report a history of ear infections, head trauma, noise exposure, or atypical drug use. Otorhinolaryngologic examination is within normal limits.

Results

The audiogram (Case 21-1A) on both ears shows normal pure tone sensitivity through 1000 Hz and a mild sensorineural loss above 1000 Hz. The audiometric configuration is sloping with greater loss in the high frequency region than in the low frequency region. The PTA scores (Case 21-1B) are 10 dB HL on the right ear and 13 dB HL on the left ear.

Speech audiometry (Case 21-1A) shows normal maximum intelligibility scores bilaterally. On the right ear, the PB max score (Case 21-1B) is 96%; the SSI max score is 90%. On the left ear, the PB max score is 100%; the SSI max score is 90%. No roll-

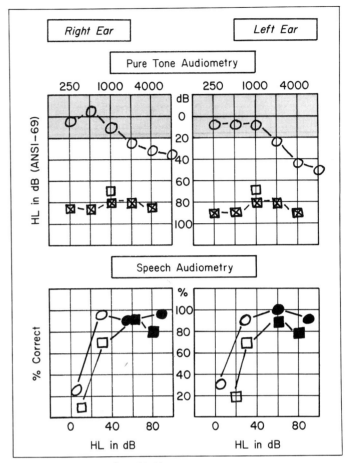

Case 21-1A

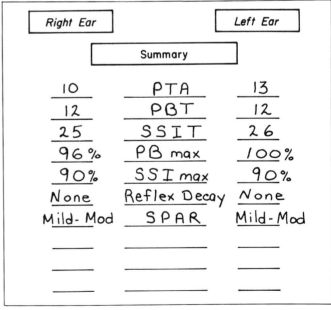

Case 21-1B

over effect is observed on either ear at high intensity levels.

The PBT scores, 12 dB HL on both ears, agree with average pure tone sensitivity results bilaterally. In contrast to PBT results, however, SSIT scores on both ears are elevated with respect to average pure tone results.

The SSIT scores are 25 dB HL on the right ear and 26 dB HL on the left ear.[11]

Impedance audiometry (Case 21-1C) shows normal, type A, tympanograms and normal static compliance measures bilaterally. On both ears, crossed and uncrossed acoustic reflexes (Case 21-1A) are present at normal HLs at all frequencies. No reflex decay (Case 21-1B) is observed on either ear at 500 Hz or 1000 Hz. SPAR results predict a mild to moderate sensitivity loss on each ear.[12]

Summary

On both ears, normal sensitivity through 1000 Hz; mild sensorineural loss above 1000 Hz. Impedance audiometry is consistent with normal middle ear function bilaterally. Relative to the PTA and PBT scores, SSIT scores show a disproportionate loss on both ears.

CASE 2. AN 81-YEAR-OLD FEMALE WITH PRESBYACUSIS.

History

The patient complains of a hearing loss in both ears. The loss has been slowly progressive for many years. She does not remember when she first noticed difficulty in hearing.

The patient reports that she can understand conversation if individuals "speak plainly and don't mumble." She denies tinnitus, dizziness, previous ear infections, head injury, atypical drug use, and noise exposure.

Otorhinolaryngologic examination is within normal limits. The patient is generally healthy except for a 1-year history of anginal syndrome due to arteriosclerotic heart disease.

Results

The audiogram (Case 21-2A) on both ears shows a mild sensorineural loss through 2000 Hz and a moderate sensorineural loss above 2000 Hz. The PTA scores (Case 21-2B) are 28 dB HL on the right ear and 33

11. On both ears, elevated SSIT scores relative to PBT scores suggest the possibility of central auditory disorder. Remember, on PI-SSI testing, patients with retrocochlear disorders may show unusually reduced maximum intelligibility scores and unusually elevated SSIT scores (see patient 2, Chapter 1, Acoustic Schwannoma).

12. The SPAR measure accurately predicts the audiogram in this patient. Remember, however, SPAR predictions are generally more accurate in young people than in elderly adults. For example, in a series of 130 children and 217 adults over 59 years old, SPAR results showed a good correlation with actual audiometric findings in 85% of children, but only 55% of adults (Jerger et al., 1978).

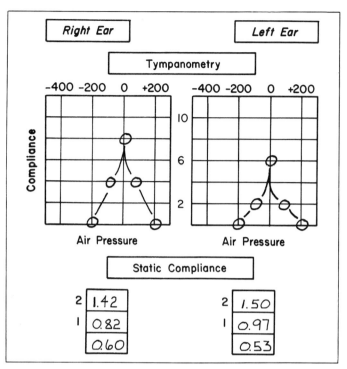

Case 21-1C

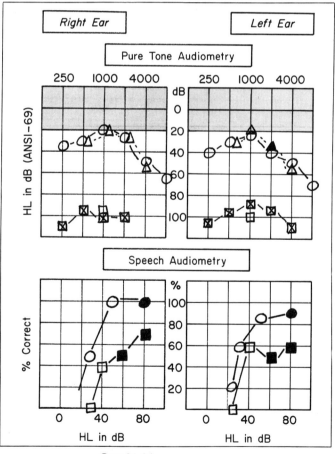

Case 21-2A

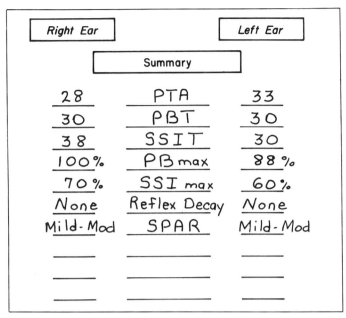

Case 21-2B

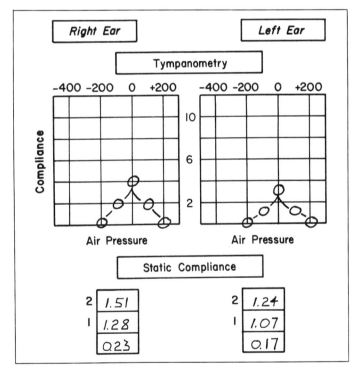

Case 21-2C

13. On both ears, notice the discrepancy between PB max and SSI max scores. A difference of 30% is too substantial to be attributed to the slightly rising audiometric contour and is interpreted as evidence of a central auditory disorder.

In a series of 204 individuals, the difference between PB max vs SSI max performance changed from 0% to about 25% as age increased from 15 to 85 years (Jerger and Hayes, 1977).

14. SSIT scores in this patient were based on a 25% intelligibility level, rather than a 50% intelligibility level. Remember, in the presence of an unusually slow rise to maximum performance (right ear) or a maximum intelligibility score near 50% (left ear), SSIT scores are more accurately obtained at a 25%, rather than a 50%, reference level.

15. In some elderly patients, results of tympanometry and static compliance may mimic the pattern found in otosclerotic ears. Notice, however, that a normal reflex time course and no air-bone gap argue against fixation of the ossicular chain in this patient (see Chapter 18, Otosclerosis).

maximum intelligibility scores bilaterally. The SSI max scores (Case 21-2B) are 70% on the right ear and 60% on the left ear. The shape of the PI functions is normal on both ears.[13]

Speech thresholds agree with average pure tone sensitivity bilaterally. On the right ear, the PBT score is 30 dB HL; the SSIT score is 38 dB HL. On the left ear, the PBT and SSIT scores are 30 dB HL.[14]

Impedance audiometry (Case 21-2C) shows shallow, type A, tympanograms and abnormally reduced static compliance measures bilaterally. Crossed and uncrossed acoustic reflexes (Case 21-2A) on both ears are present at normal HLs from 500 Hz through 2000 Hz. However, crossed reflexes are elevated or absent at 250 Hz and 4000 Hz bilaterally.

The SPAR measure (Case 21-2B) predicts a mild to moderate sensitivity loss on each ear. No reflex decay is observed at 500 Hz or 1000 Hz on either ear. The reflex time course is normal. There is no negative deflection at the offset of reflex eliciting signals.[15]

Summary

Pure tone sensitivity on both ears shows a mild sensorineural loss through 2000 Hz and a moderate sensorineural loss above 2000 Hz. The overall pattern of results suggests the presence of both peripheral and central aging effects. A peripheral disorder is documented by the pure tone sensitivity loss and decreased mobility of the middle ear system on impedance audiometry. A central disorder is supported by the substantial difference between PB max and SSI max performance.

Impression

Combined peripheral and central bilateral auditory disorder.

SELECTED READINGS

Bergman, M. Hearing and aging. *Audiology* 10:164, 1971.

Corso, J. Auditory Perception and Communication. In J. Birren and K. Schaie (eds.), *Handbook of the Psychology of Aging*. New York: Van Nostrand, Reinhold, 1977. Pp. 535–553.

Dayal, V., Kane, N., and Mendelsohn, M. Patterns of pure tone hearing loss. *Acta Otolaryngol.* 69:329, 1970.

dB HL on the left ear. Bone conduction measures are superimposed on air conduction measures bilaterally.

PI-PB functions (Case 21-2A) on both ears show normal maximum intelligibility scores. The PB max scores (Case 21-2B) are 100% on the right ear and 88% on the left ear. In contrast to PI-PB functions, PI-SSI functions (Case 21-2A) show reduced

Feldman, R., and Reger, S. Relations among hearing, reaction time, and age. *J. Speech Hear. Res.* 10:479, 1967.

Gilad, O., and Glorig, A. Presbyacusis: The aging ear. *J. Am. Audiol. Soc.* 4:195 (Part I), 207 (Part II), 1979.

Glorig, A. Some medical implications of the 1954 Wisconsin State Fair hearing survey. *Trans. Am. Acad. Ophthalmol. Otolaryngol.* 61:160, 1957.

Hall, J. Effects of age and sex on static compliance. *Arch. Otolaryngol.* 105:153, 1979.

Hayes, D., and Jerger, J. Aging and the use of hearing aids. *Scand. Audiol.* 8:33, 1979.

Hayes, D., and Jerger, J. Low frequency hearing loss in presbyacusis. *Arch. Otolaryngol.* 105:9, 1979.

Hinchcliffe, R. The anatomical locus of presbyacusis. *J. Speech Hear. Dis.* 27:301, 1962.

Igarashi, M. Pathology of Inner Ear Endorgans. In J. Minkler (ed.), *Pathology of the Nervous System* (vol. 3). New York: McGraw-Hill, 1972. Pp. 2856–2879.

Jerger, J. Audiological findings in aging. *Adv. Otorhinolaryngol.* 20:115, 1973.

Jerger, J., and Hall, J. Effect of age and sex on the auditory brain stem response. *Arch. Otolaryngol.* 106:387, 1980.

Jerger, J., and Hayes, D. Diagnostic speech audiometry. *Arch. Otolaryngol.* 103:216, 1977.

Jerger, J., Hayes, D., and Anthony, L. Effect of age on prediction of sensori-neural hearing level from the acoustic reflex. *Arch. Otolaryngol.* 104:393, 1978.

Kirikae, I., Sato, T., and Shitara, T. A study of hearing in advanced age. *Laryngoscope* 74:205, 1964.

Korsan-Bengtsen, M. The Diagnosis of Hearing Loss in Old People. In G. Liden (ed.), *Geriatric Audiology*. Stockholm: Almquist and Wiksell, 1968. Pp. 24–36.

Kronholm, A. Auditory Problems in a Home for the Aged. In G. Liden (ed.), *Geriatric Audiology*. Stockholm: Almquist and Wiksell, 1968. Pp. 58–62.

Lebo, C., and Reddell, R. The presbyacusis component in occupational hearing loss. *Laryngoscope* 82:1399, 1972.

Leske, M. 1971–1975 U.S. Health and Nutrition Examination Survey. Presented at the Seminar on Hearing Problems for the Elderly. The National Institute on Aging and The National Institute on Neurological and Communicative Disorders and Stroke, Bethesda, Md., 1979.

Lowell, S., and Paparella, M. Presbyacusis: What is it? *Laryngoscope* 87:1710, 1977.

Orchik, D., and Burgess, J. Synthetic sentence identification as a function of the age of the listener. *J. Am. Audiol. Soc.* 3:42, 1977.

Pestalozza, G., and Shore, I. Clinical evaluation of presbyacusis on the basis of different tests of auditory function. *Laryngoscope* 65:1136, 1955.

Rasmussen, A. Studies of the VIIIth cranial nerve of man. *Laryngoscope* 50:67, 1940.

Rosen, S., Bergman, M., Plester, D., El-Mofty, A., and Satti, M. Presbyacusis study of a relatively noise-free population in the Sudan. *Ann. Otol. Rhinol. Laryngol.* 71:727, 1962.

Schuknecht, H. *Pathology of the Ear.* Cambridge: Harvard University Press, 1974. Pp. 388–409.

Schuknecht, H., and Igarashi, M. Pathology of slowly progressive sensori-neural deafness. *Trans. Am. Acad. Ophthalmol. Otolaryngol.* 68:222, 1964.

Surjan, L., Devald, J., and Palfalvi, L. Epidemiology of hearing loss. *Audiology* 12:396, 1973.

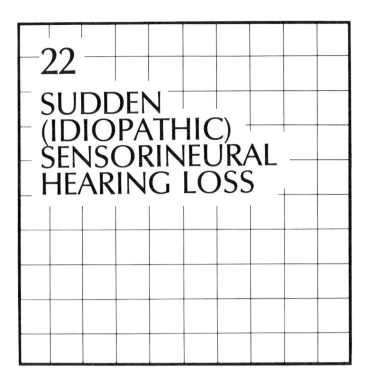

22

SUDDEN (IDIOPATHIC) SENSORINEURAL HEARING LOSS

DESCRIPTION

Sudden idiopathic sensorineural hearing loss refers to the occurrence of an abrupt loss of hearing with no discernible cause. Proposed explanations for sudden idiopathic sensorineural loss revolve primarily around viral or vascular etiologies. Suggested vascular disturbances include sludging of blood, hemorrhage, thrombosis, embolism, and spasms.[1]

The principal findings of histologic studies in patients with sudden idiopathic sensorineural hearing loss include atrophy of the organ of Corti, the tectorial membrane, and the stria vascularis. A decrease in the number of eighth nerve fibers and spiral ganglion cells may be observed. In one patient with a sudden sensorineural hearing loss of undetermined cause (Ishii and Toriyama, 1977), a complete loss of eighth nerve fibers was observed. In contrast to the severe eighth nerve abnormality, however, the structural components of the organ of Corti appeared relatively normal.

PATIENT CHARACTERISTICS

Sudden idiopathic sensorineural hearing loss may occur at any age. However, approximately 75% of patients are more than 40 years old. The condition affects males and females equally. The hearing loss is unilateral in more than 90% of individuals.

1. Sudden sensorineural loss of known causation is excluded from this chapter; see Chapter 11, Herpes Zoster Oticus; Chapter 14, Meniere's Disease; Chapter 15, Multiple Sclerosis; Chapter 16, Noise-Induced Hearing Loss; Chapter 19, Ototoxicity; Chapter 23, Syphilis; and Chapter 24, Trauma.

Of patients in the Kaiser Foundation Health Plan of Northern California, the average prevalence of sudden idiopathic sensorineural loss is 10.7 per 100,000 individuals. Prevalence appears to vary with age, ranging from 4.6 per 100,000 in children less than 15 years old to 47 per 100,000 in persons more than 64 years of age (Byl, 1978). Of new patients seen in an otologic practice over a 2-year period, ap-proximately 2% of persons had a sudden sensorineural hearing loss of undetermined origin (Sheehy, 1960).

2. In a series of 13 patients with bilateral sudden idiopathic sensorineural hearing loss, approximately 70% of persons had both ears affected simultaneously and about 30% of individuals had the second ear affected from 3 months to 20 years later (Sheehy, 1960).

3. Anesthetizing the stellate ganglion produces vasodilation and increased blood flow.

4. Physicians with sudden idiopathic sensorineural loss have a higher recovery rate (80%) than the general population.

Both ears appear to be equally vulnerable to the occurrence of sudden idiopathic sensorineural loss.

CLINICAL COURSE

Sudden idiopathic sensorineural hearing loss may occur instantaneously or may develop over a period of a few days. In many individuals, the hearing loss is first noticed on awakening in the morning. In about 50% of persons, the hearing loss is preceded, accompanied, or followed by vertigo, dizziness, or feelings of unsteadiness. Tinnitus is noted in about 70% to 85% of individuals. Some patients may report a feeling of pressure or fullness in the affected ear. On the rare occasions when sudden idiopathic sensorineural hearing loss is bilateral, both ears may be affected simultaneously or the second ear may become affected months or years later.[2]

There is no standard medical treatment for sudden idiopathic sensorineural loss. Some clinicians suggest no treatment at all. Other clinicians recommend dietary restrictions, drug therapy, bed rest or limited physical activity, and/or anesthetizing blocks of the stellate ganglion.[3]

Spontaneous recovery of sudden idiopathic sensorineural loss may occur in about 25% to 50% of individuals. In patients who receive medical treatment, recovery may be related to the time interval between the onset of the hearing loss and the initiation of medical therapy. Successful recovery is observed in about 70% of persons who are treated within 10 days of the onset of the hearing loss. However, in individuals with delayed medical treatment (initiated more than 10 days post-onset of the hearing loss) recovery is observed in only about 25% of patients (Byl, 1978).[4]

In persons with spontaneous or treatment-induced recovery of auditory function, pure tone sensitivity may return to within normal limits or some degree of hearing loss may persist. Recovery of hearing sensitivity to within normal limits is more likely in individuals without severe vertigo and without an initially profound degree of hearing loss. Approximately 90% of all improvement in hearing sensitivity occurs within the first 6 weeks after the onset of the hearing loss. On rare occasions,

5. Of patients with sudden sensorineural hearing loss, about one-third recover to normal hearing, about one-third have a permanent mild to severe hearing loss for at least one frequency, and about one-third have a permanent profound sensitivity loss for all frequencies (Snow, 1973).

Of 51 patients with sudden sensorineural hearing loss, about 12% of individuals showed progressive hearing deterioration over time (Surjan et al., 1973).

6. Of 50 patients with sudden idiopathic sensorineural hearing loss, the initial degree of loss was mild to moderate in about 30% of persons and severe to profound in about 70% of individuals (Byl, 1978).

Of 223 patients with sudden sensorineural hearing loss, the audiometric contour in persons with measurable hearing was flat in 41% of individuals, sloping in 29% of patients, and rising in 17% of patients (Sheehy, 1960).

Spontaneous recovery may be related to the configuration of the initial audiogram. In 88 patients with sudden idiopathic sensorineural hearing loss, spontaneous recovery was observed in 92% of persons with an upwardly rising audiometric contour, but only 28% of individuals with a downwardly sloping configuration (Simmons, 1978).

7. Upper respiratory infections during or a few days before the onset of hearing loss may be reported by about 25% to 30% of patients.

hearing sensitivity may show progressive deterioration, instead of recovery, over time. Substantial changes in the hearing sensitivity of patients with sudden idiopathic sensorineural hearing loss stress the importance of serial audiometric evaluations.[5]

SITE OF DISORDER

Cochlea and/or eighth nerve.

GENERAL AUDIOLOGIC PATTERN

Initial pure tone sensitivity results characteristically show a severe to profound, unilateral sensorineural loss. In some individuals, however, the degree of loss may be mild or moderate. On isolated occasions, sudden idiopathic sensorineural hearing loss may be bilateral, rather than unilateral. In persons with measurable hearing, the initial audiometric contour varies substantially. Hearing sensitivity may be depressed for a restricted range of frequencies or at all frequencies.[6]

During the initial stage of sudden idiopathic sensorineural hearing loss, pure tone sensitivity may be unstable in many persons. Recovery or deterioration of hearing thresholds may occur. In patients with improvement of hearing sensitivity, pure tone thresholds may return to within normal limits at all frequencies.

Maximum speech intelligibility scores vary depending on the site of the auditory disorder. In patients with cochlear site, maximum speech intelligibility performance is usually consistent with the degree of sensitivity loss. In patients with eighth nerve site, however, maximum speech intelligibility scores may be unusually reduced relative to the degree of sensitivity loss. The shape of the PI function may be abnormal (rollover phenomenon). In individuals with unstable pure tone sensitivity, speech intelligibility results may improve or deteriorate in a manner consistent with pure tone sensitivity fluctuation.

Impedance results characteristically show normal, type A, tympanograms and normal static compliance measures. Acoustic reflex results vary, however, depending on the site of the disorder and the degree of sensitivity loss. As a general rule, in patients with cochlear site, reflexes are present at reduced sensation levels at all frequencies. In pa-

tients with eighth nerve site, however, acoustic reflex results are generally characterized by elevated threshold HLs and/or an abnormal temporal pattern.

In individuals with profound hearing loss, reflex thresholds cannot be measured because signals cannot be presented at sufficiently high intensity levels. In patients with improvement of hearing sensitivity over time, acoustic reflex thresholds may also show systematic recovery to within normal limits at all frequencies.

If reflexes are abnormal or the PI function shows rollover or disproportionately reduced maximum intelligibility scores, further tests for the diagnostic evaluation of eighth nerve site are indicated. Appropriate tests may include Bekesy and BCL audiometry, STAT, TDT, and ABR audiometry.

In patients with hearing improvement over time, the pattern of results on diagnostic auditory tests may show concurrent change over time. In particular, individuals with an eighth nerve or cochlear pattern of results at the initial evaluation may subsequently show completely normal findings on all test procedures.

Illustrative Patient

CASE 1. A 50-YEAR-OLD FEMALE WITH A SUDDEN IDIOPATHIC SENSORINEURAL HEARING LOSS ON THE LEFT EAR.

History

Approximately 1 week ago, the patient noticed a hearing loss in the left ear upon awaking in the morning. During the following 12 hours, the patient noticed unusual fluctuations in her hearing ability. After the initial 12-hour period of fluctuation, however, she became "deaf" in her left ear.

Several days prior to the onset of the hearing loss, the patient had an isolated, momentary episode of light-headedness and a "locust" sound in her left ear. Five days before the onset of the loss, the patient had an upper respiratory infection.[7]

Physical examination, neurologic evaluation, and otorhinolaryngologic examination are essentially within normal limits except for the hearing loss on the left ear. Chest x-rays, mastoid x-rays, tomograms of the internal auditory canal, and routine labora-

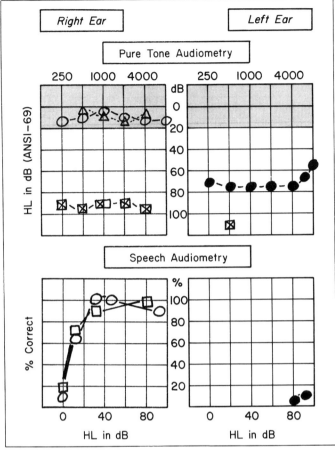

Case 22-1A

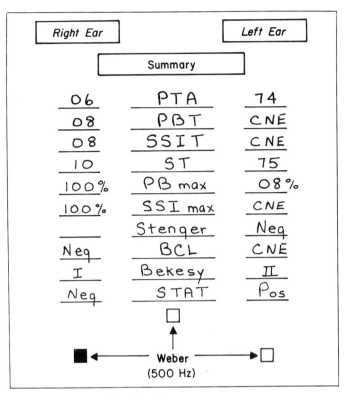

Case 22-1B

8. In some patients with sudden sensorineural hearing loss associated with physical exertion, barotrauma, or severe stress, auditory symptoms may be due to a labyrinthine membrane rupture, rather than an idiopathic etiology (Goodhill and Harris, 1979).

tory studies are normal. The patient denies previous barotrauma, exposure to loud noises, atypical or unusual drug usage, and unusual physical exertion or strain.[8] The patient has no hearing complaints about her right ear.

Results

The audiogram (Case 22-1A) shows normal sensitivity on the right ear and a severe sensorineural loss on the left ear. The PTA scores (Case 22-1B) are 6 dB HL on the right ear and 74 dB HL on the left ear. Unmasked bone conduction thresholds (Case 22-1A) are superimposed on the air conduction thresholds of the right ear. With masking noise to the right ear, bone conduction sensitivity at 500 Hz through 4000 Hz on the left ear is beyond equipment limits. The Weber test (Case 22-1B) at 500 Hz lateralizes to the right ear.

Speech audiometry (Case 22-1A) on the right ear shows normal PI-PB and PI-SSI functions. The PB max and SSI max scores

9. Remember, a severe unilateral hearing loss of sudden onset is commonly observed in patients with functional hearing disorders (see Chapter 8, Functional Hearing Disorders).

(Case 22-1B) are 100%. The PBT and SSIT scores, 8 dB HL, are consistent with pure tone sensitivity results. On the left ear, the administration of speech intelligibility tests is limited by the severity of the pure tone sensitivity loss. PB testing (Case 22-1A) shows an intelligibility score of 8% at 90 dB HL. There is no response to SSI materials presented at 80 dB HL.

Spondee thresholds (STs) (Case 22-1B) on both ears agree with average pure tone sensitivity. The STs are 10 dB HL on the right ear and 75 dB HL on the left ear. A speech Stenger test is negative for a functional hearing disorder on the left ear.[9]

Impedance audiometry (Case 22-1C) shows normal, type A, tympanograms and normal static compliance measures bilaterally. Crossed and uncrossed acoustic reflexes (Case 22-1A) with sound to the right ear are present at normal HLs at all frequencies. With sound to the left ear, crossed and uncrossed acoustic reflexes are elevated or absent at all frequencies. The reflex pattern (Case 22-1D) indicates an abnormal sound effect (diagonal configuration) on the left ear. Results are consistent with a severe sensorineural loss on the left ear.

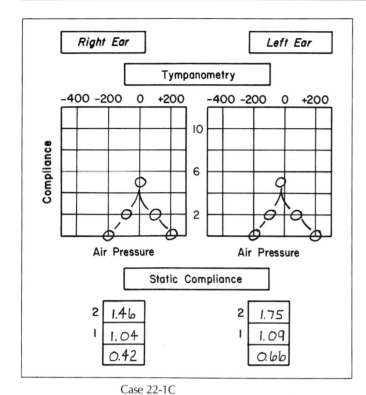

Case 22-1C

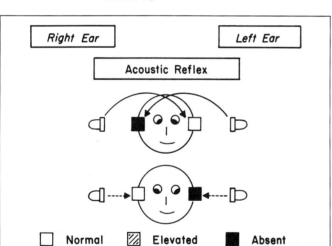

Case 22-1D

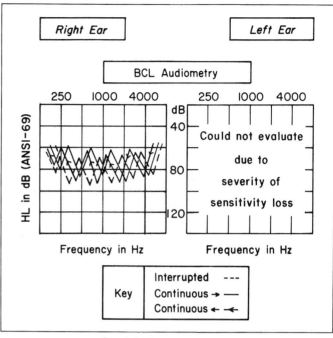

Case 22-1E

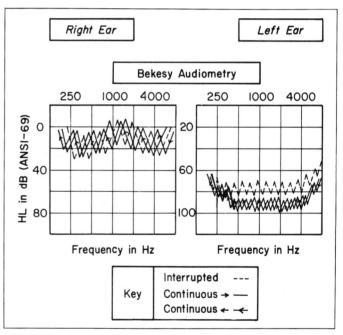

Case 22-1F

BCL audiometry (Case 22-1E) on the right ear yields a negative pattern. Results do not show any adaptation of the continuous tracing in comparison to the interrupted tracing. BCL results could not be obtained on the left ear. The patient reported that sounds at equipment limits on the left ear were never comfortably loud.

Bekesy audiometry (Case 22-1F) on the right ear yields a type I tracing with no forward vs backward discrepancy. On the left ear, the Bekesy audiogram is a type II pat-

tern with no difference between forward and backward continuous tracings.

The STAT (Case 22-1G) is negative on the right ear but shows abnormal adaptation at all frequencies on the left ear. With STAT signals to the left ear, the patient ceased responding in less than 15 seconds at all three test frequencies.

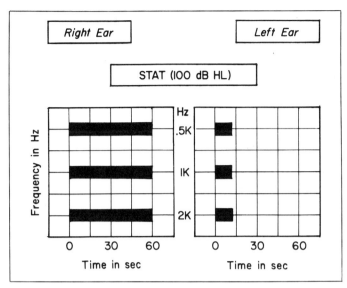

Case 22-1G

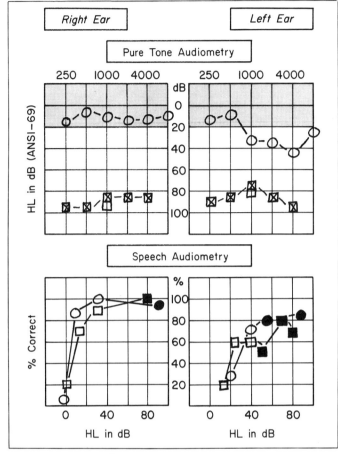

Case 22-1H

Impression

RIGHT EAR: Normal pure tone sensitivity.

LEFT EAR: Severe sensorineural loss. The administration and interpretation of diagnostic test results are limited by the severity of the pure tone sensitivity loss. However, we observed evidence of both cochlear and eighth nerve abnormality. The presence of cochlear dysfunction is supported by a type II threshold Bekesy audiogram. The presence of eighth nerve abnormality is suggested by abnormal adaptation on STAT.

Audiologic Reevaluation

HISTORY. Subsequent to the initial audiologic evaluation, the patient received drug therapy and a series of stellate ganglion blocks. She was placed on dietary restrictions.

During the administration of stellate ganglion block therapy, hearing sensitivity was monitored daily. Pure tone thresholds and speech intelligibility performance on the left ear improved substantially.[10] Subsequently, for a period of approximately 6 months, hearing on the left ear was tested at approximately 4-week intervals. During this time period, hearing threshold levels and speech intelligibility scores on the left ear appeared relatively stable. The following results were obtained about 6 months after the initial audiologic evaluation.

Results

The audiogram (Case 22-1H) shows normal pure tone sensitivity on the right ear and a

10. Of 56 patients receiving stellate ganglion blocks for sudden idiopathic sensorineural hearing loss, about 60% of persons showed an improvement of at least 20 dB in average pure tone sensitivity. About 53% of individuals had an improvement of at least 20% on speech intelligibility (PB word) tests (Haug et al., 1976).

11. Notice, on the left ear, that pure tone sensitivity is improved about 50 dB relative to results of the initial evaluation (Case 22-1A). Threshold sensitivity on the right ear is unchanged.

12. On the left ear, speech intelligibility performance for PB words and SSI materials is improved about 80% relative to results of the initial evaluation (Case 22-1A). Speech intelligibility performance on the right ear is unchanged.

mild high frequency sensorineural loss on the left ear. The PTA scores (Case 22-1I) are 9 dB HL on the right ear and 26 dB HL on the left ear.[11]

The PI-PB and PI-SSI functions (Case 22-1H) on the right ear are normal with 100% maximum intelligibility scores. On the left ear, the PI-PB and PI-SSI functions show mildly reduced maximum intelligibility scores. The PB max score (Case 22-1I) is 84%; the SSI max score is 80%. No rollover is observed.[12]

Speech thresholds on both ears agree with average pure tone sensitivity. On the right ear, the PBT is 5 dB HL; the SSIT is 9 dB HL. On the left ear, the PBT is 30 dB HL; the SSIT is 21 dB HL.

Tympanometry and static compliance measures (not shown) are within normal limits bilaterally. Results are the same as those obtained at the initial evaluation (Case 22-1C). Crossed and uncrossed acoustic reflexes (Case 22-1H) on both ears are present at normal HLs at all frequencies. No reflex

158

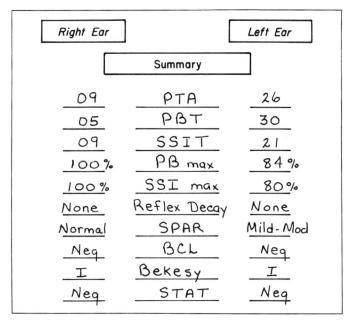

Case 22-1I

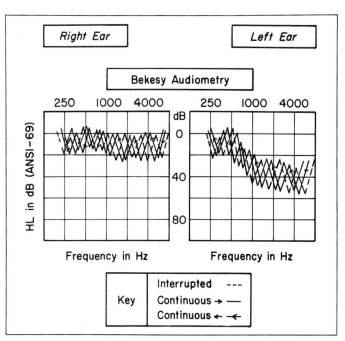

Case 22-1K

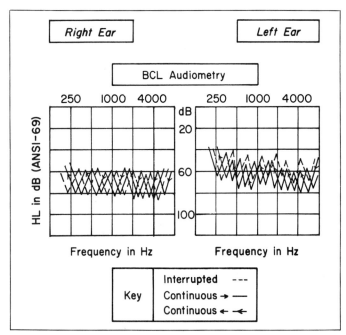

Case 22-1J

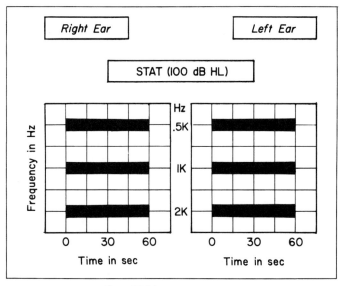

Case 22-1L

decay (Case 22-1I) is observed at 500 Hz or 1000 Hz on either ear. The SPAR procedure predicts normal sensitivity on the right ear and a mild to moderate sensitivity loss on the left ear.

BCL audiometry (Case 22-1J) yields negative results on both ears. No abnormal adaptation of the continuous tracing relative to the interrupted tracing is observed on either ear. Bekesy audiometry (Case 22-1K) on both ears shows type I tracings with no

13. On the left ear, notice the normalcy of diagnostic test results at this evaluation relative to results of the initial evaluation. STAT (Cases 22-1G and 22-1L) no longer shows evidence of abnormal adaptation. Conventional Bekesy audiometry (Cases 22-1F and 22-1K) no longer

forward vs backward discrepancy. The STAT (Case 22-1L) does not show abnormal adaptation at any frequency on either ear.[13]

Impression

RIGHT EAR: Normal pure tone sensitivity.

LEFT EAR: Mild high frequency sensorineural loss. Diagnostic test results do not show any evidence of eighth nerve disorder. No abnormal adaptation is observed on acoustic reflex testing, BCL audiometry, Bekesy au-

shows separation of interrupted and continuous tracings. Acoustic reflex thresholds (Cases 22-1A and 22-1H) are improved by more than 35 dB at some frequencies.

14. In the interpretation of test results, notice that a careful distinction is made between results that vote for or against an eighth nerve site and results that vote for or against a cochlear site. For example, a lack of abnormal adaptation on the STAT is not interpreted as evidence for a cochlear site of disorder. Instead, STAT results are more accurately reported as evidence against an eighth nerve site of disorder. Remember, on many test procedures, results that are a vote *against* an eighth nerve site *may not* automatically be a vote *for* a cochlear site.

diometry, or the STAT procedure. Maximum speech intelligibility performance is consistent with the degree of pure tone sensitivity loss. No rollover of the PI functions is observed. A cochlear site is supported by the occurrence of acoustic reflex thresholds at normal HLs and reduced sensation levels.[14]

Comment

The etiology of the hearing loss in this patient has remained undetermined during a 5-year observation period. This finding strengthens the probability of an idiopathic origin for the sensorineural disorder. According to Byl (1978), after 18 months of medical monitoring, about one-third of patients with an initial diagnosis of sudden idiopathic sensorineural loss may have a more specific diagnosis, e.g., Meniere's disease.

SELECTED READINGS

Alford, B., Shaver, E., Rosenberg, J., and Guilford, F. Physiologic and histopathologic effects of microembolism of the internal auditory artery. *Ann. Otol. Rhinol. Laryngol.* 74:728, 1965.

Beal, D., Hemenway, W., and Lindsay, J. Inner ear pathology of sudden deafness. *Arch. Otolaryngol.* 85:591, 1967.

Bosatra, A., and De'Stephani, G. The idiopathic sudden deafness. A clinical study. *Acta Otolaryngol.* Suppl. 169:7, 1962.

Byl, F. Sudden hearing loss research clinic. *Otolaryngol. Clin. North Am.* 11:71, 1978.

Goodhill, V., and Harris, I. Sudden Hearing Loss Syndrome. In V. Goodhill (ed.), *Ear Diseases, Deafness, and Dizziness.* New York: Harper & Row, 1979. Pp. 664–681.

Haug, O., Draper, W., and Haug, S. Stellate ganglion blocks for idiopathic sensori-neural loss. *Arch. Otolaryngol.* 102:5, 1976.

Igarashi, M., Alford, B., Konishi, S., Shaver, E., and Guilford, F. Functional and histopathological correlations after microembolism of the peripheral labyrinthine artery in the dog. *Laryngoscope* 79:603, 1969.

Ishii, T., and Toriyama, M. Sudden deafness with severe loss of cochlear neurons. *Ann. Otol. Rhinol. Laryngol.* 86:541, 1977.

Jerger, J., Allen, G., Robertson, D., and Harford, E. Hearing loss of sudden onset. *Arch. Otolaryngol.* 73:350, 1961.

Mattox, D., and Simmons, F. Natural history of sudden sensori-neural hearing loss. *Ann. Otol. Rhinol. Laryngol.* 86:463, 1977.

Sando, I., Harada, T., Laehr, A., and Sobel, J. Sudden deafness. *Ann. Otol. Rhinol. Laryngol.* 86:269, 1977.

Schuknecht, H. *Pathology of the Ear.* Cambridge: Harvard University Press, 1974. Pp. 473–479.

Sheehy, J. Vasodilator therapy in sensori-neural hearing loss. *Laryngoscope* 70:885, 1960.

Simmons, F. Fluid dynamics in sudden sensori-neural loss. *Otolaryngol. Clin. North Am.* 11:55, 1978.

Snow, J. Sudden Deafness. In M. Paparella and D. Shumrick, *Otolaryngology* (vol. 2). Philadelphia: Saunders, 1973. Pp. 357–364.

Stephens, M., Swisher, L., and Novotny, G. Change in response to auditory stimuli after sudden hearing loss. *Arch. Otolaryngol.* 86:72, 1967.

Surjan, L., Devald, J., and Palfalvi, L. Epidemiology of hearing loss. *Audiology* 12:396, 1973.

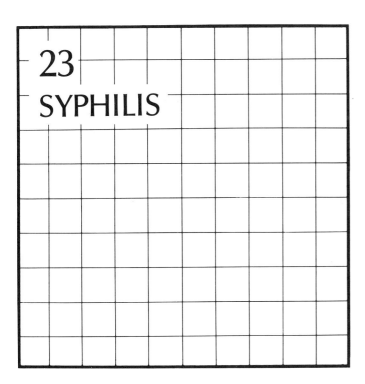

23
SYPHILIS

DESCRIPTION

1. Syphilis may be termed *lues*.

In 1972, United States public health officials estimated the incidence of syphilis to be about 80,000 to 100,000 individuals annually. The peak incidence occurred in the 20- to 24-year-old age group (Holmes, 1974).

Of pregnancies occurring in women with untreated syphilis, about 70% of infants (live births) have the disease (Dodd, 1954).

Syphilis is a chronic, systemic infection caused by the spirochete *Treponema pallidum*. In animals and humans with hearing loss due to syphilis, histologic studies show deformity and/or destruction of the bony otic capsule. Findings may include endolymphatic hydrops of the membranous labyrinth and/or atrophy of the organ of Corti. Gummatous lesions in the spiral ganglion may be observed. On rare occasions, abnormalities of the external ear, middle ear, mastoid, and petrous bone may be produced by destructive gummatous growths. Complications of syphilis may include meningitis in about 0.2% of individuals.[1]

PATIENT CHARACTERISTICS

Syphilis may be congenital or acquired. Congenital syphilis is caused by intrauterine infection as a consequence of syphilis in the mother. Individuals with a history of severe congenital syphilis during infancy usually show the stigmata of syphilis. Maldevelopment of the teeth and changes in the bone formations of the skull and face are characteristically observed.

The reported prevalence of syphilis is higher in males than in females. Serious complications of syphilis are twice as common in males as in females. In contrast to this observation, the prevalence of hearing

2. Of 19 patients with hearing loss due to congenital syphilis, the loss was bilateral in 95% of individuals (Hahn et al., 1962).

A distinction between the hearing loss due to congenital syphilis vs acquired syphilis is not emphasized in this chapter. Since the introduction of antibiotic therapy, some clinicians (Schuknecht, 1974; Smyth et al., 1976) suggest that acquired syphilis is no longer a significant cause of hearing disorders.

3. Symptomatic involvement of the central nervous system (neurosyphilis) occurs in about 7% of individuals with syphilis (Holmes, 1974). The prevalence of hearing loss in patients with symptomatic neurosyphilis is about 80% of persons (Tamari and Itkin, 1951).

The successive stages of acquired syphilis may be termed *initial, secondary*, and *tertiary syphilis*.

4. Congenital syphilis of delayed onset may be termed *tardive*.

Estimates of the prevalence of hearing loss in patients with congenital syphilis range from about 20% to 40% of individuals.

loss due to congenital syphilis is greater in females (65% to 75%) than in males. In females, the hearing loss may be more pronounced premenstrually (Hahn et al., 1962) and during or shortly after pregnancy (Perlman and Leek, 1962).

In persons with syphilis, the onset of hearing loss may occur at any age. In about one-third of individuals with congenital syphilis, the onset of hearing loss occurs during childhood. However, the onset of auditory symptoms due to congenital syphilis may be noted in patients as old as 60 years of age. The hearing loss is characteristically bilateral.[2]

CLINICAL COURSE

In general, syphilis is characterized by a fluctuating, although relentlessly progressive, course. In patients with acquired syphilis, the clinical course is usually marked by three distinct stages: an initial period of infection, a latent period, and a subsequent period of active symptomatology. The initial stage of infection is generally not accompanied by disturbing signs or symptoms. In the later active stage of the disease, however, disorders of the auditory system, cardiovascular system, and central nervous system may be observed.[3]

In patients with congenital syphilis, the onset of demonstrable symptomatology may be early or delayed. In general, when symptoms begin during infancy, congenital syphilis is a severe, and sometimes fatal, disease. Auditory problems, if present, may be overshadowed by pronounced life-threatening disorders. In contrast, when symptoms begin in later life, congenital syphilis may be characterized by mild or severe symptomatology. Clinical manifestation of congenital syphilis (of either early or delayed onset) may include disorders of the skin, bones, eyes, ears, and central nervous system. Auditory symptoms may develop long after other active manifestations of the infection have subsided.[4]

In patients with syphilis, the initial onset of hearing loss and auditory symptomatology may vary. As a general rule, in persons with congenital syphilis and an onset of auditory symptoms during childhood, the onset of hearing loss is characteristically abrupt. In contrast, in persons

5. Notice that the auditory symptomatology of patients with syphilis may mimic the symptoms of Meniere's disease. In a series of patients originally diagnosed as having Meniere's disease, 7% of persons were subsequently diagnosed as having syphilis (Pulec, 1972).

Syphilis is termed *the great imitator*. In addition to Meniere's disease, luetic symptomatology may imitate the symptoms of toxic or viral labyrinthitis and of intracranial tumors.

with congenital syphilis and an onset of auditory symptoms during adulthood, the onset of hearing loss may be gradual or sudden. In these latter individuals, the initial degree of loss may fluctuate. However, over time, the degree of loss is usually progressive. The rate of progression may vary substantially within a patient and among patients. The fluctuating hearing loss may be accompanied by episodic vertigo. Tinnitus may be reported by about 50% of individuals.[5]

Treatment of patients with syphilis involves drug therapy. During therapy, at least 50% of individuals may notice improvement or stabilization of hearing. In some persons, improvement in speech intelligibility performance may be more dramatic than changes in pure tone sensitivity. Patients with a profound hearing loss before treatment may not show measurable changes in hearing ability. Many patients may require prolonged, often lifetime, treatment to maintain hearing. Early diagnosis and treatment are important for maximal recovery of auditory function.

The observation of unstable pure tone sensitivity in some patients before, during, and after treatment stresses the importance of serial audiometric evaluations of individuals with luetic hearing deficits.

SITE OF DISORDER

Cochlea. In some individuals, the external ear, middle ear, eighth nerve, seventh nerve, and central auditory pathways may be involved.

GENERAL AUDIOLOGIC PATTERN

In persons with an onset of hearing loss during childhood, pure tone sensitivity results characteristically show a bilateral, symmetric, sensorineural loss. The degree of loss is generally severe to profound.

In persons with an onset of hearing loss during adulthood, pure tone sensitivity results generally show bilateral, asymmetric fluctuating sensorineural loss. The degree of loss may vary substantially. In some individuals, the hearing loss may progress rapidly to a profound impairment.[6]

During the initial stages of auditory symptomatology, a unilateral, rather than

bilateral, sensorineural loss may be observed. In this circumstance, a hearing loss on the uninvolved opposite ear usually occurs in a few years.[7] On rare occasions, a conductive component may be observed if the external ear or middle ear systems become involved.

The audiometric contour is characteristically flat. However, during the initial course of the hearing impairment, a rising configuration with greater loss in the low frequency region than in the high frequency region may be observed in many patients.

Results of speech audiometry vary during the course of the disease. In the initial stages of hearing loss, maximum speech intelligibility scores are frequently normal, even in the presence of sensorineural hearing loss. Subsequently, however, speech intelligibility performance may decrease dramatically. Substantial fluctuations in speech understanding ability may occur. In some patients, an unusual decrement in speech intelligibility results may occur without a concurrent decrease in pure tone sensitivity. In the later stages of luetic hearing loss, speech intelligibility performance may be disproportionately poor relative to the degree of pure tone sensitivity loss. In patients with improvement of auditory function during drug therapy, the improvement in speech intelligibility may be more marked than the improvement in pure tone sensitivity.

Impedance results characteristically show normal, type A, tympanograms and normal static compliance measures. Acoustic reflexes are characteristically present at normal HLs and reduced sensation levels. However, in patients with severe to profound hearing loss, reflex thresholds cannot be measured because signals cannot be presented at sufficiently high intensity levels.[8]

During drug therapy, pure tone sensitivity and speech understanding may improve to within normal limits. After the termination of drug therapy, however, auditory function may deteriorate in some patients.

DIAGNOSIS OF SYPHILIS

The diagnosis of syphilis generally involves serologic tests and microscopy. Serologic tests may be divided into two categories. One category consists of tests based on the identification of treponemal antibodies. The antibodies are formed by the host against the *T. pallidum* spirochete. An example of a treponemal antigen test is the fluorescent treponemal antibody absorption (FTA-ABS) test. Some clinicians consider the FTA-ABS technique to be the most sensitive and reliable method in use today for diagnosing syphilis.

The second basic category of serologic tests involves methods for identifying nontreponemal reagins. Reagins are reactive substances produced by the host in response to the breakdown of cells and the formation of breakdown products at the sites of syphilitic lesions. Reagins are nonspecific to syphilis and are produced during the course of many nonsyphilitic diseases. Of the reagin procedures, the most universally accepted is the Venereal Disease Research Laboratory (VDRL) test.

Although serodiagnostic tests for syphilis are widely used, it should be stressed that all current procedures may yield false-positive and false-negative findings.

In addition to serologic tests, microscopy may be used for the direct visualization of the *T. pallidum* spirochete. In general, the spirochete is visualized from scrapings of syphilitic lesions.

Illustrative Patients

CASE 1. A 42-YEAR-OLD MALE WITH LUETIC HEARING LOSS ON BOTH EARS.

History

Approximately 20 years ago, the patient was diagnosed as having syphilis. He received penicillin therapy. Approximately 10 years ago, the patient began to notice fluctuating hearing ability in both ears. At the same time, he began to experience visual difficulties. His hearing and visual problems slowly increased. However, the hearing and visual symptoms did not bother him sufficiently to seek medical attention until the present time.[9]

Physical examination, otorhinolaryngologic evaluation, and neurologic studies are within normal limits except for bilateral hearing and visual abnormalities. X-rays of the skull and internal auditory canals are within the normal range. VDRL and FTA-ABS studies are positive for syphilis.

The patient denies a history of head trauma and unusual or atypical drug use,

9. Visual disorders, particularly interstitial keratitis, a lesion of the cornea, are the most frequent manifestation of late-onset congenital syphilis. The combination of interstitial keratitis, malformed teeth, and sensorineural hearing loss are three classic signs of syphilis referred to as *Hutchinson's triad.*

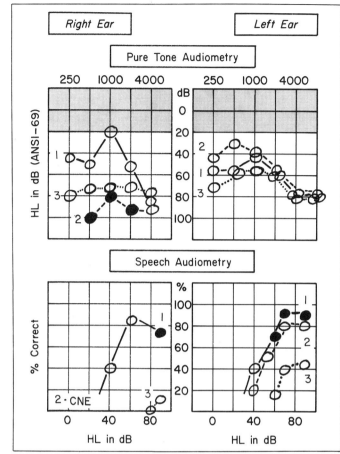

Case 23-1A. *Pure tone audiogram and speech audiometry. "1" initial evaluation, approximately 20 years after first diagnosis of syphilis; "2" audiologic reevaluation 3½ years after initial evaluation; "3" audiologic reevaluation approximately 10½ years after initial evaluation.*

except for the previous antibiotic therapy. He has a history of noise exposure from industrial equipment. He reports a roaring tinnitus in both ears. On occasion, the patient has spontaneous dizzy spells of short duration. He denies nausea.

The patient thinks that his hearing sensitivity has slowly deteriorated with noticeable periods of fluctuation in both ears over the past 10 years. He thinks his hearing is better in the right ear than in the left ear.

Results

Case 23-1A summarizes results for three audiometric evaluations. Notice the results labeled "1." The audiogram ("1," Case 23-1A) on both ears shows a moderate sensorineural loss in the low frequency region, and a severe to profound sensorineural loss

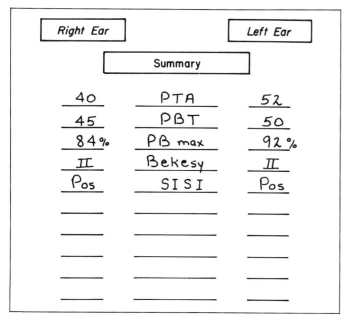

Case 23-1B. *Summary of test results for initial evaluation ("1").*

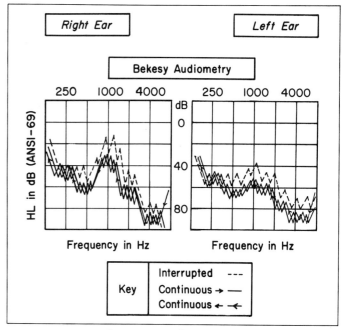

Case 23-1C. *Bekesy audiometry at initial evaluation ("1").*

in the high frequency region. On the left ear, the audiometric contour is mildly sloping. On the right ear, the audiogram shows an unusual rising configuration in the low to mid frequency regions with relatively normal sensitivity at 1000 Hz. The PTA scores (Case 23-1B) are 40 dB HL on the right ear and 52 dB HL on the left ear. Masked bone conduction thresholds (not shown) are superimposed on air conduction sensitivity bilaterally.

PI-PB functions ("1," Case 23-1A) show maximum intelligibility scores of 84% on the right ear and 92% on the left ear. Significant rollover is not observed on either ear. The PBT scores on both ears agree with average pure tone sensitivity results. The PBT is 45 dB HL on the right ear and 50 dB HL on the left ear.[10]

Conventional threshold Bekesy audiometry (Case 23-1C) on both ears shows a type II pattern with interweaving forward vs backward continuous tracings. The SISI test (Case 23-1B) yields positive results on both ears.

Impression

A bilateral sensorineural loss of moderate degree in the low frequency region and of severe to profound degree in the high frequency region. An exception is the island of relatively normal sensitivity at 1000 Hz in

10. Speech intelligibility scores in this patient, particularly on the left ear, support the frequent observation (Hendershot, 1978) that speech understanding ability during the initial stages of auditory symptomatology may be unusually good relative to the degree of pure tone sensitivity loss.

the right ear. Bekesy audiometry and the SISI test are consistent with a cochlear site on each ear. No evidence of eighth nerve disorder was observed. PB max scores are within normal limits on both ears and no rollover is observed.

Audiologic Reevaluation—3½ Years Later

HISTORY. Two weeks ago, the patient awoke in the morning with a feeling of fullness and a complete loss of hearing in the right ear. The hearing has not returned during the past 2 weeks. He does not notice any hearing change on his left ear.

For the past 3 years, the patient has continued to have intermittent episodes of dizziness. His hearing does not change during the dizzy attacks. He notices a high pitched ringing tinnitus in both ears.

Physical examination and neurologic evaluation are essentially within normal limits except for decreased hearing and vision bilaterally. During the past 3 years, the patient has received corneal transplants on both eyes for interstitial keratitis. X-rays of the skull and internal auditory meatus are within the normal range. The patient denies any serious illnesses or additional noise exposure since the last audiometric evaluation.

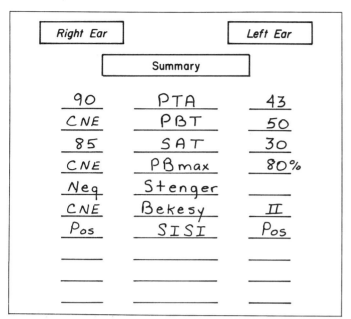

Case 23-1D. *Summary of test results for audiologic reevaluation ("2").*

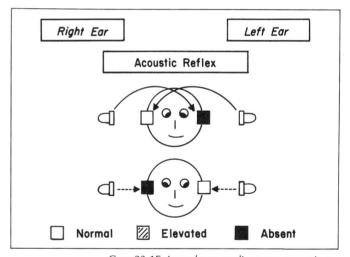

Case 23-1E. *Impedance audiometry: tympanometry and static compliance measures (in cc) at audiologic reevaluation ("2").*

Results

The audiogram (labeled "2," Case 23-1A) shows a severe sensorineural loss on the right ear and a moderate sensorineural loss on the left ear. The PTA scores (Case 23-1D) are 90 dB HL on the right ear and 43 dB HL on the left ear. Unmasked bone conduction sensitivity (not shown) at 500 through 2000 Hz is superimposed on the air conduction thresholds on the left ear. With masking to the left ear, there is no response to bone conducted signals at equipment limits on the right ear.

The PI-PB function ("2," Case 23-1A) on the left ear shows a maximum intelligibility score of 80%. The PBT score, 50 dB HL, agrees with average pure tone sensitivity. No rollover is observed.[11] PI-PB testing on the right ear could not be carried out (CNE) due to the severity of the pure tone sensitivity loss.[12] Speech awareness thresholds (SATs) (Case 23-1D) agree with pure tone results bilaterally. The SAT scores are 85 dB HL on the right ear and 30 dB HL on the left ear. A speech Stenger test is negative for a functional hearing disorder on the right ear.

Impedance audiometry (Case 23-1E) shows normal, type A, tympanograms and normal static compliance measures bilaterally. The reflex pattern (Case 23-1F) is characterized by a diagonal configuration. With sound to the right ear, crossed and un-

11. Relative to results of the first evaluation, the left ear shows slightly improved pure tone sensitivity and slightly decreased speech intelligibility. Remember, over time, speech understanding ability in individuals with luetic hearing disorders generally becomes disproportionately poor in relation to the degree of sensitivity loss.

12. Notice that the SSI procedure was not administered to this patient. SSI testing was not possible due to the patient's visual acuity problem. Re-

Case 23-1F. *Impedance audiometry: acoustic reflex pattern (crossed vs uncrossed conditions) at audiologic reevaluation ("2").*

member, the SSI test requires the patient to identify the sentence that he hears from a list of 10 alternatives.

13. More specifically, with sound to the right ear, acoustic reflexes are

crossed reflexes are absent at equipment limits. With sound to the left ear, crossed and uncrossed reflexes are present at normal HLs. No reflex decay is observed. Results are consistent with a severe sensorineural loss on the right ear.[13]

Conventional threshold Bekesy audiometry (Case 23-1D) on the left ear shows

absent at all frequencies. With sound to the left ear, reflexes are present at normal HLs (80 to 90 dB) at 250 through 2000 Hz and elevated (105 dB) at 4000 Hz.

a type II pattern with no difference between continuous forward vs backward tracings. Bekesy audiometry could not be administered on the right ear due to the severe hearing loss. The SISI test (Case 23-1D) was positive on both ears.

Impression

RIGHT EAR: Severe sensorineural loss. Sensitivity is markedly poorer, about 50 dB, than results of the first evaluation. The administration and interpretation of diagnostic tests is limited by the severity of the pure tone sensitivity loss.

LEFT EAR: Moderate sensorineural loss. Relative to results of the first evaluation, pure tone sensitivity below 2000 Hz is slightly improved (about 10 dB) and speech intelligibility performance is slightly decreased (about 12%). Diagnostic test results are consistent with a cochlear site. A cochlear site is supported by the presence of a type II Bekesy audiogram, positive SISI test, and acoustic reflex thresholds at normal HLs and reduced SLs.

Comment

The patient received drug therapy at this time. Hearing was monitored frequently. Pure tone sensitivity and speech intelligibility performance on the right ear improved. After medical therapy, the PTA scores were 58 dB HL on the right ear and 48 dB HL on the left ear.

Audiologic Reevaluation—Approximately 7 Years Later

HISTORY. The patient complains of fluctuating hearing sensitivity on both ears. The fluctuation is more pronounced on the left ear. He continues to experience intermittent dizzy spells. He does not report nausea or vomiting, however. He complains of a ringing tinnitus bilaterally. The pitch of the tinnitus fluctuates widely.

The patient reports no serious illnesses since the last evaluation. Physical examination, otorhinolaryngologic examination and neurologic evaluation are essentially normal except for the hearing loss and visual difficulties. X-rays of the internal auditory meatus are within normal limits. EEG findings are within the range of normal variation. Brain scan and blood flow studies are nor-

Right Ear		Left Ear
	Summary	
68	PTA	59
CNE	PBT	65
72	ST	65
12%	PB max	48%

Case 23-1G. *Summary of test results for audiologic reevaluation ("3")*

14. Relative to previous findings following medical therapy (see Comment above), pure tone sensitivity shows slight change, a decrease of about 10 dB on both ears. In contrast to a slight change in hearing sensitivity, speech intelligibility performance on the left ear has dropped substantially, about 30%.

mal. The VDRL and FTA-ABS tests are positive for syphilis.

Results

The audiogram (labeled "3," Case 23-1A) shows a moderate sensorineural loss on both ears. The PTA scores (Case 23-1G) are 68 dB HL on the right ear and 59 dB HL on the left ear. Unmasked bone conduction sensitivity (not shown) is superimposed on the air conduction thresholds of the left ear. With masking to the left ear, there is no response to bone conducted signals at equipment limits on the right ear.

PI-PB functions ("3," Case 23-1A) show reduced maximum intelligibility scores on both ears. The PB max scores (Case 23-1G) are 12% on the right ear and 48% on the left ear. No rollover is observed.[14]

Speech thresholds for PB words and spondee words (Case 23-1G) agree with average pure tone sensitivity. On the left ear, the PBT and ST scores are 65 dB HL. On the right ear, the ST score is 72 dB HL. A PBT score on the right ear could not be established (CNE) due to the severity of the speech intelligibility loss.

Impedance audiometry shows normal, type A, tympanograms and normal static compliance measures on both ears. Results are essentially identical to findings of the

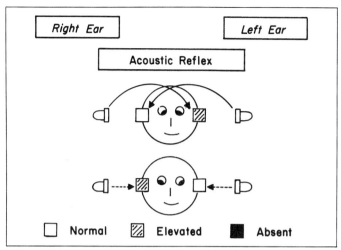

Case 23-1H. *Impedance audiometry: acoustic reflex pattern (crossed vs uncrossed conditions) at audiologic reevaluation ("3").*

15. Specifically, crossed and uncrossed reflexes with sound to the right ear are elevated (105 to 110 dB HL) at 250 Hz through 2000 Hz and absent (greater than 110 dB HL) at 4000 Hz. With sound to the left ear, crossed and uncrossed reflexes are present at normal HLs (90 to 100 dB HL) at all frequencies.

previous evaluation (Case 23-1E). Acoustic reflex testing (Case 23-1H) yields a diagonal pattern. Crossed and uncrossed reflex thresholds are elevated with sound to the right ear and present at normal HLs with sound to the left ear.[15]

Impression

Moderate sensorineural loss on both ears. On the right ear, sensitivity is slightly improved relative to results of the previous evaluation. On the left ear, pure tone sensitivity and speech intelligibility performance are poorer than any previous results obtained during the past 7 years.

Comment

During the 5 years following this evaluation, hearing sensitivity appears to have stabilized on the two ears. At the end of the 5-year monitoring period, the PTA scores are 67 dB HL on the right ear and 59 dB HL on the left ear.

SELECTED READINGS

Dawkins, R., Sharp, M., and Morrison, A. Steroid treatment in congenital syphilitic lesions. *J. Laryngol.* 82:1095, 1968.

Dodd, K. Spirochetal Infections. In W. Nelson (ed.), *Textbook of Pediatrics* (6th ed.). Philadelphia: Saunders, 1954.

Hahn, R., Rodin, P., and Haskins, H. Treatment of neural deafness with prednisone. *J. Chron. Dis.* 15:395, 1962.

Hendershot, E. Luetic deafness. *Laryngoscope* 83:865, 1973.

Hendershot, E. Luetic deafness. *Otolaryngol. Clin. North Am.* 11:43, 1978.

Holmes, K. Syphilis. In M. Wintrobe, G. Thorn, R. Adams, E. Braunwald, K. Isselbacher, and R. Petersdorf (eds.), *Harrison's Principles of Internal Medicine* (7th ed.). New York: McGraw-Hill, 1974. Pp. 876–887.

Igarashi, M. Pathology of the Inner Ear Endorgans. In J. Minkler (ed.), *Pathology of the Nervous System* (vol. 3). New York: McGraw-Hill, 1972. Pp. 2856–2879.

Karmody, C., and Schuknecht, H. Deafness in congenital syphilis. *Arch. Otolaryngol.* 83:44, 1966.

Kerr, A., Smith, G., and Cinnamond, M. Congenital syphilitic deafness. *J. Laryngol.* 87:1, 1973.

Patterson, M. Congenital luetic hearing impairment. *Arch. Otolaryngol.* 87:378, 1968.

Perlman, H., and Leek, J. Late congenital syphilis of the ear. *Laryngoscope* 62:1175, 1962.

Pulec, J. Meniere's disease: Results of a two and one-half year study of etiology, natural history and results of treatment. *Laryngoscope* 82:1703, 1972.

Schepers, G. Laboratory diagnosis of venereal disease. *Med. Ann. Dist. Col.* 35:357, 1966.

Schuknecht, H. *Pathology of the Ear.* Cambridge: Harvard University Press, 1974. Pp. 262–266.

Schulman, J. Syphilis of the Temporal Bone. In V. Goodhill (ed.), *Ear: Diseases, Deafness, and Dizziness.* New York: Harper & Row, 1979. Pp. 682–690.

Smyth, G., Kerr, A., and Cinnamond, M. Deafness due to syphilis. *J. Otolaryngol. Soc. Austral.* 4:36, 1975–1976.

Tamari, M., and Itkin, P. Penicillin and syphilis of the ear. *Eye Ear Nose Throat Mon.* 30:252, 1951.

Willcox, R., and Goodwin, P. Nerve deafness in early syphilis. *Br. J. Vener. Dis.* 47:401, 1971.

Zoller, M., Wilson, W., Nadol, J., and Girard, K. Detection of syphilitic hearing loss. *Arch. Otolaryngol.* 104:63, 1978.

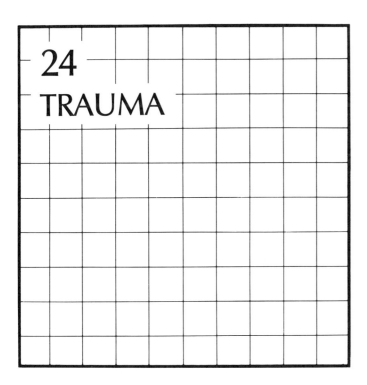

24

TRAUMA

DESCRIPTION

1. More than 500,000 head injuries occur annually in England (Barber, 1969).

In the general population, head injury from blows to the skull is more common than penetrating head wounds and barotrauma.

The United States Navy estimates that barotrauma occurs in about 5% to 20% of individuals involved in diving or flight operations (Behnke, 1944).

Trauma to the auditory system from noise or ototoxic drugs is not considered in this chapter (see Chapter 16, Noise-Induced Hearing Loss and Chapter 19, Ototoxicity).

2. Of temporal bone fractures, approximately 80% are longitudinal, about 15% are transverse, and about 5% are mixed.

Trauma to the auditory system may result from direct blows to the head, penetrating wounds to the head, and sudden severe pressure changes in the atmosphere (barotrauma). In animals and humans with auditory abnormality due to trauma, histopathologic studies and surgical or autopsy findings have noted disorders at every level of the auditory system from the external auditory canal to the central auditory pathways.[1]

Complications of trauma to the head may include meningitis, cholesteatoma and mastoiditis. Specific characteristics of head blows, penetrating wounds, and barotrauma are briefly summarized below.

Direct blows to the head. Consequences of direct head trauma frequently include skull fractures with or without fracture of the temporal bone. From an otologic viewpoint, fractures of the temporal bone are classified into two types. Classification depends on the location of the fracture line relative to the long axis of the petrous bone. The two categories of temporal bone fractures are termed *longitudinal* and *transverse*.[2]

Longitudinal fractures characteristically occur from blows to the side of the head. The fracture runs lengthwise through the petrous pyramid and may extend through the external auditory canal, the middle ear, and the mastoid bone. Rupture of the tym-

3. For an in-depth discussion of auditory findings in patients with ossicular chain interruption, see Chapter 6, Discontinuity of the Ossicular Chain.

4. Estimates of the prevalence of temporary or permanent hearing loss due to head trauma vary depending on the type of injury. Of patients with temporal bone fractures, about 65% to 85% may have hearing loss. Of patients with skull fractures not involving the temporal bone, about 45% may have hearing loss. Of patients with head trauma without skull fracture, about 18% may have hearing loss (Proctor et al., 1956; Podoshin and Fradis, 1975).

Of patients with head injuries severe enough to produce unconsciousness, a hearing loss may be observed in about 50% of individuals (Schuknecht and Davidson, 1956).

panic membrane, laceration of the mucous membranes of the middle ear cavity, accumulation of blood in the middle ear space, tearing of ossicular ligaments, and ossicular chain derangement may occur.[3]

Classic symptoms of longitudinal temporal bone fractures are tympanic membrane laceration and bleeding from the external ear canal. Longitudinal fractures characteristically do not extend through the cochlea.

In contrast to longitudinal fractures, transverse fractures of the temporal bone run horizontally across the petrous pyramid. The fracture characteristically occurs from blows to the front or the back of the head. The fracture line may extend through the otic capsule and, on occasion, through the internal auditory canal. Injury to the inner ear may result from tearing of the membranous labyrinth, hemorrhage, and rupture of the oval or round windows. Blood and/or cerebrospinal fluid may collect in the middle ear cavity.

In patients with cochlear damage from head trauma, histopathologic findings may show a proliferation of fibrous tissue and bone within the inner ear and degeneration of hair cells and cochlear neurons. Degenerative changes in the organ of Corti may be more pronounced in the basal coil of the cochlea than in the apical region.

In individuals with eighth nerve damage from head trauma, injury to the nerve may result from hemorrhage and tearing or stretching of eighth nerve fibers.

In patients without evidence of a skull fracture or in ears opposite a temporal bone fracture, damage to the inner ear (a sensorineural hearing loss) may be observed. A precise mechanism of cochlear damage in these patients is unknown. Proposed theories suggest that the loss may be due to a disturbance of the cochlear blood supply or to mechanical injury from pressure waves transmitted through the skull to inner ear fluids.[4]

In patients with damage to the central auditory system from head trauma, hemorrhage, edema, and softening of brain tissue may occur. Findings at autopsy may include degeneration and necrosis of auditory pathways and nuclei.

Penetrating wounds to the head. Penetrating wounds of the skull may occur from gunshot wounds or from direct injury by objects, such as pencils, placed into the external auditory canal. Foreign objects that directly injure the auditory system from the external auditory canal may perforate the tympanic membrane, dislocate the ossicular chain, and introduce foreign matter into the middle ear cavity. Gunshot wounds to the temporal bone area may produce all degrees and combinations of auditory injury depending on the degree and site of the trauma.

Barotrauma. Barotrauma commonly occurs in patients during descent from high altitudes in airplane flight or during ascent from underwater diving. Barotrauma is caused by a failure of the Eustachian tube to open sufficiently to permit equalization of middle ear pressure and atmospheric pressure. Barotrauma may be associated with distention, stretching, or rupture of the tympanic membrane; edema of the mucous membrane of the middle ear space; excretion of fluid into the middle ear cavity; dislocation of the ossicular chain; and rupture of blood vessels in the middle ear space. Cochlear damage may also be observed. A cause of cochlear damage is not clearly defined. Proposed theories suggest inner ear hemorrhage and rupture of the oval or round window membranes.[5]

PATIENT CHARACTERISTICS

Of patients with middle ear injury due to head trauma, approximately 50% are children less than 13 years of age and about 70% are individuals less than 22 years old. Only about 4% of individuals are more than 59 years of age. Of persons with middle ear injury due to a penetrating wound, about 75% are children.

Approximately 75% of persons with otologic trauma are male. The hearing loss is unilateral in about 80% of persons with middle ear injury from head trauma.[6]

CLINICAL COURSE

The onset of hearing loss is characteristically acute. However, on rare occasions, in individuals with traumatic sensorineural hearing loss, the onset of the loss may be delayed relative to the injury. The initial degree of loss may be unstable. Fluctuation, recovery,

5. For an example of auditory findings in a patient with hearing loss due to barotrauma, see patient 2, Chapter 6, Discontinuity of the Ossicular Chain.

6. In a state fair survey of 1741 males and 1724 females, blows to the head were reported by 24% of the males, but by only 12% of the females. Of these individuals, the insult had been severe enough to produce unconsciousness in 15% of males, but in only 7% of females (Glorig, 1957).
Of persons with

longitudinal temporal bone fractures, the fracture is unilateral in about 77% of individuals (Grove, 1947).

7. Of 44 persons with sensorineural hearing loss due to head injury, hearing sensitivity improved in about 14%, deteriorated in about 4%, and remained unchanged in about 82% of individuals (Podoshin and Fradis, 1975).
Of 120 persons with traumatic conductive hearing loss, hearing ability spontaneously returned to normal in 80% of individuals (Tos, 1971).

or deterioration of pure tone sensitivity may occur.[7]

As a general rule, recovery of auditory function occurs during the first 3 weeks following the injury. However, improvement in hearing sensitivity has been observed for as long as 6 months after the traumatic insult (Schulman, 1979). Unstable hearing sensitivity stresses the importance of serial audiometric evaluations of patients with posttraumatic hearing deficits.

Of patients with a fracture of the temporal bone, facial nerve paralysis may occur in about 10% to 20% of individuals with longitudinal fractures and in about 40% to 50% of individuals with transverse fractures. The onset of the facial paralysis may be immediate or may be delayed for a few days. The paralysis may be partial or complete. The facial nerve disorder may be temporary or permanent.

Tinnitus may be present in about 25% to 45% of individuals. Dizziness may be observed in about 45% to 65% of patients. Nausea and vomiting may occur. Any dizziness, nausea, and vomiting usually subside in 2 to 3 weeks. However, feelings of unsteadiness may persist for months.

Patients with head trauma may have variable degrees of psychiatric and intellectual impairment. Symptoms may include impairment of recent memory, loss of emotional control, a decreased ability to perform intellectual tasks, depression, hysteria, and unusual fatigability.

Treatment of otologic disorders due to head trauma may include bed rest, strict asepsis, and surgery.

SITE OF DISORDER

External ear, middle ear, and/or cochlea. In some individuals, the eighth nerve or central auditory pathways may be the primary site of involvement.

GENERAL AUDIOLOGIC PATTERN

Pure tone sensitivity results may show a wide variety of findings in patients with head trauma. The audiogram may show a conductive, mixed, or sensorineural loss. The type of loss varies depending on the site of the head injury. As a general rule, a conductive or mixed hearing loss is present in patients with longitudinal temporal bone fractures. In contrast, a sensorineural loss is usually observed in patients with transverse temporal bone fractures, with skull fractures not involving the temporal bone, and with head blows without fracture of the skull.

In patients with conductive disorders, the loss is usually unilateral. In patients with sensorineural disorders, the loss may be unilateral or bilateral. The degree of loss is characteristically mild, but may range to profound in some individuals.[8]

In patients with bilateral hearing loss, the degree of loss may be asymmetric. In most individuals, the hearing loss is more severe on the side of the head that received the injury. However, on rare occasions, the degree of loss may be more severe on the ear contralateral to the side of the head that received the injury.

The audiometric contour varies substantially. The hearing loss may occur in a restricted range of frequencies or at all frequencies.

In patients with unstable pure tone sensitivity, hearing may show improvement or deterioration over time. Improvement of auditory sensitivity may be observed in patients with conductive or sensorineural hearing loss. Persons with conductive hearing loss may show recovery of pure tone sensitivity to within normal limits at all frequencies. In contrast, patients with sensorineural hearing loss rarely recover to within normal limits. In particular, a high frequency sensorineural deficit may persist.

Maximum speech intelligibility scores vary depending upon the severity and site of the auditory disorder. In patients with middle ear site, maximum speech intelligibility scores are typically within normal limits. In patients with cochlear site, maximum speech intelligibility performance is usually consistent with the degree of sensitivity loss.

In the occasional patient with eighth nerve site, maximum speech intelligibility performance may be unusually poor relative to the degree of sensitivity loss. The performance-intensity (PI) function for speech materials may be abnormal (rollover effect). In patients with unstable pure tone sensitivity (middle ear, cochlear, or eighth nerve sites), speech intelligibility results may improve or deteriorate in a manner consistent with the pure tone sensitivity fluctuation.

In patients with traumatic involvement of the central auditory system, pure tone sensitivity and monosyllabic speech intelligibility performance may be normal. In contrast, performance for degraded speech intelligibility tests may be strikingly abnormal. Speech signals may be degraded by filtering, temporal alteration, and competing noise or speech messages.

In patients with posttraumatic hearing disorders, the administration of auditory tests for the evaluation of central auditory disorder may be limited. Limitations may be a result of the patient's young age, the patient's malaise, or concurrent abnormality of the peripheral auditory system.[9]

Results of tympanometry and static compliance measures are typically abnormal in patients with middle ear site and normal in patients with cochlear or retrocochlear sites. Acoustic reflex results vary depending on both the site of disorder and the degree of sensitivity loss. The possible sites of disorder affecting acoustic reflex results are the middle ear, the cochlea, the eighth nerve, the seventh nerve, and the brain stem.

As a general rule, in patients with middle ear or seventh nerve abnormalities, reflexes are absent for both crossed and uncrossed conditions with probe to the affected ear. The abnormal reflex pattern is characterized by a vertical configuration. In patients with cochlear disorder, reflexes are generally present at normal HLs and reduced sensation levels for all frequencies. A normal reflex pattern is produced. In patients with eighth nerve disorder, reflexes are absent for both crossed and uncrossed conditions with sound to the affected ear. This reflex abnormality yields a diagonal reflex pattern. In patients with brain stem site, reflexes on both ears are abnormal in the crossed condition and normal in the uncrossed condition. The abnormal reflex pattern is characterized by a horizontal configuration. In patients with profound hearing loss, reflex thresholds cannot be measured because signals cannot be presented at sufficiently high intensity levels.[10]

Illustrative Patients

CASE 1. A 17-Year-Old Female with a Hemotympanum in the Right Ear.

---

8. In a series of 88 patients with hearing loss due to head trauma, the average degree of loss was mild (less than 40 dB HL) in 75% of persons with sensorineural disorders and in 100% of individuals with conductive disorders (Podoshin and Fradis, 1975).

9. Remember, results of central auditory tests are equivocal in the presence of peripheral hearing loss. In this circumstance, abnormal results may be reflecting either the peripheral or central auditory dysfunction.

A notable feature of patients with trauma is that auditory disorders may involve more than one site.

10. For further information on audiometric findings in middle ear, cochlear, eighth nerve, seventh nerve, and central auditory disorders, see Chapter 1, Acoustic Schwannoma; Chapter 6, Discontinuity of the Ossicular Chain; Chapter 7, Facial Nerve Disorders; Chapter 12, Intracranial Tumors Affecting the Central Auditory System; and Chapter 14, Meniere's Disease.

History

Approximately 4 weeks ago, the patient was admitted to the hospital with a fracture of her right jaw and bloody drainage from her right ear. She had been kicked on the right side of the face by a horse. She was reportedly unconscious for a few minutes immediately after the accident.

At hospitalization, otorhinolaryngologic examination of the left ear was within normal limits. On the right side, examination noted a localized mass of extravasated blood within the external auditory canal (hematoma), blood within the middle ear space (hemotympanum), and a condylar fracture. Radiographic studies documented a fracture of the sub-condyle on the right side. X-ray studies were negative for a fracture of the external auditory canal wall.

The audiometric evaluation was carried out 12 days after the accident. Otorhinolaryngologic evaluation at this time indicated that the external auditory canal wall hematoma had resolved and that the hemotympanum was in the process of resolving.

Presently, the patient complains of a hearing loss in the right ear. She thinks her hearing in the right ear was normal before the accident. She reports some feelings of unsteadiness. She does not notice tinnitus on either ear. She has no hearing complaint about her left ear.

Results

The audiogram (Case 24-1A) shows a moderate conductive loss on the right ear and normal pure tone sensitivity on the left ear. The PTA scores (Case 24-1B) are 48 dB HL on the right ear and 9 dB HL on the left ear. Bone conduction and SAL audiometry on the right ear show a conductive component of about 40 dB to 50 dB. On the left ear, bone conduction and SAL results are essentially superimposed on air conduction thresholds.

The Weber test at 500 Hz (Case 24-1B) is referred to the right ear, the side of the conductive hearing loss. The Bing test at 500 Hz (not shown) on the right ear shows no difference between occluded and unoccluded thresholds. On the left ear, an occlusion effect of 10 dB is observed.

PI-PB and PI-SSI functions (Case 24-1A) on both ears show normal maximum intel-

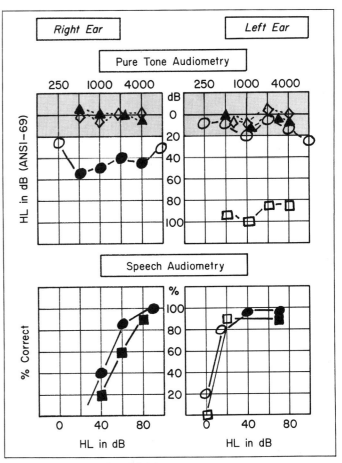

Case 24-1A

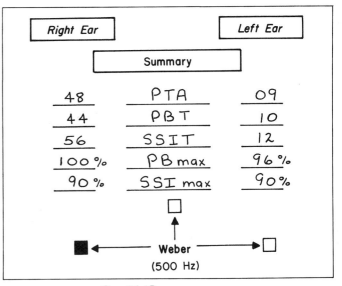

Case 24-1B

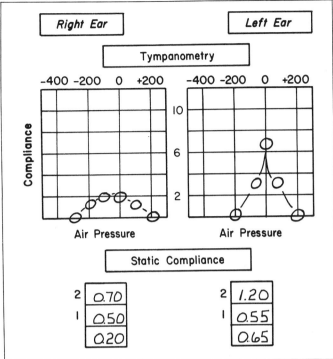

Case 24-1C

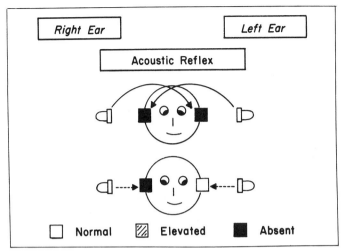

Case 24-1D

ligibility scores and no rollover. The PB max scores (Case 24-1B) are 100% on the right ear and 96% on the left ear. The SSI max scores are 90% on both ears.

Speech thresholds agree with average pure tone sensitivity results bilaterally. PBT scores are 44 dB HL on the right ear and 10 dB HL on the left ear. SSIT scores are 56 dB HL on the right ear and 12 dB HL on the left ear.

Impedance audiometry (Case 24-1C) on the right ear shows a type B tympanogram and an unusually reduced static compliance measure. Tympanometry and static compliance are normal on the left ear.[11]

Crossed and uncrossed acoustic reflexes (Case 24-1A) on the right ear are absent at all frequencies. With sound to the left ear, crossed acoustic reflexes are absent at equipment limits at all frequencies. However, uncrossed reflexes at 500 Hz through 4000 Hz are within normal limits. The reflex pattern (Case 24-1D) is characterized by an inverted L-shaped configuration. Only uncrossed reflexes on the left ear are present at normal HLs. All other crossed and uncrossed reflexes are absent at equipment limits. An inverted L-shaped pattern indicates a combined probe effect (vertical pat-

11. Contrast impedance results, especially the ear canal volume (1) measure, in this patient to findings in a patient with perforation of the tympanic membrane (see patient 1, Chapter 3, Cholesteatoma).

12. Remember that clinically, the inverted L-shaped pattern is a nonspecific finding. It may result from either a unilateral middle ear disorder, a combined seventh and eighth nerve disorder, or an intraaxial brain stem disorder eccentric to one side.

tern) and sound effect (diagonal pattern) on the right ear.[12]

Impression

RIGHT EAR: Moderate conductive loss. A middle ear site is supported by the presence of an air-bone and air-SAL gap, abnormal type B tympanogram, unusually low static compliance, and absent acoustic reflexes. Impedance results suggest unusually reduced mobility of the ossicular chain.

LEFT EAR: Normal pure tone sensitivity.

CASE 2. A 21-YEAR-OLD MALE WITH A TEMPORAL BONE FRACTURE ON THE RIGHT SIDE.

History

Approximately 3 weeks ago, the patient was involved in a motorcycle accident. He was unconscious for 2 weeks following the accident. After he regained consciousness, he noticed that he could not hear out of his right ear. He had tinnitus on the right ear and severe vertigo.

Cranial nerve evaluation indicated normal sensory and motor function except for a hearing loss on the right ear. Skull x-rays, mastoid x-rays, and polytomography of the right temporal bone showed a fracture of the right temporal bone and an apparently comminuted fracture of the right petrous mastoid bone. One fracture line extended from the middle fossa into the roof of the attic of the middle ear. An additional component or a separate fracture line extended across the bony labyrinth and the internal auditory canal.

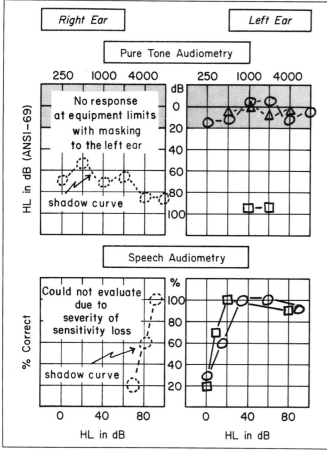

Case 24-2A

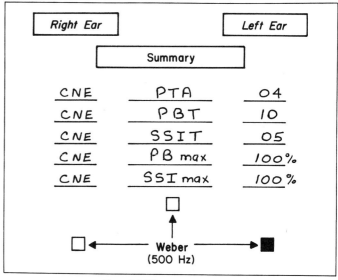

Case 24-2B

At the time of audiologic evaluation, otorhinolaryngologic examination on the right ear indicated a slightly retracted tympanic membrane. Otologic examination on the left ear was within normal limits. The patient does not think he can hear any sounds out of his right ear. He reports that he had normal hearing in the right ear before the accident. The patient has no hearing complaints about his left ear. His chief complaint is a feeling of unsteadiness, particularly when he changes position.

Results

13. Remember, a test signal presented by air conduction to the right (bad) ear without masking noise in the left (good) ear may travel around or through the skull to the left (non-test) ear and be heard. Such false thresholds are called shadow curves (Case 24-2A)

The audiogram (Case 24-2A) on the left ear shows normal pure tone sensitivity. With masking noise in the left ear, the audiogram on the right ear shows no response to air conducted or bone conducted signals at equipment limits. Without masking noise in the left ear, pure tone signals presented to the right ear are heard at about 60 to 80 dB HL.[13] The PTA score (Case 24-2B) on the left ear is 4 dB HL. A PTA score could not be established (CNE) on the right ear.

because they "shadow" the auditory curve on the good (left) ear, attenuated by the amount of sound lost in the trip around or through the head. The difference between the intensity level of the signal and the threshold sensitivity of the good (left) ear defines the amount of interaural attenuation. The presence of a shadow curve is a strong vote against a functional hearing loss on the right ear.

14. The unusual W-shaped tympanogram on the right ear is a rare occurrence. In a series of about 1000 ears with varying types and degrees of hearing disorders, a W-shaped tympanogram at 220 Hz was observed in only 3% of ears (Alberti and Jerger, 1974). The W-shaped pattern at a probe frequency of 220 Hz is associated with ossicular chain discontinuity.

Unmasked bone conduction thresholds (Case 24-2A) are superimposed on the air conduction thresholds of the left ear. With masking to the left ear, there is no response to bone conducted signals presented to the right ear at equipment limits. The Weber test (Case 24-2B) at 500 Hz lateralizes to the left ear.

Speech audiometry (Case 24-2A) on the left ear shows normal maximum intelligibility scores of 100% correct for both PB word and SSI materials. No rollover is observed. Speech thresholds on the left ear agree with average pure tone sensitivity. The PBT score is 10 dB HL; the SSIT score is 5 dB HL.

On the right ear, there is no response to masked speech signals at equipment limits. However, unmasked speech signals (PB words) show a normal speech "shadow curve" with an interaural attenuation of about 65 dB.

Tympanometry (Case 24-2C) shows an unusual W-shaped tympanogram on the right ear and an abnormally deep, type A, tympanogram on the left ear. Static compliance measures are abnormally high on both ears.[14] Crossed and uncrossed acoustic reflexes (Case 24-2A) on the right ear are absent at equipment limits at all frequencies. With sound to the left ear and probe to the right ear, crossed acoustic reflexes are absent at all frequencies at equipment limits. However, uncrossed reflexes on the left ear at 1000 Hz and 2000 Hz are within normal limits. The reflex pattern (Case 24-2D) is

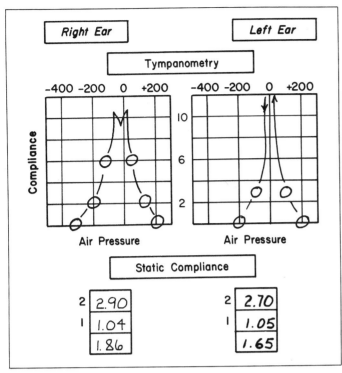

Case 24-2C

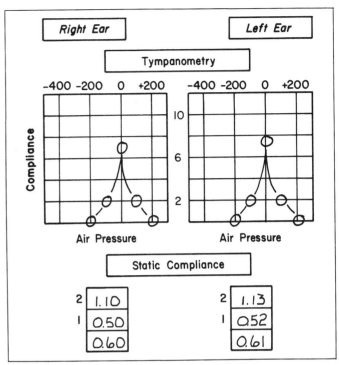

Case 24-3A

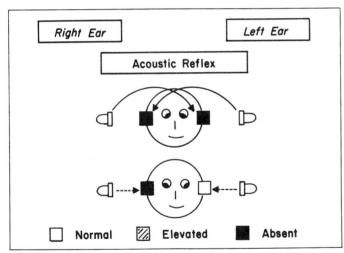

Case 24-2D

characterized by an inverted L-shaped configuration. Results suggest a combined probe effect (vertical pattern) and sound effect (diagonal pattern) on the right ear.

Impression

RIGHT EAR: No measurable hearing by air conduction or bone conduction. Impedance audiometry indicates a middle ear disorder characterized by an unusual W-shaped tympanogram and absent acoustic reflexes with probe to the right ear. This pattern of

results is consistent with discontinuity of the ossicular chain. The presence of a normal "shadow curve" for pure tone and speech signals is evidence against the possibility of a functional hearing disorder.[15]

LEFT EAR: Normal pure tone sensitivity.

CASE 3. A 7-YEAR-OLD FEMALE WITH BRAIN STEM CONTUSION.

History

At admission to the hospital, the patient was comatose due to head trauma suffered in an automobile accident. Severe neurologic deficits secondary to brain stem contusion were observed.

At the time of the audiologic evaluation, the patient was semicomatose.

Results

No behavioral audiometric results could be obtained due to the patient's malaise. However, impedance audiometry was carried out. Tympanometry and static compliance measures (Case 24-3A) show normal, type A, tympanograms and normal static compliance measures on both ears.

Acoustic reflexes (Case 24-3B) on both ears are abnormal to crossed stimulation and normal to uncrossed stimulation. With

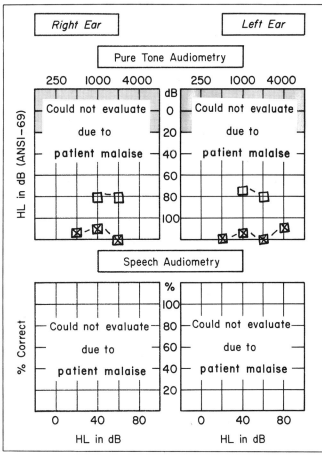

Case 24-3B

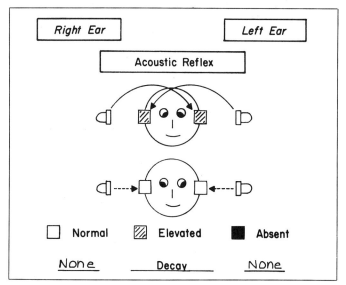

Case 24-3C

16. Remember, with the horizontal reflex pattern, the possibility of measurement error is troublesome. In the crossed condition, reflexes are elicited via earphones. In the uncrossed condition, however, reflexes are elicited with a probe tip sealed into the ear canal. Any occlusion of the ear canal will affect crossed reflexes, but not uncrossed reflexes. In this patient, we carefully ruled out the possibility of a collapsing ear canal on each ear.

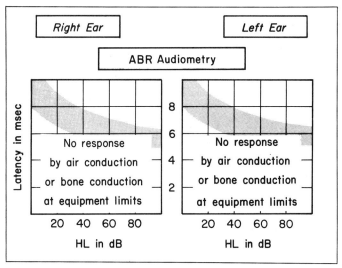

Case 24-3D

sound to the right ear, crossed acoustic reflexes are elevated or absent at all frequencies. However, uncrossed reflexes at 1000 Hz and 2000 Hz are within normal limits. With sound to the left ear, the same pattern of results is obtained. Reflex decay testing, measured in the uncrossed condition at 1000 Hz, showed a normal reflex time course on both ears.

The reflex pattern (Case 24-3C) is characterized by a horizontal configuration. Reflexes are abnormal on both ears to crossed stimulation only. Auditory brain stem response (ABR) audiometry (Case 24-3D) yields no recognizable waves (I through V) on either ear to air conducted or bone conducted signals at the intensity limits of the equipment.

Impression

Behavioral audiometric results could not be obtained due to the patient's malaise. Tympanometry, static compliance measures, and uncrossed acoustic reflexes suggest normal middle ear function in both ears. The relation between crossed vs uncrossed reflex thresholds and ABR audiometry is consistent with an intraaxial brain stem disorder.[16]

SELECTED READINGS

Alberti, P., and Jerger, J. Probe tone frequency and the diagnostic value of tympanometry. *Arch. Otolaryngol.* 99:206, 1974.

Barber, H. Head injury audiological and vestibular findings. *Ann. Otol. Rhinol. Laryngol.* 78:239, 1969.

Behnke, A. Physiologic effect of pressure changes with reference to otolaryngology. *Trans. Am. Acad. Ophthalmol. Otolaryngol.* 48:63, 1944.

Glorig, A. Some medical implications of the 1954 Wisconsin State Fair hearing survey. *Trans. Am. Acad. Ophthalmol. Otolaryngol.* 61:160, 1957.

Grove, W. Skull fractures involving the ear. A clinical study of 211 cases. *Laryngoscope* 49:678, 1939.

Grove, W. Hearing impairment due to craniocerebral trauma. *Ann. Otol. Rhinol. Laryngol.* 56:264, 1947.

Hough, J. Otologic Trauma. In M. Paparella and D. Shumrick (eds.), *Otolaryngology* (vol. 2). Philadelphia: Saunders, 1973. Pp. 241–262.

Igarashi, M. Pathology of Inner Ear Endorgans. In J. Minkler (ed.), *Pathology of the Nervous System* (vol. 3). New York: McGraw-Hill, 1972. Pp. 2856–2879.

Kirikae, I., Eguchi, K., Okamoto, M., and Nakamura, K. Histopathological changes in the auditory pathway in cases of fatal head injury. *Acta Otolaryngol.* 67:341, 1969.

Lamkin, R., Axelsson, A., McPherson, D., and Miller, J. Experimental aural barotrauma. *Acta Otolaryngol.* Suppl. 335:1, 1975.

Podoshin, L., and Fradis, M. Hearing loss after head injury. *Arch. Otolaryngol.* 101:15, 1975.

Proctor, B., Gurdjian, E., and Webster, J. The ear in head trauma. *Laryngoscope* 66:16, 1956.

Schuknecht, H. A clinical study of auditory damage following blows to the head. *Ann. Otol. Rhinol. Laryngol.* 59:331, 1950.

Schuknecht, H. *Pathology of the Ear.* Cambridge: Harvard University Press, 1974. Pp. 292–317.

Schuknecht, H., and Davidson, R. Deafness and vertigo from head injury. *Arch. Otolaryngol.* 63:513, 1956.

Schulman, J. Traumatic Diseases of the Ear and Temporal Bone. In V. Goodhill (ed.), *Ear Diseases, Deafness, and Dizziness.* New York: Harper & Row, 1979. Pp. 504–516.

Tos, M. Prognosis of hearing loss in temporal bone fractures. *J. Laryngol.* 85:1147, 1971.

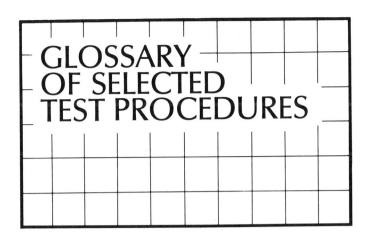

GLOSSARY OF SELECTED TEST PROCEDURES

Acoustic Reflex. Acoustic reflex thresholds are routinely measured for broadband noise and for pure tones at octave intervals between 250 and 4000 Hz. Reflex threshold is defined as the lowest HL in dB that produces reliable changes in acoustic immittance time-locked to the reflex-eliciting signal. In standard clinical practice, the maximum intensity used to elicit reflex contractions is 110 dB HL. This rule may be violated, however, on rare occasions in patients with middle ear or central auditory disorder.

Acoustic reflex threshold is interpreted as normal if the HL is 100 dB or less. Threshold is considered abnormally elevated if the HL is 105 dB HL or more. The reflex sensation level (SL), defined by the difference between the reflex threshold HL and the behavioral threshold HL, normally ranges from about 70 to 100 dB. SLs of less than about 55 dB are abnormally reduced (a cochlear sign), and SLs of more than 100 dB are abnormally large (a retrocochlear sign).

If the reflex threshold at 500 and/or 1000 Hz is noted at 100 dB HL or less, reflex decay testing is routinely administered. For this procedure, a sustained tone of 500 and/or 1000 Hz is presented at a reflex SL of 10 dB for at least 10 seconds. Results of reflex decay testing are considered positive for eighth nerve site if reflex amplitude declines to less than one-half the initial magnitude within a 10-sec test period (Jerger et al., 1974). If reflex amplitude does not decay over time to less than the one-half of initial amplitude criterion, results are reported as negative.

Ordinarily, reflex decay is considered a retrocochlear sign at frequencies of 500 or 1000 Hz. On rare occasions, however, useful information may be provided at 2000 Hz, but results must be interpreted cautiously because of the high false positive rate of reflex decay at this frequency.

The 4-reflex array summarizing relations among crossed and uncrossed reflex thresholds of the two ears yields distinct patterns useful in differentiating site of disorder (J. Jerger, 1975). Refer to J. Jerger (1975) or S. Jerger (1980) for a detailed discussion of the diagnostic significance of each pattern.

Auditory Brain Stem Response *(ABR)* Audiometry. The auditory brain stem response is a sequence of six vertex positive waves occurring within the first 10 msec after the presentation of a click or click-like signal. The presumed physiologic generators of the component waves are: wave I, eighth nerve; wave II, cochlear nucleus; wave III, superior olivary complex; wave IV, ventral nucleus of the lateral lemniscus; wave V, inferior colliculus; and wave VI, medial geniculate body.

ABR potentials are commonly recorded with surface electrodes on the vertex and mastoid. The amplified electrical activity is signal averaged and displayed graphically on a strip chart or X-Y recorder. The ABR waveform typically represents the average response to 1000 to 2000 clicks. The standard click rate is 10 to 20 per sec. However, higher repetition rates are routinely used in individuals with suspected retrocochlear disorder to stress the auditory system. In patients with suspected middle ear disorder, latency-intensity functions for bone-conducted clicks, as well as air-conducted clicks, are characteristically obtained.

Clinically, ABR audiometry is used for threshold sensitivity estimation (Jerger and Mauldin, 1978), for quantifying the approximate degree of conductive component (Mauldin and Jerger, 1979), and for the evaluation of neuro-otologic disorders (Stockard and Rossiter, 1977; Jerger et al., 1980). For diagnostic purposes, absolute latencies, interwave latencies, interwave amplitude ratios, binaural vs monaural amplitude ratios, and latency variation with click rate provide useful indices.

Bekesy Audiometry. Bekesy audiometry refers to a tracking technique in which the patient tracks his own auditory threshold by means of a self-recording audiometer. The frequency of the threshold tracking signal is constantly changing, usually at a rate of one octave per minute. The signal train may be either continuous or periodically interrupted in time. Signal intensity changes at a constant rate, usually 2.0 to 2.5 dB per sec. The patient determines the direction of intensity change by alternately pressing and releasing a key that reverses the direction of a motor-driven attenuator. Patients are instructed to press the key when signals are just audible and to release the key when signals are just inaudible. A pen-writing system connected to the attenuator yields a graphic representation, or tracing, of the patient's successive threshold crossings.

In clinical practice, three sweep-frequency tracings are obtained in the following order: (1) forward-interrupted (signal periodically interrupted; frequency changing from 200 to 8000 Hz), (2) forward-continuous (signal continuous; frequency changing from 200 to 8000 Hz), and (3) backward-continuous (signal continuous; frequency changing from 8000 to 200 Hz).

Results of Bekesy audiometry are classified according to the relation between forward-interrupted and forward-continuous tracings (J. Jerger, 1960) and between continuous-forward and continuous-backward tracings (Jerger et al., 1972).

Bekesy Comfortable Loudness (BCL) Audiometry. Sweep-frequency tracings for forward-interrupted, forward-continuous, and backward-continuous signals are obtained over the frequency range from 200 to 8000 Hz. Rate of frequency and intensity change is the same as for conventional Bekesy audiometry. The patient is instructed to press a manual response button when the signals are just more than comfortably loud and to release the button when the signals are just less than comfortably loud.

Results of BCL audiometry are divided into six patterns on the basis of the relation between forward-interrupted vs continuous tracings and the relation between continuous-forward vs backward tracings (Jerger and Jerger, 1974).

Bing Test. For the Bing test, the difference between unoccluded and occluded bone conduction sensitivity is measured at 500 Hz. When the occluded bone conduction threshold is better than the unoccluded threshold by at least 10 dB, results are interpreted as consistent with normal middle ear function. If occluded and unoccluded thresholds are the same (a difference of less than 10 dB), results are interpreted as consistent with a middle ear disorder. The non-test ear must·be masked during the testing procedure.

Impedance (Immittance) Audiometry. A test battery consisting of (1) tympanometry, (2) static immittance, and (3) acoustic reflex thresholds for both crossed and uncrossed signals. For a detailed discussion of the diagnostic significance of the various outcomes of the impedance battery, see Jerger and Northern (1980).

PI (Performance vs Intensity) Functions. PI functions are obtained by presenting monosyllabic word (PB) or sentence (SSI) materials at several different intensity levels. Performance is characteristically defined from that intensity level yielding 0 to 20% correct up to a maximum speech intensity of 90 dB HL. The PI-PB function is obtained in quiet. The PI-SSI function is obtained in the presence of a competing speech message. The competing message is presented to the same ear that receives the test sentences at a message-to-competition ratio (MCR) of 0 dB. The diagnostic value of PI functions has been discussed in detail in the literature (Jerger and Jerger, 1975a; Jerger and

Hayes, 1977). For an explanation of speech threshold estimation from the PI function, please see PBT and SSIT, Glossary of Selected Terms and Abbreviations.

SAL (Sensorineural Acuity Level) Test. The SAL test measures the threshold shift of an air conducted pure tone signal produced by a bone conducted broadband noise signal. The patient's sensorineural acuity level may be calculated either from threshold shift measures or from the patient's absolute threshold-in-noise relative to the normal absolute threshold-in-noise. The former approach yields the patient's bone conduction sensitivity level; the latter approach yields the conductive component. In patients with no benefit from occlusion on the Bing test, SAL results must be corrected by the amount of the normal occlusion effect before plotting SAL results onto the audiogram. For a discussion of the SAL test and the occlusion effect, please see Jerger and Jerger (1965).

SISI (Short Increment Sensitivity Index) Test. This procedure measures an individual's ability to detect the presence of 1.0 dB increments superimposed on a continuous tone presented at 20 dB sensation level. SISI scores between 70 and 100% are considered positive for cochlear disorder. SISI scores between 0 and 20% are interpreted as negative for cochlear disorder. The test is limited to frequencies where the patient's hearing threshold level is at least 40 dB HL (at least a moderate degree of sensitivity loss).

SSI-CCM (Synthetic Sentence Identification [SSI] materials in the presence of a Contralateral Competing Message [CCM]). The sentences are presented at 50 dB SPL (30 dB HL). The message-to-competition ratio (MCR) is varied from 0 to −40 dB. The SSI-CCM score is obtained by averaging performance at 0, −20, and −40 dB. Normal performance for the SSI-CCM procedure remains at 100% for all MCRs.

The SSI-CCM score is sensitive to central auditory disorder, especially at the temporal lobe level (Jerger and Jerger, 1975a).

SSI-ICM (Synthetic Sentence Identification [SSI] materials in the presence of an Ipsilateral Competing Message [ICM]). The SSI materials are presented at 50 dB SPL (30 dB HL). The message-to-competition ratio is varied from +10 dB to −20 dB. The SSI-ICM score is obtained by averaging performance at 0, −10, and −20 dB. Average normal performance for the SSI-ICM procedure is about 75% correct.

The SSI-ICM score is sensitive to central auditory disorder, especially at the brain stem level (Jerger and Jerger, 1975a).

SSW (Staggered Spondaic Word) Test. The SSW test requires the listener to repeat spondee words. The words are presented to both ears in competing (dichotic) and noncompeting conditions. The time sequence of the spondee word presentation to each ear may be illustrated as follows: the first syllable is presented to the right ear in isolation; the second syllable on the right ear is presented simultaneously with the first syllable on the left ear; and the final syllable on the left ear is presented in isolation. The SSW test is sensitive to central auditory disorder, especially at the temporal lobe level. The diagnostic interpretations and the various scoring techniques of the SSW test have been discussed previously (Brunt, 1972; Jerger and Jerger, 1975).

STAT (Supra Threshold Adaptation Test).

The STAT test (Jerger and Jerger, 1975b) records the presence or absence of abnormal decay for continuous tones presented for 60 sec at 100 dB HL. The patient is asked to respond as long as he hears the sound. If he responds for the full 60-sec period, the result is negative. If, however, he fails to respond for the full 60-sec period, the result is considered positive for eighth nerve site. One constraint on test administration is that the presentation level (100 dB HL) must represent a sensation level of at least 20 dB at each test frequency.

Stenger Test.

A test for evaluating the possibility of a functional unilateral hearing loss. Voluntary spondee thresholds (STs) are first determined for each ear. Spondee words are then presented to both ears at about 10 dB above the voluntary ST on the uninvolved ear. The level on the "bad" ear is increased in 10-dB steps until the speech intensity equals the patient's voluntary ST. If the patient ceases to respond before his voluntary ST level is reached, the Stenger test is considered positive for a functional component to the apparent hearing loss on the "bad" ear. If the patient continues to respond as the speech intensity on the "bad" ear is increased to the voluntary ST level, the Stenger test is considered negative for a functional component to the hearing loss. However, as a control measure for patients who continue to respond, the spondee words must, on occasion, be removed from the uninvolved "good" ear and presented to the "bad" ear in isolation at levels below the voluntary "bad" ear ST. In this control condition, we assure ourselves that the patient is not responding to speech intensities below his voluntary ST determined prior to administering the Stenger test. The administration and interpretation of the Stenger test have been summarized by Martin (1975).

TDT (Threshold Tone Decay Test).

The TDT measures the minimum intensity increases required to maintain audibility for 60 sec. Testing begins at threshold. Results are considered positive for eighth nerve site if the difference between the patient's threshold and the 60-sec audibility level is more than 30 dB at any test frequency (Tillman, 1969). In a modification proposed by Olsen and Noffsinger (1974), testing begins not at threshold, but at 20-dB sensation level.

Tympanometry.

A graphic plot (tympanogram) of the change in immittance of the middle ear mechanism as air pressure is varied in the external canal. Results and interpretation of tympanometry are discussed in detail by Harford (1980).

Weber Test.

For the Weber test, the patient is asked to indicate the location of a bone conducted 500-Hz tone presented at a comfortable listening level. The pure tone is presented via a bone vibrator placed on the patient's forehead. If the tone is lateralized to the ear with poorest sensitivity, results are interpreted as consistent with conductive loss on the poorer side. If the tone is lateralized to the ear with the best sensitivity, results are interpreted as consistent with sensorineural loss on the poorer side. The clinical value of the Weber test has been discussed by Dirks (1973).

REFERENCES

Brunt, M. The Staggered Spondaic Word Test. In J. Katz (ed.), *Handbook of Clinical Audiology*. Baltimore: Williams & Wilkins, 1972. Pp. 334–356.

Dirks, D. Bone-conduction Measurements. In J. Jerger (ed.), *Modern Developments in Audiology* (2nd ed.). New York: Academic Press, 1973. Pp. 1–36.

Harford, E. Tympanometry. In J. Jerger and J. Northern (eds.), *Clinical Impedance Audiometry* (2nd ed.). Acton, Mass.: American Electromedics Corp., 1980. Pp. 40–64.

Jerger, J. Bekesy audiometry in the analysis of auditory disorders. *J. Speech Hear. Res.* 3:275, 1960.

Jerger, J. Diagnostic Use of Impedance Measures. In J. Jerger (ed.), *Handbook of Clinical Impedance Audiometry*. New York: American Electromedics Corp., 1975. Pp. 149–174.

Jerger, J., Harford, E., Clemis, J., and Alford, B. The acoustic reflex in eighth nerve disorders. *Arch. Otolaryngol.* 97:92, 1974.

Jerger, J., and Hayes, D. Diagnostic speech audiometry. *Arch. Otolaryngol.* 103:216, 1977.

Jerger, J., and Jerger, S. Critical evaluation of SAL audiometry. *J. Speech Hear. Res.* 8:103, 1965.

Jerger, J., and Jerger, S. Diagnostic value of Bekesy comfortable loudness tracings. *Arch. Otolaryngol.* 99:351, 1974.

Jerger, J., and Jerger, S. Clinical validity of central auditory tests. *Scand. Audiol.* 4:147, 1975a.

Jerger, J., and Jerger, S. A simplified tone decay test. *Arch. Otolaryngol.* 101:403, 1975b.

Jerger, J., Jerger, S., and Mauldin, L. The forward-backward discrepancy in Bekesy audiometry. *Arch. Otolaryngol.* 72:400, 1972.

Jerger, J., and Mauldin, L. Prediction of sensorineural hearing level from the brain stem evoked response. *Arch. Otolaryngol.* 104:456, 1978.

Jerger, J., Neely, J., and Jerger, S. Speech, impedance, and auditory brain-stem response audiometry in brainstem tumors. Importance of a multiple-test strategy. *Arch. Otolaryngol.* 106:218, 1980.

Jerger, J., and Northern, J. (eds.). *Clinical Impedance Audiometry* (2nd ed.). Acton, Mass.: American Electromedics Corp., 1980.

Jerger, S. Diagnostic Application of Impedance Audiometry in Central Auditory Disorders. In J. Jerger and J. Northern (eds.), *Clinical Impedance Audiometry* (2nd ed.). Acton, Mass.: American Electromedics Corp., 1980. Pp. 128–140.

Martin, F. *Introduction to Audiology*. Englewood Cliffs, N.J.: Prentice-Hall, 1975. Pp. 339–341.

Mauldin, L., and Jerger, J. Auditory brain stem evoked responses to bone-conducted signals. *Arch. Otolaryngol.* 105:656, 1979.

Olsen, W., and Noffsinger, D. Comparison of one new and three old tests of auditory adaptation. *Arch. Otolaryngol.* 99:94, 1974.

Stockard, J., and Rossiter, V. Clinical and pathologic correlates of brain stem auditory response abnormalities. *Neurology* 27:316, 1977.

Tillman, T. Special hearing tests in otoneurologic diagnosis. *Arch. Otolaryngol.* 89:51, 1969.

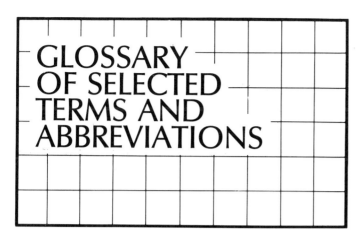

GLOSSARY OF SELECTED TERMS AND ABBREVIATIONS

CT *(Computerized Axial Tomographic)* **Scan.** X-ray beams are passed through a desired structure and digitized. The digitized beam quantifies the attenuation of the primary x-ray beam by the structure being studied. Attenuation varies as a function of different tissue types. The digital values yield a reconstructed image of the area being examined. Computerized tomography is discussed in depth by Davis and Alper (1977).

dB(A). The overall sound pressure level (SPL) as measured on the A scale of a sound level meter. The A scale is weighted so that very low and very high frequencies receive less emphasis than the mid frequency region.

EEG *(Electroencephalographic)* **Test.** Records the spontaneous electric activity of the brain by means of surface scalp electrodes.

Occlusion Effect. Enhancement of low frequency bone conduction threshold sensitivity accompanying occlusion of the external auditory canal.

PB-K *(PB-Kindergarten)* **Words.** A list of monosyllabic, phonemically balanced (PB) words that use a restricted vocabulary appropriate for children.

PB Max. The maximum percent correct score for phonemically balanced (PB) monosyllabic word testing; the highest point on the performance-intensity (PI) function for PB words.

PBT *(PB Word Threshold).* Speech threshold obtained from the performance-intensity (PI) function for PB words. The threshold is based on the 50% correct point if the maximum PB score is between 71% and 100% correct and on the 25% correct point if the maximum PB score is between 31% and 70% correct. In individuals with maximum PB scores of less than 31%, a PBT cannot be established.

PTA *(Pure Tone Average).* The PTA is a common index for quantifying degree of pure tone sensitivity loss. It is usually obtained by averaging threshold levels at 500, 1000, and 2000 Hz. More recently, however, the average of threshold levels at 1000, 2000, and 4000 Hz has been found useful in connection with estimates of threshold sensitivity based on ABR audiometry and on acoustic reflex thresholds.

Reflex Decay. Please see Acoustic Reflex, Glossary of Selected Test Procedures.

Rollover. A decrease in speech intelligibility performance as the intensity of the speech signal is increased above the level yielding the maximum percent correct score. The amount of rollover is defined by the difference between maximum speech intelligibility (PB max) performance and the lowest speech intelligibility score (PB min) occurring above the speech level yielding PB max. In general, rollover of more than 20% is suggestive of retrocochlear disorder. A rollover index may be computed by the following equation: (PB max − PB min) ÷ PB max. A rollover index of more than 0.40 is considered positive for eighth nerve disorder. A rollover index of less than or equal to 0.40 is interpreted as negative for eighth nerve disorder.

SAT *(Speech Awareness Threshold).* The hearing level at which a defined speech sample is correctly detected about 50% of the time.

SPAR *(Sensitivity Prediction from the Acoustic Reflex).* A prediction of hearing sensitivity based on the difference between acoustic reflex thresholds for pure tone vs broadband noise signals. The major alternative methods of hearing loss prediction from AR thresholds have been recently detailed and critiqued by Hall (1980).

SSI Max. The maximum percent correct score obtained on the synthetic sentence identification (SSI) task; the highest point on the performance-intensity (PI) function for SSI materials in the presence of a competing speech message at a message-to-competition ratio of 0 dB. The diagnostic significance of the SSI max lies in its relation to the PB max (Jerger and Hayes, 1977).

SSIT *(Synthetic Sentence Identification Threshold).* Speech threshold obtained from the performance-intensity (PI) function for synthetic sentence identification (SSI) materials in the presence of a competing speech message at a 0 dB message-to-competition ratio. The threshold is based on the 50% correct point if maximum performance is more than about 70% correct and on the 25% correct point if maximum performance is between about 30% and 70% correct. In individuals with maximum SSI scores of less than 30%, an SSIT cannot be established. On occasion, an SSIT may be obtained from the PI function for SSI materials presented in quiet (SSIT-quiet), instead of in competition.

ST *(Spondee Word Threshold).* The hearing level yielding 50% correct performance for spondee words. On occasion, the ST may be obtained with selected pictures. In this circumstance the speech threshold is referred to as the STP (Spondee Word Threshold with Pictures).

REFERENCES

Davis, D., and Alper, N. Computerized Tomography of the Orbit and Orbital Lesions. In P. Arger (ed.), *Orbit Roentgenology.* New York: Wiley, 1977. Pp. 195–214.

Hall, J. Predicting Hearing Loss from the Acoustic Reflex. In J. Jerger and J. Northern (eds.), *Clinical Impedance Audiometry* (2nd ed.). Acton, Mass.: American Electromedics Corp., 1980. Pp. 141–163.

Jerger, J., and Hayes, D. Diagnostic speech audiometry. *Arch. Otolaryngol.* 103:216, 1977.

INDEX